Second Edition — Textbook of

Pharmacognosy

Volume I

Second Edition

Textbook of
Pharmacognosy

Volume I

P Suresh Narayana MSc
Principal (Retired)
SSBN Junior College
Anantapur, AP

T Pullaiah MSc PhD
Professor of Botany (Retired)
Sri Krishnadevaraya University
Anantapur, AP

D Varalakshmi MSc MPhil
Head, Department of Biotechnology (Retired)
Government Degree College
Anantapur, AP

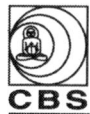

CBS

CBS Publishers & Distributors Pvt Ltd

New Delhi • Bengaluru • Chennai • Kochi • Kolkata • Mumbai
Bhopal • Bhubaneswar • Hyderabad • Jharkhand • Nagpur • Patna • Pune
Uttarakhand • Dhaka (Bangladesh)

Second Edition Textbook of
Pharmacognosy
Volume 1

ISBN 978-81-94125-48-8

Copyright @ Authors and Publisher

Second Edition: 2020
Reprint: 2023, **2025**
First Edition: 2010

Published by **Satish Kumar Jain** and produced by **Varun Jain** for

CBS Publishers & Distributors Pvt Ltd

4819/XI Prahlad Street, 24 Ansari Road, Daryaganj, New Delhi 110 002, India.
Ph: 011-23266838, 23289259   Website: www.cbspd.com
                                                      e-mail: delhi@cbspd.com

Corporate Office: 204 FIE, Industrial Area, Patparganj, Delhi 110 092
Ph: 011-4934 4934   Fax: 011-4934 4935
                                    e-mail: publishing@cbspd.com; publicity@cbspd.com

Branches

- **Bengaluru:** Seema House 2975, 17th Cross, KR Road, Banasankari 2nd Stage, Bengaluru 560 070, Karnataka, India
  Ph: +91-80-26771678/79   Fax: +91-80-26771680   e-mail: bangalore@cbspd.com
- **Chennai:** 18/8B, Subbarayan Street, Shenoy Nagar, Chennai 600 030, Tamil Nadu, India
  Ph: +91-44-42032115, 26681266   e-mail: chennai@cbspd.com
- **Kochi:** 42/1325, 1326, Power House Road, Opp KSEB, Power House, Ernakulum Kochi 682 018, Kerala, India
  Ph: +91-484-4059061-65,67   Fax: +91-484-4059065   e-mail: kochi@cbspd.com
- **Kolkata:** 147, Hind Ceramics Compound, 1st Floor, Nilgunj Road, Belghoria, Kolkata-700056, West Bengal, India
  Ph: +033-25633055, 033-25633056   e-mail: kolkata@cbspd.com
- **Lucknow:** Basement, Khushnuma Complex, 7 Meerabai Marg (Behind Jawahar Bhawan), Lucknow-226001, UP, India
  Ph: +0522-4000032   e-mail: tiwari.lucknow@cbspd.com
- **Mumbai:** PWD Shed, Gala no 25/26, Ramchandra Bhatt Marg, Next to JJ Hospital Gate no. 2, Opp. Union Bank of India, Noorbaug,
  Mumbai-400009, Maharashtra, India
  Ph: 022-66661880/89   e-mail: mumbai@cbspd.com

Representatives

- Hyderabad   0-9885175004   • Jharkhand   0-9811541605   • Nagpur   0-8692091830
- Patna   0-9334159340   • Pune   0-9664372571   • Uttarakhand   0-9716462459

Printed at Glorious Printers, Jhilmil Industrial Area, Delhi, India

Preface to the Second Edition

The first edition of *Textbook of Pharmacognosy: Volume I* was warmly received by the students and teachers and it exhausted within no time. Many useful suggestions were received by the readers and it necessitated the printing of this second revised edition. The general plan of the book remains unchanged in this edition, except the additional information added in different chapters where it is essential. Besides, addition of a new appendix, the entire text has been thoroughly revised and updated. We hope this edition will be more useful to the readers and will continue to serve the purpose more effectively. The constructive suggestions from the readers for the purpose of further improvement of this book are cordially invited.

We express our thanks to CBS Publishers & Distributors Pvt. Ltd, New Delhi, for their continued cooperation in bringing out this edition in a highly presentable form within a short time. Finally, we express our deep sense of gratitude to our family members for their continued cooperation, encouragement and best support in times of stress during the preparation of this volume.

P Suresh Narayana
T Pullaiah
D Varalakshmi

Preface to the First Edition

Pharmacognosy is an "interdisciplinary science of therapeutically active drugs and a large number of them are the natural products, either from vegetable, animal or mineral sources" being widely used at present in Allopathy as well as other alternate systems of medicine like Ayurveda, Unani, Naturopathy, etc. Keeping in mind the importance of such drugs, this book on Pharmacognosy is prepared and every attempt has been made to consolidate all the details to provide the students of pharmacy the relevant information all at one place.

The products from plants, animals and minerals were in use since times immemorial in the treatment of not only human ailments but also the domestic animals. It is only in recent times, the constituents from the bodies of plants and animals have been scientifically processed for use in the required form and dosage.

The object of this publication is to provide a standard and useful 'Textbook of Pharmacognosy' to the students of Pharmacy, and every sincere effort has been made to incorporate all the details as per their requirement, with a sincere hope that this publication removes the lacuna of a text that will be useful for the diploma and degree students of pharmacy in colleges and universities of JNTU area of Andhra Pradesh, where pharmacognosy is being taught.

The content of the book is organized in 8 chapters: 1. Pharmacognosy—History and development, 2. Natural sources of drugs, 3. Classification of crude drugs, 4. Cultivation of medicinal plants, 5. Good agricultural practices and strategies, 6. Systematic study of carbohydrates, 7. Pharmacognostic study of lipids and 8. Systematic study of volatile oils. Each chapter covers introductory details of the concerned category, classification, biological and geographical sources, methods of collection and preparation, macroscopic and microscopic characters, properties of the drug, chemical constituents and pharmaceutical uses of the drug. The readers will find in this book the synonyms (for the binomials), the vernacular names of the drugs (in different languages) and the etymology as well as the derivation of the generic and specific names of the source of the drug for easy identification of the concerned drug. In addition to the medicinal uses of the drugs, non-medicinal uses like the culinary uses, industrial uses, the uses of the parts of the plants other than the main drug and adulterants have also been added. The history of the drug has been added as far as possible to make the student follow the time line of use and historical development. The questions have been prepared by carefully going through the entire text and incorporated at the end of each chapter for the benefit of the students to help prepare for their final examination. A detailed glossary of the medical terms used in the text has been provided along with an account of the general tests for easy detection of the components of the drug as appendices at the end of the text. We have also included a detailed index at the end of the book.

We have done our best to incorporate all the details as far as possible and the book has run longer than we have expected. We wish to state that every care has been taken to bring out an error-free volume, and some errors and omissions if any might have crept in without our knowledge, they will be rectified in future editions. The suggestions for the improvement of the quality of this publication are welcome.

Our sincere thanks are due to authors and publishers of Wikipedia and other sources of web, books, materia medica, magazines, periodicals, monographs, bulletins, research reports, etc. Finally, we express our thanks to IKON Books, Hyderabad, for their continued cooperation in bringing out this publication in a highly presentable form within a short time.

Finally, we express our deep sense of gratitude to our family members for their continued cooperation, encouragement and best support in times of stress during the preparation of this volume.

P Suresh Narayana
pathiki.dharani@gmail.com

T Pullaiah
pullaiah.thammineni@gmail.com

Contents

Appendix

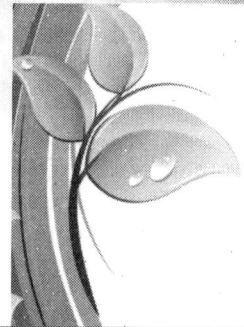

Chapter 1

Definition, History, Scope and Development of Pharmacognosy

INTRODUCTION

Mother nature has provided all the needs of human being including the medicines for better health. It includes a complete cure for almost all the types of ailments of the mankind. The knowledge and the experience accumulated over 1000s of years have given birth to today's modern medicine system. More than 60% of world population, directly or indirectly still uses the natural products for their primary healthcare needs. Nature is a symbiotic complex of the interdependent biotic and abiotic components. In the biotic component, the plants remain indispensable for human life, and provide a complete storehouse of remedies to all human ailments along with animals and other natural components. Very early man sought to alleviate his sufferings from injury and disease by growing plants around him and using them. But today, we have an accumulation of knowledge about the therapeutic properties of different plants. It is estimated that over 3 lakh species of plants yield many products of medicinal importance derived from over 300 families of flowering plants. The plant kingdom still holds many species of plants containing substances of medicinal value which have yet to be discovered and large numbers of plants are constantly being screened for their possible medicinal value.

A large number of crude drugs consist of entire plants or animals like Irish moss and cantharides, of parts of plants or animals like leaflets of senna and thyroid gland, of minerals like kaolin and chalk, of substances derived by extraction from plants or animals like catechu, resins, etc. are included in pharmacognosy. In addition to these, others like fibres and fabrics used for surgical dressings, materials such as diatomite and asbestos used as strainers for filtration and clarification of liquids, substances such as agar, gelatine, wax used as remedial agents and vehicles for the preparation of ointments, culture media, substances like pyrethrum used for the destruction of the insect pests are also included. The earliest books that contained the descriptions of the above materials were referred to as 'herbals' while the more recent ones are called the 'materia medica'. The herbals are represented by 'Ortus Sanitatis' (the Garden of Health – 1491), 'De Historia Stirpium' (1542) by Leonhart Fuchs and 'A New Herbal' (1551) by William Turner. Ortus Sanitatis contained an account of materia medica of animal, vegetable and mineral kingdoms arranged in an alphabetical order along with the illustrations and were used as a standard textbook of medicine in the 16th century England. It also contained many quotations from the Arabian writings of Rhazes and Avicenna, from the Greek writings of Dioscorides and Galen and from Roman writings of Pliny and Cato. De Historia Stirpium consisted of vegetable drugs arranged alphabetically with their Latin names and provided reliable descriptions and illustrations with which the medicinal plants could be correctly identified. 'A New Herbal' was a notable and earliest English herbal of the 16th century which provided a true scientific account of plants. The plants (simples) are arranged alphabetically under their Latin names which replaced 'The Great Herbal' (Ya Grete Herball) similar to 'Ortus Sanitatis'.

Later, an increasing amount of the details were gradually added onto the accounts contained in the earlier textbooks like their action, the preparation and an arrangement based on the accepted botanical and zoological classifications. This can be exemplified by the treatise of Pereira's Materia Medica (1839). As such an inclusion of the details became unwieldy; the study on the basis of different points of view was divided into four distinct branches, viz. 'Pharmaceutical Chemistry'—dealing with theory and fundamentals of scientific chemistry of the substances of pharmaceutical importance, 'Pharmaceutics' or 'Pharmacy'—dealing with the modes of treatment of chemicals and crude drugs in the preparation of medicines in a form suitable for administration, 'Pharmacodynamics' or 'Pharmacology' (synonymous with the older materia medica, still used under the same name in USA) concerned with the study of responses of organisms when they are subjected to treatment by drugs and 'Pharmacognosy'—dealing with structural, physical, chemical and sensory characters of crude drugs of animal, vegetable and mineral origin including their history, cultivation and collection, and other particulars related to their passage from the producer to the distributor or pharmacist. In the earlier days, the crude drugs were referred to as 'simples' or 'simple drugs' as their occurrence was natural and the terms 'simples' and 'Simplicia' were used in French books such as Guibourt's 'Histoire des Drogues Simples' and London pharmacopoeia as a general heading.

PHARMACOGNOSY–DEFINITION

The term, 'Pharmacology', may be defined as 'a branch of biology which deals in detail with crude medicinal and related products derived from plant, animal or mineral sources, and is concerned with the responses of the organisms to drugs *after their administration'*. The 'drug' on the other hand, is *'a substance used to modify the physiological system or the pathological state for the benefit of the receiver'*. This is the systematic study of the crude drugs obtained from natural origin like plants, animals and minerals. This involves the detailed study of the drugs obtained through natural sources including the name, habitat, collection, cultivation, macroscopy, microscopy, physical properties, chemical constituents, therapeutic actions, uses and adulterants. The drug science (pharmacology) is divided into three branches, *viz.* *'Pharmacy'* (*'Pharmacy'* is a Greek word which means *'Poison'* or *'Drug'*) dealing with the procurement, testing, storage and conversion into suitable medicinal forms of drugs, *'Pharmacodynamics'* concerned with the action of drugs upon the organism and *'Pharmacotherapy'* dealing with the use of drugs in the disease treatment. The drugs may be organic or inorganic and the organic drugs may be synthetic or of biological origin. Pharmacognosy deals with the drugs of biological origin. The term, *Physiopharmcognosy* proposed by Wasicky is a more appropriate name. The American Society of Pharmacognosy defines pharmacognosy as: *'the study of the physical, chemical, biochemical and biological properties of drugs, drug substances or potential drugs or drug substances of natural origin as well as the search for new drugs from natural sources'*.

In the 19th century, the term, *'Materia Medica'* was used for *'Pharmacognosy'*. Even though the science of pharmacognosy was practiced since a very early period, the term, *'pharmacognosy'* formed from the Greek words was used for the first time by the Austrian Physician, Johann Adam Schmidt (1811), in his handwritten manuscript *'Lehrbuch der materia medica'*, which was posthumously published in Vienna (1811), to describe 'the study of medicinal plants and their properties'. It was in 1815, during his studies with Sarsaparilla, it was Crr. Anotheus Seydler, a German scientist, coined the term, *'pharmacognosy'* in his work, *'Analecta Pharmacognostica'*, a small work. The term *'Pharmacognosy'* is derived from two Greek words, *'pharmakon'* meaning a *'drug'* (derived from Latin term—*Droog* meaning 'dried'—when dried plants were commonly used as medicine in the earlier times) and *'gnosis'* meaning *'knowledge'*, meaning the *'knowledge of drugs'*, as recorded by Dr. K. Ganzinger. Pharmacognosy may be defined as *'the study of those natural substances principally plants that find use in medicine'*. During the 19th century and the beginning of the 20th century, pharmacognosy was used to define the branch of medicine or commodity sciences (*Warenkunde*, in German) which deals with 'the drugs in their crude or unprepared form'. The crude drugs are dried, unprepared material of plant, animal or mineral origin, used for medicine. Such study under the name, *'pharmacognosie'* was first developed in German speaking areas of Europe, while the other language areas often used the older term, *'materia medica'* and in German, the term *'drogenkunde'* (science of crude drugs) is also used synonymously.

PHARMACOGNOSY-HISTORY

The history of herbal medicine is as old as human civilisation. The primitive man, who went in search of food, ate at random the plants or plant parts like leaves, fruits, seeds, roots, tubers, etc. He categorised them as edible (for food) if he found no ill effects after eating, and inedible if he was subjected to any ill effect and according to the nature of the symptoms observed, he used them to cure the diseases. For example, a plant was used as a purgative, if it caused diarrhoea, as an emetic, if it caused vomiting, as an arrow–poison if it caused death. This knowledge was obtained as a trial and error. He used these drugs as infusions and decoctions. The results were passed on from generation to generation and knowledge was added on in the same way. The antiquity documents reveal that the plants were used as medicine in China, India, Egypt and Greece long before the Christian era. The Egyptians were familiar with the medicinal properties of plants and animals in addition to human anatomy and embalming the dead and preserving their bodies as mummies. The earliest reference to the use of the medicinal herbs and a cure for disease as well as the method of embalming the dead was described in the most famous manuscript of 'Papyrus Ebers', an ancient book (150 BC), 60 feet long and 1 foot wide scroll found in one of the mummies dating back to 16th century BC. It contained 800 formulae and 700 different drugs such as acacia, castor oil, fennel, iron oxide, sodium chloride, sodium carbonate and sulphur. The ancient Egyptians documented their knowledge about medicine on paper made from *Cyperus aquaticus*, commonly called *Papyrus*, or *Aquatic sage*. *Papyrus Ebers* (around 1500 BC), *Berlin Papyrus, Edwin Smith Smith Papyrus, Kahum Medicak Papyrus* are some of the oldest handbooks which contain the information of illness and treatments. In ancient Egypt and Mesopotamia, clay tablets were used to document the knowledge of drugs which date back to 3000 BC. The people in the prehistoric times used plants quite intuitively for food, shelter and even curing their many bodily disorders and thereby kept their health in perfect state of fitness and lived a long-life. The medicinal plants played a very important role from times immemorial. The medicinal properties of plants were almost certainly known to the Chinese as long ago as 5000 BC although not until the Egyptians in the reign of Khufu around 4500 BC had documentary proof of the exploitation of such materials is seen. The oldest known herbal is *Pen-tsao* written by the Emperor Shen Nung around 3000 BC. It contained 365 drugs, one for the each day of a year. The Ayurvedic texts of the Indian Healers (of Ancient India) around 1000 BC list many hundreds of plant extracts and their use for medicinal and spiritual purposes. The information about the drugs of Ancient India was documented in several Ayurvedic texts which still exist (such as *Atharvaveda, Charak Samhita, Sushrut Samhita, Madhav Nidan* and *Bhava Prakash*).

Greeks also contributed much to the knowledge of natural history. About 4000 BC, Hippocrates (460–370 BC), the *'Father of Medicine'*, rejected magico-ritual treatment of the disease and advocated that medicine was a science and not a myth. Following Hippocrates, Aristotle (384–322 BC), a student of Plato and a philosopher, wrote authoritatively on animal kingdom. Theophrastus (30–287 BC), a student of Aristotle, wrote in detail about the plant kingdom and Dioscorides (40–80 AD), a physician described medicinal plants like belladonna, ergot, opium and colchicum which are in use even today. Pliny wrote natural history in 37 volumes and Galen (131–200 AD), the first pharmacist, devised *'galenicals'*, the methods of preparation of the plant and animal drugs. He was also known for a number of pain relieving preparations including opium. The early Arabians have also contributed much to herbal medicine. Paracelsus (1493–1541) developed mineral salts as potential curative agents. The early writings on the clay tablets by the Sumarians show that their medicines included opium, liquorice, thyme and mustard. Babylonians used senna, saffron, coriander, cinnamon, garlic, etc. in their medicinal concoctions, wines, and poultices. A perusal of ancient Sanskrit texts dating back to the vedic periods reveal that Indians have a sound knowledge of *'Vrikshayurveda'*, the *'science of medicinal plants'*. Varahamihira in his *'Brihatsamhita'* and *'Agnipurana'* and Sarangadhara in his *'Vrikshayurveda'* have dealt with the subject in a greater detail. Parasara, Uddalaka and Yajnavalkya have also written on *'Vrikshayurveda'*. Atreya (1st century AD), a famous medical practitioner, wrote *'Atri Samhita'*. During the middle ages, the knowledge of medicinal plants was further developed by the European monks who studied and grew drug plants and also translated the Arabic herbals. The Central and South American natives also possessed extensive knowledge of the indigenous traditional herbs. One important inclusion is *Uncaria tomentosa* (*Una de Gato* or Cat's Claw herb) from the Peruvian rain forest which has become very popular in USA as an immune-stimulant. *Prunus africana* (pygeum) beneficial for the prostate gland was discovered from native Africans, tea tree oil from the leaves of *Melaleuca* tree was discovered from the Australian aborigines and was used by the British soldiers as an antiseptic during World War II and *Morinda citrifolia* (noni), an immune-stimulant and *Piper methysticum* (Kava kava) were discovered from the natives of South Pacific.

The evidence for the knowledge of medicinal plants in India is very old as the medicinal properties of plants for a wide range of purposes were described in Rigveda and Atharvaveda, during 3500–1500 BC from which the science of Ayurveda developed. They have been in fact used in a continuous unbroken tradition for over 4 millennia. *'Rig veda'*, the oldest repository of human knowledge written between 4500 and 1500 BC mentions the use of 67 plants for the therapeutic use and *'Yajurveda'* enlists 81 plants whereas the *'Athrva veda'* written during 1200 BC describes 290 plants of medicinal value. In Ayurveda, the well known treatises are 'Charaka Samhitha' (900 BC) which dealt with mostly plants wherein 500 medicinal plants were described in 50 groups of 10 herbs each sufficing the ordinary needs of a physician and 'Sushrutha Samhitha' (600 BC) in which surgery was also included contained 760 medicinal herbs in 7 distinct sets on the basis of their common properties.

Pharmacognosy was more a descriptive science even up to the beginning of the 20th century which made a rapid stride thereafter. A century ago, the objective of pharmacognosy was limited primarily to the recognition of crude plant and animal drugs and their sources. The pharmacist then was concerned with the procurement of drugs and manufacturing galenical preparations from them. The species of Capsicum did not enter the European pharmacognosy until Columbus and his crew encountered them on the island of Hispanola, the modern Greater Antilles (1494). Garcia da Orta (1563) of the Portuguese Colonial Services practiced medicine and studied pharmacognosy with particular reference to the plants of Southern Indian peninsula and tropical medicine. During the rule of Ming Dynasty (1368–1644), a monumental work on materia medica, 'Compendium of Materia Medica' (Bencao Gangmu) was compiled by a doctor and a pharmacist, Li Shizhen and published in 52 volumes (1590). It contained the details of 1892 drugs, 1160 pictures and 11096 prescriptions and was a multidisciplinary book of botany, pharmacognosy, pharmacology and therapeutics. The importance of alcohol in the extraction of medicines was reported by Le'mery (1645–1715). W. Withering (1785) published an account of the medicinal properties of foxglove leaves. Derosne, the French, Pharmacist (1803), isolated narcotine from opium. Serttuerner (1806) isolated morphine from opium and recognised its role in alleviating pain. In the coming years (1817–1820), strychnine, emetine, brucine, piperine, quinine and colchicine were isolated. Pelletier, the French Pharmacist, was the first to report the isolation of strychnine from Ignatius Beans and later from seeds of Nux vomica. Martius (1825) delivered the first lecture on pharmacognosy. Dr King (1835) developed a resinous Cimicifuga alcohol-based extract which he called cimicifugin (macrotin), which was the first resinous concentrates of Eclectics and described the obstetric uses. Stass and Otto (1852) developed a new extraction process for the alkaloids. Posselt and Reimann (1828) isolated nicotine from the leaves of tobacco, Neumann (1860) isolated cocaine, Hardy and Gallows (1867) isolated ouabain, Gerrard and Hardy (1875) isolated pilocarpine, Nagai (1887) isolated ephedrine and Kuersten (1891) isolated podophyllotoxin. Other significant discoveries in the 20th century are the isolation of ergometrine, digitoxin, reserpine, theophylline and quinidine. The first laboratory manual on pharmacognosy, 'Pharmacy and Prescription Writing', was published in 1902 as its second edition. The first published American Materia Medica, 'Therapeutics and Pharmacognosy' (1919) lists lemon as the primary citrus plant to have the medicinal properties and citric acid in the lemon juice is a very useful therapy. It is mentioned that lemon juice can be used in the treatment of malaria and some cases of chronic rheumatism and gout in addition to prevention of scurvy and to control postpartum.

Jakob Schleiden (1857) discovered that various types of Sarsaparilla root can be distinguished by means of their endodermal cells. Since then, drug histology was recognised as an important means of detecting impurities and adulterants in the crude drugs. Commerce made more foreign drugs available and the adulterants also became more common. With the rise of drug houses, drugs became available not only in whole form but also in cut and powdered from. The powders could not be identified with certainty by visual inspection only and as a result, the identification of some drugs and the testing of their purity became much more complicated.

The period between 1930 and 1960 refers to the development of modern pharmacognosy by the simultaneous application of any disciplines as well as the methods and techniques of analytical chemistry like chromatography and spectrophotometry. During this period, many substances were isolated and elucidated from plants. These included the isolation of penicillin by W. Fleming (1928) and its large scale production by Florey and Chain (1941),

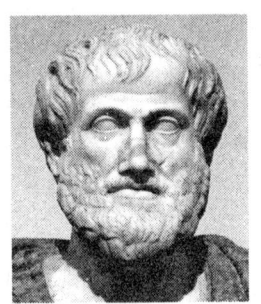
Aristotle

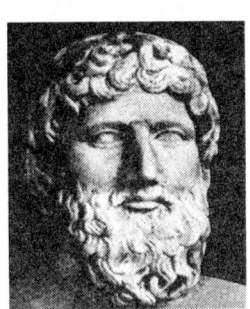
Plato

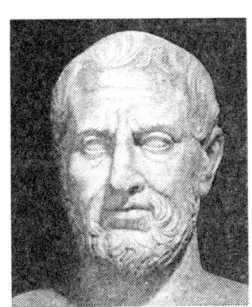
Theophrastus

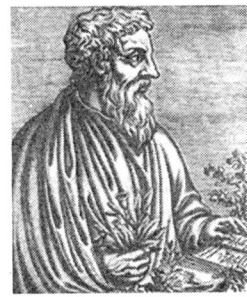
Dioscorides

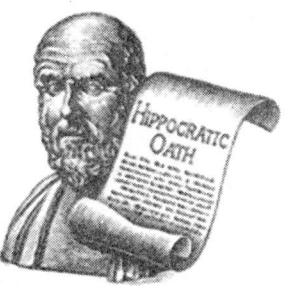
Hippocrates

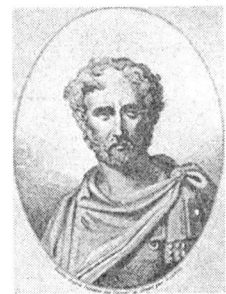
Pliny—the Elder

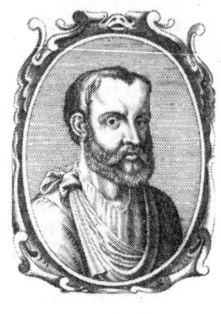

Galen

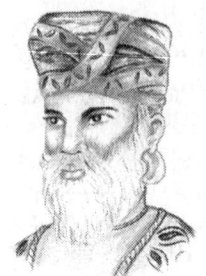

Charaka

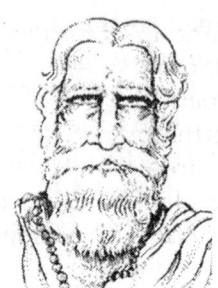

Sushrutha

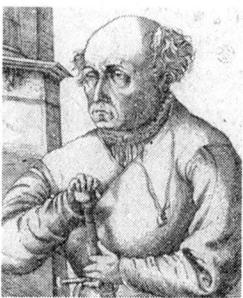

Paracelsus

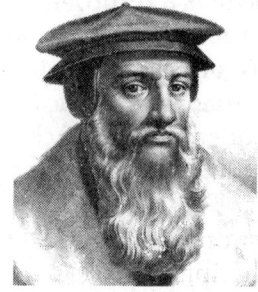

Leonhart Fuchs

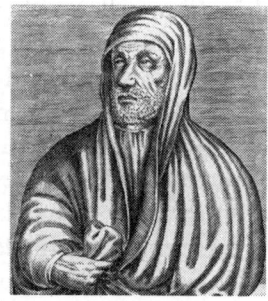

Avicenna

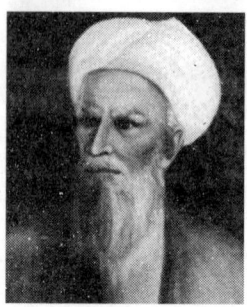

Rhazes

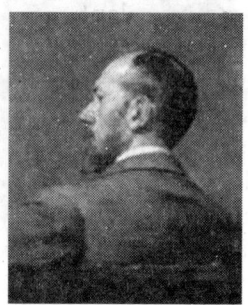

William Turner

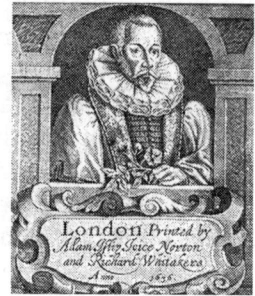

John Gerard

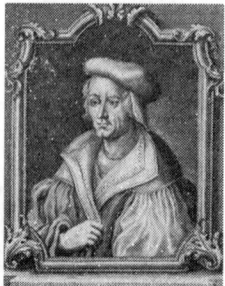

Otto Brunfels

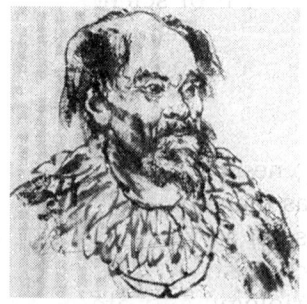

Emperor Shen Nung

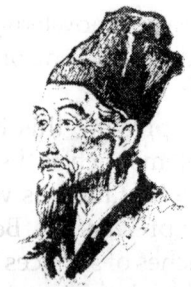

Li Shizhen-Physician

isolation of reserpine and confirmation of its tranquilising properties, isolation of vincristine and vinblastine with proven anticancerous properties and many steroid hormones. As such, this period was referred to as the antibiotic age due to isolation and studies of other active antibiotics like streptomycin, chloramphenicol, tetracycline, etc. During 1980–1990s, new plant drug development programmes are traditionally undertaken by random screening or ethnobotanical approach.

PHARMACOGNOSY-SCOPE AND DEVELOPMENT

Pharmacognosy encompasses the knowledge of the history, distribution, cultivation, collection, processing and preservation, the study of sensory, physical, chemical and structural characters and the use of crude drugs. It also includes the study of other materials used in pharmacy such as suspending, disintegrating and flavouring agents, filtering aids, etc. and substances like antibiotics, allergens, hallucinogenic and poisonous plants, immunising agents, pesticides, raw materials for the production of oral contraceptives, etc.

This branch is the oldest of all pharmacy science, and is critical in the development of different disciplines of science. A pharmacognosist should possess a sound knowledge of the terms used to describe the vegetable and animal drugs in botany and zoology respectively. The knowledge of plant taxonomy, plant breeding, plant pathology and plant genetics is helpful in the development of cultivation technology for the medicinal and aromatic plants. Phytochemistry has undergone significant development in recent years as a separate discipline, and is concerned with an enormous variety of substances that are synthesised and accumulated by the plants as well as their structural elucidation. The extraction, isolation, purification, and characterisation of a variety of phytochemicals from the natural sources are important for the advancement of the medicine system. In addition, the knowledge of chemotaxonomy, the biogenetic pathways (for the formation of medicinally active primary and secondary metabolites), plant tissue culture and other related fields is also essential for the complete understanding of this branch of science. Similarly, one should have the basic knowledge of the biochemistry and chemical engineering for the development of collection, processing and storage technology of the crude drugs.

At present, this interdisciplinary branch of science is concerned with problems such as the biogenesis of drug products, drug resistance, mutation and adaptation as well as the effect of the environment on organisms of drug production. Because of a wider scope, it shares ground with other branches of sciences like chemistry, biochemistry, physiology, enzymology, food technology, bacteriology, and other fields of specialisation like taxonomy, anatomy, morphology, plant physiology, genetics, biochemistry, phytochemistry, microbiology and several others. It also supplies the general information to the pharmacists. Because of these reasons, pharmacognosy has become a discipline of increasing significance.

Nowadays, this has become a kind of multidisciplinary subject which embraces phytochemistry, analytical pharmacognosy, pharmacotherapy, medicinal plant biotechnology, herbal formulations and nutraceuticals. *Zoopharmacognosy* is a branch of pharmacognosy which involves the observation of the animal behaviour for the discovery and the development of new drugs. At present, drugs from the natural origin are studied, formulated and regulated in the framework of allopathy.

REVIEW QUESTIONS

1. **Essay and Short Answer Questions**
   1. What is 'pharmacognosy'? Write an account of its historical development.
   2. Write an account of the history, development and the scope of 'pharmacognosy'.
   3. Define 'pharmacognosy'. What is its scope in the studies of drug development? Discuss the development of pharmacognosy in recent years.

2. **Choose the Correct Alternative**
   1. The term 'pharmacognosy' was first used by: [ ]
      a. Theophrastus   b. JA Schmidt
      c. K Ganzinger   d. Wasicky
   2. The term 'pharmacognosy' was coined by: [ ]
      a. Gannzinger   b. Guibourt
      c. Seydler   d. Leonhart Fuchs
   3. The medicinal properties of Foxglove leaves were first published by: [ ]
      a. Lémery   b. Derosne
      c. Withering   d. Serttuerner
   4. Ephedrine was isolated by: [ ]
      a. Posselt and Reimann   b. Hardy and Gallows
      c. Stass and Otto   d. Nagai
   5. Cocaine was isolated by: [ ]
      a. Neumann   b. Kuersten
      c. Hardy   d. Reimann

3. **Fill in the Blanks:**

   1. The earliest reference of the use of the herbs and a cure for the disease was ....

   2. The oldest known herbal written by Shen Nung (3000 BC) was ....

3. The mineral salts were developed as potential curative agents by ....

4. .... isolated morphine from opium and recognised its role in pain alleviation.

5. The isolation of strychnine from Ignatius Beans was first reported by ....

4. True or False Statements:

1. Diatomite is used as a strainer for filtration and clarification of liquids. [True/False]

2. *Ortus Sanitatis* was not a standard textbook of medicine in England during the 16th century. [True/False]

3. The earliest English herbal of the 19th century was *A New Herbal*. [True/False]

4. Pharmacology deals with the study of responses of the organisms during treatment. [True/False]

5. In the olden days, the crude drugs were called *simples*. [True/False]

5. Match the following:

1. Leonhart Fuchs [ ]   a. *A New Herbal*
2. CA Seydler [ ]   b. *Physiopharmacognosy*
3. Wasicky [ ]   c. *De Historia Stirpium*
4. Hippocrates [ ]   d. *Analecta Pharmacognostica*
5. William Turner [ ]   e. *Father of Medicine*

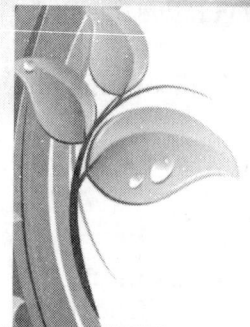

Chapter **2**

Brief Introduction to Natural Sources of Drugs with Examples

The ecosystems of earth which abound in plant, animal and mineral substances are the main source of very many drugs used by humans to cure their ailments. Ever since man dominated the Mother Earth, he has been exclusively relying on nature for his sustenance and survival. Instinctive urge, intuition and accumulated knowledge have guided him to use natural products as remedies for his short-term and chronic ailments. The natural drugs obtained from plants and animals are called the drugs of biological origin which are produced in the living cells of their bodies.

It is estimated that 265,000 flowering plants inhabit the earth. Of these, less than 1% has been studied for their chemical composition and medicinal values. As it is impossible to screen each of the species for their biological activity, researchers gather the vegetation at random in any area with rich biodiversity and this results in only few new drug possibilities. Hence, other methods are adopted and the best possible approach is ethno-botanical approach which seems to be more productive. The ethnobotanists interested in drug discovery mainly rely on elderly healers to identify the plants likely to contain potential bioactive chemicals by conducting long-term field work in the remote areas of the world. The plant collection surveys may be phylogenetic during which close relatives of plants known to produce useful compounds are chosen, ecological in which the plants living in particular habitats capable of exerting an effect on animals are selected, and/or they may focus their attention on specimens which are immune from predation by the insects.

As on today there are at least 120 distinct chemical substances derived from plants considered to be important and currently in use in many countries of the world. Many of the drugs sold in the market are simple synthetic modifications of the naturally obtained crude drugs. For example, ipecac from the tropical *Cephaelis ipecacuanha* now is referred to as emetine and taxol from the species of *Taxus brevifolia* is now marketed as Paclitaxel and quinidine from *Cinchona pubescens* bark as cardioquin. Plants have been a rich source of medicines because they produce a host of bioactive molecules most of which probably evolved as potential chemical defences against predators or infection within their bodies.

The drugs are obtained from seven major sources: Plant/vegetable, animal, mineral/earth, marine, microorganisms/microbiological, semi-synthetic/synthetic and from genetic engineering/recombinant DNA technology.

PLANT (VEGETABLE) SOURCE

Today, the plant medicines are the most widely used medicines in the world. About 85% of world population employs herbs as their primary medicines. The plant-based remedies are used for both acute and chronic health problems, from common cold (coryza) to controlling blood pressure and cholesterol. Such medicines are made available in tablet, liquid or ointment form. Physical evidence of the use of herbal medicines dates back some 60,000 years to a burial site at Shanidar Cave in Iraq in which a Neanderthal man was uncovered (1969). The archaeologists collected 8 species of plants from the burial site, 7 of which are used for medicinal purposes even today. The most extraordinary of the century was the discovery of an ice mummy preserved by freezing in Otzal Alps, Austria (1991) by two hikers. The analysis of the samples of organic tissues has determined that the Ice Man lived between 3350 and 3100 BC. The man who suffered from a number of medical conditions died approximately 5200 years ago at an age of 40–50 years. He turned into a mummy almost immediately by the freezing weather conditions and was turned into the Ice Man. He belonged to the Neolithic age in Europe and his most valuable possession was his 'medicine kit' which contained 2 walnut-sized lumps of a birch fungus used as a laxative and as a natural antibiotic.

Medicines from plants are safer, gentler and better for human health than the synthetic drugs because humans have co-evolved with plants over the past a few millions of years. Human beings eat plants, drink their juices and consume them in many forms and their ingredients from carbohydrates to vitamins and minerals are a part of our body composition and chemistry. Some compounds of our body perform the same functions in plants. For example, naturally occurring antioxidant phenols in plants protect their cells from oxidation and carry out the same function in our bodies. The human body can easily recognise the substances that occur in plants and also possess a highly evolved mechanism for metabolising them. At the same time, plants can also be dangerous to human health. For example, the drinking of a decoction of oleander leaves or chewing a handful of foxglove results in death. But, if the herbs can be used in specific dosage range as has been determined by centuries, we are likely to be benefited without any side effects. Hence, plant medicines remain indispensable to modern pharmacology and clinical practice.

Folk medicines are the primary source of crude drugs as they are already being subjected to human screening by trial and error method by the primitive society. But, folk medicine in aboriginal societies is rapidly declining due to the change of mode of life of the people. Ethnobotanists are desperate to gather valuable information from them before they fade out. By scanning thousands of herbarium specimens at Harvard University, it was possible to document an extensive record of plants used in the treatment of cancer. This is being followed up by a collaborative team work of botanists, phytochemists, pharmacologists and clinicians at National Cancer Institute, USA, who could screen thousands of plant extracts for antineoplastic and cytotoxic activity.

A perusal of list of drugs derived from natural sources reveals that most of the dicotyledons provide a number of useful drugs. Arab physicians in the 9th century introduced *Senna alexandrina* to Europe where its pods are still widely used as laxatives even today. The species of *Mentha* are the natural sources of menthol (peppermint camphor) commonly used in lozenges for sore throats and in inhalers to treat upper respiratory disorders and also as a mild anaesthetic to ease muscular tension. Peppermint oil is an age-old remedy for relieving an upset stomach. *Gaultheria procumbens* (wintergreen) is a source of methylsalicylate used in topical ointments to relieve muscular pain, for lumbago, sciatica and rheumatism. *Papaver somniferum* (opium poppy) yields narcotic opium from which morphine, the potent painkiller is made. This is known since 8th century and it was Belon (1546), a French naturalist, who drew European attention to its abuse among Turks. *Digitalis purpurea* (purple foxglove) is a source of digitoxin which increases the strength of the heart beat while decreasing it rate. The plant first appeared in the French pharmacopoeia since its first printing (1818). This is used in the treatment of congestive heart failure and other disorders of the heart. Manal, an Indian on a trip to Burma (1930) discovered that the wild elephants in captivity fed by the elongated snake-like roots of a plant were surprisingly very calm. As such, he collected the samples and brought them back to India to conduct tests on its properties. The plant showed tranquilising and antihypertensive properties. It proved to be *Rauwolfia serpentina* (after Leonhart Rauwolf, 16th century German physician). The effects were due to the alkaloid reserpine (drug serpina was launched in 1934) which as a sedative relieves some psychiatric disorders. *Cinchona pubescens* (Ecuador Cinchona) stands among the greatest life saving medicines of all time. This was brought to light when Juan Del Vega (Ecuadorian physician, 1620) used a Quichua remedy known as 'quina bark' on the Countess of Chinchon, wife of the Viceroy of Peru, who contracted malaria which is potentially fatal at that time. She recovered from the illness and the bark became to be known as the 'Countess bark'. This spread and cinchona got popularised by Robert Talbor, an assistant to an apoethecary, in late 1660s. The bark is the source of alkaloids namely quinidine, cinchonine and cinchonidine. The source of curare, a poison on the tips of arrows which killed the animals and humans immediately was *Chondodendron tomentosum*. This came to light in 1493 during the second trip of Columbus to Americas in the forests of Amazon. Richard Gill (1938), an American, successfully identified the plant which is a source for the drug tubocurarine used as an adjunct in general anaesthesia and in cases of spastic paralysis and plastic muscular rigidity. In cancer chemotherapy, taxol, a derivative of *Taxus brevifolia* (Pacific Yew) is used while *Catharanthus roseus* (Madagascar Periwinkle) is the source of vinblastine and vincristine used in the treatment of Hodgkin's disease and pediatric leukemia.

Other important drugs of vegetable origin include: khellin, a bronchodilator from *Ammi visnaga*, berberine, an antidiarrhoeal from species of *Berberis*, and caffeine, a stimulant of central nervous system from *Camellia sinensis*. Vincristine, an anticancerous agent from *Catharanthus roseus*, sennoside, a laxative from species of *Cassia*, emetine, an antiamoebic drug from *Cephaelis ipecacuanha*, and drugs like ergometrin, ergotamine and ergotoxine used as vasodilators, antimalarials, vasoconstrictors from *Claviceps purpurea* are the products of plants. Quinine and quinidine which are antimalarial and antiarrhythmic are extracted from the species of *Cinchona*, hyoscyamine, hyoscine and atropine used as parasympatholytic have been isolated from the species of *Datura*, *Hyoscyamus* and *Atropa belladonna*. The species of *Dioscorea* yield diosgenin which is anti-inflammatory. Ephedrine, a sympathomimetic comes from the species of *Ephedra*, cocaine used as a local anaesthetic from *Erythroxylon coca*, lobelline an antiasthmatic from *Lobelia inflata* and morphine, codeine, papaverine used as sedatives, antitussives, muscle relaxants from *Papaver somniferum* are the products of plants. Similarly, pilocarpine used as a para-sympathomimetic, podophyllotoxine used as an anticancerous drug, reserpine as a vasodilator and solasodine as a hormone have been isolated from *Pilocarpus jaborandi*, species of *Podophyllum*, *Rauwolfia serpentina* and species of *Solanum* respectively. Flowers too form an important source of drugs to cure many ailments. This has been clearly explained by Dr. Edward Bach in his homoeopathic flower remedies. During 1930 – 1935, he collected about 38 wild forest flowers with which he formulated a plan of their usage as potential remedies. These include agrimonia, aspen, beech, centaurium, berry plum, chestnut, chicory, clematis, elm, gentian, heather, holly, larch, mimulus, mustard, oak, olive, red chestnut, walnut, willow, etc.

Many substances of plant origin are being used as pharmaceutical aids in medicine. To mention a few are: gums from *Acacia*, *Sterculia* and Guar used for binding, suspending, emulsification and thickening. Mucilages like ispaghol and linseed are used as demulcents and soothing agents. Saponins like qrulaia are used as emulsifying agents in culture media. Fixed oils like olive oil, sesame seed oil, cotton seed oil, almond oil and castor oil are used in the preparation of coal tar emulsion. Volatile oils like caraway oil, cardamom oil, cinnamon oil, clove oil and coriander oil, oil from fennel, lemon oil, orange oil and peppermint oil are being used as the ointment bases and as flavouring agents in drug industry. Similarly, chlorophyll and saffron are used as natural dyes. Pyrethrum is used as a suspending agent and also for the production of capsules.

ANIMAL SOURCE

The drugs are also obtained from different classes of animals of the animal kingdom. These drugs are used in allopathic, homoeopathic and unani systems. The marine creatures have a major potential though their quantity is much limited than that of the plants. The drugs used traditionally in Africa, India and other countries of the oriental region come from the invertebrate and vertebrate animal groups like porifera, coelenterata, mollusca, annelida, arthropoda, echinodermata and chordata.

In porifera, sponges contain the metabolites like bromophenols which are antibacterial, cyclic peroxides and peroxyketols which are antimicrobial, ichthyotoxic and cytotoxic and sesquiterpenes which are antimalarial, antifungal, antibacterial and anticancerous. In coelenterata, jelly fishes, sea anemones and corals are the source for prostaglandin A_2 (occurs in the soft coral, *Plexaura homoomalla*). *Sacrophyton glaucum* is the source for dipterpenoids, and sarcophytols A and B which are tumour inhibitory. In mollusca, the cuttlefish bone from *Sepia officinalis* is used in dentifrices and also as an antacid. In annelida, the Japanese species of *Lumbriconereis heteropoda* produces a potent neurotoxin, nereistoxin. Similarly, bivalirudin engineered from the saliva of the leech, *Haementeria officinalis*, is an antiplatelet protein which stops blood clotting and is used in unstable angina and to open blocked arteries in the heart. In arthropoda, beetles (Order: Coleoptera) of the genera *Cantharis* and *Mylabris* possess vesicant properties and cause blisters. The preparations of *Cantharis vesicatoria* are used as rubefacients and vesicants as plasters, collodions, etc. Cantharidin is the active principle of the cantharides, the dried bodies of the blister beetles of family Meloidae, associated with the elytra, eggs and ovaries. In small quantities, these stimulate sexual desire, stop sterility in women, incontinence of urine, spermatorrhoea, etc. On external application, it excites inflammation of the skin. These are imported into India and Pakistan for medicinal purpose. Honeybee, *Apis mellifera* (Order Hymenoptera) produces honey, bees wax, royal jelly, etc. The bony fishes (Class: Osteichthyes) like sharks, cod fishes and halibut are the important sources of liver oils which contain vitamin A and eicosapenteanoic acid used as dietary supplements. Cod liver oil is a fixed oil prepared from the fresh liver of the cod fish, *Gadus callarias*, *G. morrhua* and other species of *Gadus* (Family: Gadidae) containing due proportion of vitamins. Cod liver oil is the source of vitamins A and D. Shark liver oil is a fixed oil obtained from the fresh or carefully preserved livers of various species of Sharks, mainly *Hypoprion brevirostris* and *Galeorhinus zygopterus*. The oil is a rich source of vitamin A and is used in the treatment of xerophthalmia (abnormal dryness of the surface of conjunctiva of the eye) which occurs as a result of deficiency of vitamin A. In class amphibia, toad skin is the source of a cardioactive principle used for treating dropsy. The significance of class reptilia is well known for snake venom. The first insulin mimetic, exenatide has been isolated from the saliva of *Gila monster, Heloderma suspectum*. The class mammalia is the source for spermaceti, gelatine, musk, insulin, hormones, products of blood and liver, vaccines and sera, cat gut, wool, wool fat, etc. Spermaceti is a waxy substance obtained from the head of sperm whale, *Physeter macrocephalus* L. spermaceti is used as an emollient and also in the preparation of ointments, especially cold creams. At present, the collection of whales is illegal.

The important drugs used in homoeopathy are derived from animals of different groups of invertebrates and vertebrates. Allantoin is a product of metabolism associated with allantoic fluid, amniotic fluid, foetal urine and maggots of blowfly which are used for treating various conditions of decaying tissues. Amber is derived as a secretion from sperm whale, *Ambra grisea* used as a drug for the brain, heart and symptoms of premature old age. Craw fish, *Astacus fluviatilis* produces a drug used for urticaria and other skin diseases. Red star fish, *Asterias rubens* gives a drug useful in neuralgia, cholera, hysteria and cancer. The fresh water sponge, *Badiaga* is the source of a drug useful in the soreness of muscles and swollen glands. The poison of *Bufo*, a toad, is a drug for rheumatism and epilepsy. Thumbnail of horse, *Castor equi*, is a drug that acts on the nails, bones and warts and also helps as a cure in cracked and ulcerated nipples. The drug from beaver, *Castoreum* is a powerful remedy for hysteria. The venom of the copperhead snake, *Cenchris contortrix* is a potent drug for dyspnoea and increased sexual desire in both the sexes. The coral snake, *Elaps corallinus* is a source of a drug used in paralysis. Ox gall is used in intestinal disorders like diarrhoea, obstruction of gall ducts, biliary calculi and jaundice. Saliva of the rabid dog (hydrophobinum) is a potent drug for hydrophobia. Snake venom (lachesis) is an antidote for snake bite, haemorrhage, melancholy and paralysis. The drug from the medusa of jelly fish helps in the diseases of the eyes, nose, ears and lips. Purple fish, *Murex* is a source of medicine for diseases of the female sexual system. The drug from Black Cuba spider, *Mygale lasiodora* helps in palpitation, nervousness, fear and cholera. The cobra venom from *Naja tripudians* is known for marked dyspnoea and bulbar paralysis. Cod liver oil is a nutrient and a hepatic and pancreatic remedy and also helps in emaciation, lassitude and atrophy in infants. Similarly, Dippel's animal oil is associated with migraine and neuralgia of spermatic cord and burning pains and stitches.

The drug from wood louse, *Oniscus asellus millipedes* has distinct diuretic properties and used in dropsy as well as in bronchial catarrah. Inky juice of cuttle-fish, *Sepia*, is an important uterine remedy as it acts on the portal system with venous congestion and also has a tendency for abortion and menopause. The potent constituent from Cuban spider, *Tarantula cubensis* is associated with septic conditions, diphtheria, pruritus and bubonic plague while that from the Spanish spider, *Tarantula hispania* is a drug for hysterias, dysmenorrhoea, spinal irritability, hysterical epilepsy and intense sexual excitement. The orange spider, *Theridion* produces a drug for tubercular diathesis, rachitis, caries, necrosis and vertigo and the drug from the German viper, *Vipera* has special action on the kidneys, cardiac dropsy, liver enlargement, menopause ailments, oedema of glottis, polyneuritis and poliomyelitis.

Insects too are the source for many homoeopathic drugs. The common bed bug, *Cimex*, is a remedy for intermittent fever with weariness while the honeybee, *Apis*, is used in oedema, stinging pains and inflammation of kidneys. American cockroach, *Blatta americana*, is used in many forms of dropsy, pain in urethra on urination while Indian cockroach, *Blatta orientalis*, is a remedy for asthma when associated with bronchitis. The plant lice from *Chenopodium*, *Chenopodi glauci aphis*, is used as an anthelmintic. The ladybird beetle, *Conccinella septempunctata*, is a homeo remedy in neuralgia, toothaches, cold sensation in the mouth, pain in kidneys and loins and symptoms of hydrophobia. The Colorado potato bug, *Doryphora*, is used for gonorrhoea, gleet, and urethritis in children, prostration, body swelling and burning sensation. Yellow locust, *Robina*, is a source of the remedy for hyperchlorhydria and acidity while live wasp, *Vespa crarbo*, is a remedy for fainting, numbness and blindness, nausea and vomiting followed by creeping chills, cramping pain in bowels and swollen axillary gland. There are many more to be mentioned.

Substances like wool fat, bees wax, spermaceti and carnuba wax from animals are used as pharmaceutical aids, as emollients and as vehicles for other drugs. The animal protein gelatine is a natural dye.

MINERAL (EARTH) SOURCE

The substances of mineral origin have been used for various pharmaceutical purposes ranging from therapeutic agents to nutritional supplements to pharmaceutical necessities. The drugs from mineral sources comprise of metals and nonmetals like zinc, aluminium, mercury, etc. with their salts and mineral acids. Calamine is used in skin ointments and lotions as a topical protective agent. It is largely used in dusting powders, ointments and lotions. Calamine lotion USP is one of the most widely used preparations of calamine. Bentonite is used for the preparation of gels used for producing emulsions, ointments and creams. This is also used in many cosmetic preparations such as lip sticks, rouges, etc. Purified talc is used as a filtration and purification agent. It is also used as a lubricant in tablets and for the preparation of dusting powders and for coating and dusting pills. Fuller's earth is used as a filtering and clarifying agent. It is used in the preparation of dusting powder due to its water absorbing properties. Kieselguhr or diatomaceous earth (ooze) is employed in the manufacture of tooth powders, talcum powders, nail paints, pills and soaps. Prepared chalk is used in the preparation of talcum powder and tooth powder. Chalk is also used an antacid and in the treatment of diarrhoea. Shilajit is prescribed in ayurveda for the treatment of diabetes. It is laxative and pungent in its digestive action. It is reported to improve the strength and complexion of the body and has been considered as a potent anti-stress agent. It is used as an aphrodisiac and geriatric agent. Carbohydrates like starches, sodium alginate, glucose, sucrose, honey and agar are used pharmaceutically as aids in disintegrating agents, for stabilising thickening, as emulsifying, and deflocculating, gelling and filming agents, as sweetening agents and as laxatives.

The materials used as drugs in Indian systems of medicine from the mineral kingdom are represented by diamond, alumen, china clay, silver, oxides and salts of ammonium, arsenic, mineral pitch, gold, calcium, copper, iron, mercury, mica, lead, potassium, silica, sodium, tin, sulphur and zinc, etc.

MARINE (AQUATIC) SOURCE

The oceans on the globe provide not only food but also many more products which are useful to mankind as medicines and other substances. The compound called carrageenan comes from a sugar in red algae of the seas and oceans finds its way into the peanut butter and toothpastes which we use as it helps in spreading of the butter and gives much consistency for the toothpaste. Some of the products from the marine environment are also used in the cosmetic industry. Scientists of the US Sea Grant extracted a compound from Caribbean Sea Whip, a soft coral, capable of reducing inflammation of the skin in sunburn and reducing skin deterioration which is now being used in skin creams and ointments. The ocean is an important source of novel drugs with proven anticancer, antiviral and antibacterial ability as well as industrially important proteases and lipases. Researchers have also isolated marine actinomycetes highly resistant to toxic metals like mercury, cadmium, cobalt and zinc and the use of such strains may help in bioremediation of soil and water that is contaminated. The well known marine products that are in use include fish liver oils, spermaceti, protamine sulphate, agar, carrageenan, alginic acid, etc. The sea weeds are known to be source of drugs used in diseases of iodine deficiency like goitre, hypothyroidism and are also the source of additional vitamins and in the treatment of anaemia during pregnancy. They have an ability to cure many intestinal disorders and can be used as vermifuges. Sea weeds are also used as dressings and ointments.

The low cost broad-spectrum antiviral agents are represented by heparin-like sulphated polysaccharides from the red algae, ascidians like *Lissoclinum patella*, sponges like *Tethya crypta* and *Disidea ovata*, tunicates like *Eudistoma olivaceum* and species of *Trididemnum*. Many antitumour compounds have been isolated from marine organisms of the coral reef ecosystems such as didemnin B, diazonomide A, dolastatin 10 and discodermolide. The bluegreen alga, *Lyngbya majuscula* produces antiproliferant curacin A, while the bryozoan, *Bugula neritina* produces a bryostatin. *Digenia simplex*, a red alga is being used as a vermifuge as it is effective against parasitic round-worms, whipworms and tapeworms due to its active component alpha-kainic acid. The anthelmintic domoic acid has been isolated from *Chondria armata* and *Alsidium corallinum*. The sea anemone, *Rhodacitis howesii* and *Fucus vesiculosus* are the source of anticoagulants like fucoidan. The source of cephalosporin C, a potential antimicrobial, is the fungus, *Cephalosporium acremonium*. *Flustra foliacea*, a bryozoan, produces an antibiotic, dihydroflustramine. The pseudopterosins which are anti-inflammatory are derived from the Caribbean Sea Whip, *Pseudopterogorgia elisabethae*. Similarly, prostaglandins have been discovered from the soft coral, *Plexauria homomalla*, endotoxins from the horseshoe crab, *Limulus polyphemus* and the potent haemagglutinins, lectins are derived from the horseshoe crab. Many enzymes like D-glucanases, glycosidases, glucans, alfa-amylases, endonucleases, phosphatases, reductases, etc. have been derived from an array of marine organisms, such as embryos of *Strongylocentrotus intermedius* (sea urchin), hepatopancreas of *Paralithodes camtschatica* (crab), etc.

The early civilisations of Greece, Japan, China and India utilised marine life as a source of drugs. Agar, alginic acid, carrageenin, etc. are very much exploited from marine life by the Western World. *Digenia simplex* is a red alga used as an anthelmintic in Japanese folk medicine. It is effective against tapeworm, whipworm, roundworm, etc. Antibiotics like cephalosporin are obtained from a marine fungus, *Cephalosporium acremomum*. Cephalothin sodium, a semisynthetic derivative of the above is used mainly when infecting organism becomes resistant to benzyl penicillin and to ampicillin. Extracts of various marine algae contain vitamin C, folic acid, vitamin B, etc. There is a potential commercial value for these substances by algal cultures. Likewise, if proper investigation is made into marine life, they will be the source of several active principles like anticoagulants, carcinogens, toxins, etc.

Marine macroalgae like sea weeds have been used as crude drugs in the treatment of iodine deficiency states such as goitre, Basedow's disease and hypothyroidism. Some sea weeds have also been utilised as the sources of additional vitamins and in the treatment of anaemia during pregnancy. They are also utilised in the treatment of various intestinal disorders such as vermifuge and hypocholesterolaemic and hypoglycaemic agents. The hypoglycaemic property has been claimed by the sea weeds such as *Cystoseria barbata, Sargassum confusum* and *Jania rubens,* but the mechanism involved in lowering the levels of blood sugar by these algae are not known. Sea weeds have been employed as dressings, ointments and also in gynaecology. *Porphyra atropurpurea* has been used in Hawaii to dress up the wounds and burns and *Durvillaea antarctica* has been used by the Maoris of New Zealand in scabies. Prepared and sterilised stipes of *Laminaria digitata* have been utilised in conjunction with prostaglandins, to dilate the cervix, as they have the property of swelling up several times their original diameter upon moistening.

MICROORGANISMS (MICROBIOLOGICAL) SOURCE

The microbes too form a source of synthetic drugs. Microorganisms such as bacteria and fungi have been invaluable for drug discovery as they produce a large variety of antimicrobial agents evolved to give their hosts an advantage over their competitors. The Chinese have used a particular caterpillar fungus as a tonic for many years. The traditional Chinese medicine includes different types of mushrooms like *Agaricus, Ganoderma* and *Cordyceps* among their therapies. Microbes and fungi living in soil are easy to collect and culture and as such they provided many of the antibiotics. The microorganism screening became popular only after the discovery of penicillin. The samples of water and soil were collected from the different parts of the world and studied which led to the discovery of an array of antibacterial agents like cephalosporins, tetracyclines, aminoglycosides, rifamycins and chloramphenicol. Most of the drugs are secondary in nature as they are the products of metabolism. Many enzymes like D-glucanases, glycosidases, glucans, alpha-amylases, endonucleases, phosphatases, reductases, etc. have been derived from an array of marine microorganisms, such as species of *Alteromonas, A. macleodii, A. haloplanktis* and *Deleya marina* (marine bacteria) and species of *Vibrio. Claviceps purpurea* (Ergot) is a toxic fungus that grows on rye kernels and yields many alkaloids including ergotamine used for treating migraine. It also yields lysergic acid from which LSD (lysergic acid diethylamide), the cornerstone drug of psychedelic revolution in 1960s, is produced. Lysergic acid was first made by Albert Hofmann (1938) in the laboratories of Sandoz Pharmaceuticals, Basel, Switzerland, who accidentally discovered the effects of LSD in 1943. Similarly, the antibiotic erythromycin comes from tropical fungi. The breast cancer growth can be halted by the extracts of the mushroom, *Phellinus linteus.* Similarly, *Ganoderma lucidum* (Reishi mushroom) along with green tea enhances the immune functions of the body and is a potent drug to prevent many types of cancer. *Agaricus blazei* is capable of stimulating the human immune system and can be used in cancer treatment. Cyclosporin from the fungus, *Beauveria nivea* lowers the risk of transplanted organ rejection. Lentilan is derived from Shiitake mushroom and is used in cancer chemotherapy. Penicillin from *Penicillium chrysogenum*, cephalosporin from *Acrermonium* and griseofulvin from *Penicillium griseofulvum* and other fungal antibiotics are used in treating tuberculosis, syphilis, leprosy, etc.

As all the areas of nature and sources are not completely unfathomed and investigated, much remains to be explored with reference to production of natural drugs as well as synthetic drugs from different materials around us. This requires a continuous search for the drugs against lethal diseases such as bacterial, viral, infectious, AIDS, swine flu, etc.

SEMISYNTHETIC/SYNTHETIC SOURCE

The term *'drug'* was derived from the French word *'drogue'* meaning *dried herbs*, and a *crude drug* is any naturally occurring unrefined substance derived from biological or mineral sources intended for use in the diagnosis, cure, mitigation, and prevention of diseases. A crude drug contains pharmacologically active ingredients and requires no additional processing for use. An *official drug* is included in pharmacopoeia or in national formulary or in recognised books like pharmacopoeia, national formulary or pharmaceutical codex (such as BP or USP).

Semisynthetic drugs are the drugs that are formed through the chemical reaction of naturally occurring starting materials to form new products. The natural drugs may be improved by a semisynthetic process where the chemical structure is altered without any change in the nucleus (semisynthetic drug), e.g. apomorphine, diacetyl morphine, ethinyl estradiol, homatropine, ampicillin, methyl testosterone, bromoscopolamine, insulin, 6-aminopenicillanic acid derivatives, etc.

Synthetic drugs are the drugs with properties and effects similar to a known hallucinogen or a narcotic but having a slightly altered chemical structure, created (using man-made chemicals) but not natural ingredients, especially in order to evade restrictions against illegal substances. When the nucleus of the drug from natural source as well as its chemical structure is altered, we call it synthetic. The best example is emetine bismuth iodide. Synthetic drugs are prepared in the lab with the help of inorganic and organic drugs. Many drugs which were obtained from the plants originally are now prepared synthetically, e.g. ether and chloroform (volatile anaesthetics), sulfonamides and quinolones (antimicrobials), paracetamol (analgesic and antipyretic), pentorbitol and thiopental (hypnotic), etc. The common examples are: Synthetic phenethylamines (PEA), synthetic cathinones (synthetic stimulants) or synthetic hallucinogens (commonly known as bath salts), synthetic cannabinoids (called synthetic marijuana), synthetic LSD, synthetic PCP (phyencyclidine) and methoxamine (MXE). The drugs are also prepared synthetically, e.g. aspirin, oral antidiabetics, antihistamines, amphetamine, chloroquine, chlorpromazine, general and local anesthetics; Paracetamol, phenytoin, synthetic corticosteroids, sulfonamides and thiazide diuretics are synthetic products. Most of the drugs we use today such as antianxiety drugs, anticonvulsant drugs are synthetic.

GENETIC ENGINEERING/r-DNA TECHNOLOGY SOURCE

Recombinant DNA technology involves the cleavage of DNA by enzyme restriction endonucleases. The desired gene is coupled to rapidly replicating DNA (viral, bacterial or plasmidial). The new genetic combination is inserted into the bacterial cultures which allow production of vast amount of genetic material. Genetic engineering or r-DNA technology is the latest technique for the preparation of certain drugs such as human insulin and insulin analogs. Human insulin and insulin analogs can be prepared by the insertion of human or modified proinsulin gene into *E. coli* or *Saccharomyces,* and treating the extracted proinsulin to form the insulin or insulin analogs.

Modern biotechnology has led to a resurgence of interest in obtaining new medicinal agents from botanical sources. Through genetic engineering (GE), plants can now be used to produce a variety of proteins, including mammalian antibodies, blood substitutes, vaccines and other therapeutic entities. Research now underway will almost certainly result in GE plants designed to produce other therapeutic agents including hormones (e.g. insulin, somatotropin, erythropoietin), blood components, coagulation factors, and various interferons. In medicine, genetic engineering has been used to mass-produce insulin, human growth hormones, follistim (for treating infertility), human albumin, monoclonal antibodies, antihemophilic factors, vaccines, and many other drugs. Biochemical products of recombinant DNA technology in medicine and research include: human recombinant insulin, growth hormone, blood clotting factors, hepatitis B vaccine, and diagnosis of HIV infection. Genetically engineered drugs include hepatitis-B vaccine, recombinant-DNA engineered insulin, interferon-α-2a, and interferon-α-2b.

The main advantages of r-DNA technology are that a vast amount of drugs can be generated, the drugs can be obtained in their pure form, and the new drug is less antigenic. The disadvantages are: a well-equipped laboratory is required to carry out the process, to carry out the experiment, well-trained skilled staff is required, and the technique is complex and complicated.

The first commercially produced biopharmaceutical, r-human insulin from the bacteria, was produced in 1982; and the later development was followed with the demonstration of the potential for pharmaceutical production with the expression of human growth hormone fusion protein, interferon, MABs and serum albumin. This was followed by the production of three categories of therapeutics—antibodies, vaccines and other substances. The important antibodies are: IgG1, IgM, IgA/G, IgG, etc. The antiodies are: Hepatitis virus B antigen, malaria parasite antigen, rabies virus glycoprotein, HRV-14 epitope, HIV-1 epitope, hepatitis B surface protein, *E. coli* heat-labile enteroprotein, human cytomegalovirus glycoprotein B, diabetes-associated antoantigen, and respiratory syncytial virus, etc. The other therapeutic agents are: somatotropin (human growth hormone), human serum albumin (HSA), enzymes, interleukins (interleukin-2 and interleukin-4), interferons (human alpha-interferon), erythropoietin, human alpha- and beta- HB, etc.

The biological medicines from biological sources (including GMOs and GM products) are regulated as registered medicines, such as: vaccines, antivenoms, toxins derived from bacteria, immunoglobulins, MABs, allergens, blood products and clotting factors, hormones (insulin and growth hormone), enzymes (pancreatins) and heparins. Similarly, GMO medicines include: live attenuated vaccines (viral or bacterial), the viral vectors and modified somatic cells.

The future directions include the use of plants as factories for the production of novel vaccines, antibodies and other proteins will continue to develop. The molecular farming may become the premier expression system for new biopharmaceuticals and plant bodies. The important economic advantages will be realised and efforts will need to focus on increasing yield, scale-up production, distribution and handling of the transgenic plant material, and development and validation of the techniques of production to isolate effectively the production of pharmaceuticals for human and animal food. The biopharmaceuticals from plants will need to meet the safety and efficacy standards of the products from nonplant sources.

REVIEW QUESTIONS

1. **Essay and Short Answer Questions:**
    1. Write an account of various sources of crude drugs with examples. Describe the different sources of crude drugs with suitable examples.
    2. Write short notes on the antimicrobial drugs from marine source. Mention various sources of crude drugs with examples.
    3. Write short notes on the sources of synthetic drugs from microbes. Mention various sources of crude drugs from marine source with examples.

4. Write short notes on the sources of animal drugs with examples. Add a note on the drug sources from minerals with examples.

5. Write an account of various vegetable sources of crude drugs with examples. Mention a few important animal sources of drugs with examples.

2. Choose the Correct Alternative:

1. An age old remedy for relieving an upset stomach is: [ ]
   a. Senna pod
   b. Peppermint
   c. Wintergreen
   d. Opium

2. The plant with tranquilizing and antihypertensive properties is: [ ]
   a. *Gaultheria*
   b. *Cinchona*
   c. *Rauwolfia*
   d. *Papaver*

3. The source of tubocurarine, the arrow-poison is: [ ]
   a. *Taxus brevifolia*
   b. *Chondodendron tomentosum*
   c. *Cinchona pubescens*
   d. *Rauwolfia serpentina*

4. Anticancerous drug, vincristine is derived from: [ ]
   a. *Catharanthus roseus*
   b. *Camellia sinensis*
   c. *Ammi visnaga*
   d. *Atropa belladonna*

5. The cuttlefish bone used as a dentifrice and an antacid comes from: [ ]
   a. *Sacrophyton glaucum*
   b. *Cantharis vesicatoria*
   c. *Sepia officinalis*
   d. *Plexaura homomalla*

3. Fill in the Blanks:

1. The sea weeds are the sources of drugs used in .... deficiency like goitre and hypothyroidism.

2. Expand LSD ....

3. .... is the source of ergotamine for migraine.

4. The source of antibiotic penicillin is ....

5. LSD was first made by .... in the laboratories of Sandoz Pharmaceuticals, Basel, Switzerland.

6. Source of emetin (ipecac) is ....

4. True or False Statements:

1. Amber is not a secretion from sperm whale, and is used as a drug for the brain and the heart. [True/False]

2. The poison of *Bufo* is a potent drug for epilepsy and rheumatism. [True/False]

3. Calamine is a topical protective agent used in dusting powders and lotions. [True/False]

4. Fuller's earth is not a clarifying and filtering agent.   [True/False]

5. Bivalirudin from the saliva of leech is antiplatelet protein which promotes clotting of blood.   [True/False]

6. Paclitaxel comes from the species of *Taxus brevifolia*. [True/False]

5. **A. Match the following:**

1. Atropine	[ ]	a. Parasympatholytic
2. Wintergreen	[ ]	b. Bronchodilator
3. Ergometrin	[ ]	c. *Catharanthus roseus*
4. Hodgkin's disease	[ ]	d. Methylsalicylate
5. Khellin	[˙]	e. Vasodilator

B. Match the following:

1. Quillaia	[ ]	a. *Pilocarpus jaborandi*
2. Pyrethrum	[ ]	b. Cantharidin
3. Solasodine	[ ]	c. Edward Bach
4. Blister beetle	[ ]	d. Emulsifying agent
5. Flower remedies	[ ]	e. Suspending agent

C. Match the following:

1. Saliva of a rabid dog	[ ]	a. Saliva of leech
2. Poison of *Bufo*	[ ]	b. Cod liver oil
3. Bivalirudin	[ ]	c. Hydrophobia
4. Vitamins A and D	[ ]	d. Talcum powders
5. Kieselguhr	[ ]	e. Epilepsy

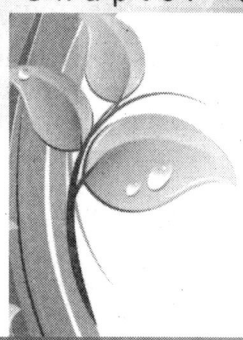

Chapter 3

Classification of Crude Drugs

The crude drugs are the drugs in a raw form that have their origin from organic or inorganic sources like vegetable, animal, mineral kingdoms. They have undergone the process of collection and drying without any further processing; and bacteria, either organs or whole organisms intended for use in the cure, treatment or prevention of a disease in man or other animals. They contain more amounts of active constituents. They do not have any side effects or fewer effects on the body which can be ignored. The use of the crude drugs is advantageous because at times their constituents have synergistic, additive or potentiating effects when they are together and are well-tolerated. Such drugs are to be recognised in the official pharmacopoeias and must affect the structure or any other bodily function of man and other animals. The advantages being crude is that they are convenient for the practical purposes, give an idea about the morphological and biological characters of the drug, their addition in a system is easy along with easier methods of location and traceability and easy identification of the adulterants.

Pharmacognosy is mainly concerned with naturally occurring substances of medicinal importance. But, it is not entirely limited to such materials and surgical dressings prepared from natural fibres, flavouring agents, suspending agents, disintegrating agents, filtering agents and supporting media, etc. are also included within the subject in addition to poisonous plants and hallucinogenic plants and the raw materials used for the preparation of oral contraceptives too. The most important natural sources are the higher plants, microbes, animals and marine organisms. Some products, both organic and inorganic in nature are also obtained from the minerals too. In order to study the individual drugs, we must adopt a particular sequence of arrangement. Such a classification must be simple, easy to use and must be free from any confusion. Each system has its own merits and demerits. In earlier days, when the study of crude drugs was not scientifically geared up, they were treated as independent units and were arranged in an alphabetical order for ready reference. Gradually as the information on various aspects of crude drugs was pouring in different types of classification procedures were framed. The drugs are classified in different ways like: Alphabetical classification, morphological classification, taxonomic classification, pharmacological classification, chemical classification, chemotaxonomical classification and serotaxonomical classification in addition to biochemical and geographical classifications.

ALPHABETICAL CLASSIFICATION

This is the simplest way of classification for disconnected materials. The crude drugs are generally arranged in an alphabetical order of their Latin and English common names or local language (vernacular) names. This system is found in Indian Pharmacopoeia, British Pharmacopoeia (in English – 1993), British Herbal Pharmacopoeia (1990), British Herbal Compendium (1992), United States Pharmacopoeia and National Formulary, British Pharmaceutical Codex, European Pharmacopoeia (in Latin – 1980) and Encyclopedia of Common Natural Ingredients used in Drugs and Cosmetics. The merits of this classification are: this method is easy and very quick to use, entries are not repeated thus avoiding confusion and location of the drug, traceability and addition of new entries becomes easier. This system has its own demerit that it lacks relationship between the previous and successive entries into it. This system is the most little disputed system. This method has been adopted in some modern books of materia medica like Reutter's 'Traite de Matiere Medicale et de Chimie Vegetale' published in Paris (1923).

The alphabetical arrangement of drugs can be exemplified by: Acacia, agar, alumina, belladonna, benzoin, cinchona, cinnamon, cod liver oil, Colchicum, cuprum (copper), Datura, Digitalis, ergot, fennel, ferrum (iron), gentian, henna, honey, hydragyrum (mercury), Hyoscyamus, Ipecacuanha, jalap, kaolin (china clay), kurchi, kalium (potassium), linum, liquorice, musk, myrrh, nux vomica, opium, ox gall, Podophyllum, Rauwolfia, rhubarb, saffron, senna, tobacco, vasaka, white wax, wool fat, yellow bees wax, etc.

MORPHOLOGICAL CLASSIFICATION

The crude drugs are arranged according to the external characters of the different parts of the plants or animals which are to be used as a drug. These may be organised or unorganised drugs. The *organised drugs* are the direct parts of the plants or the animals containing the cellular tissues which can be easily identified by their appearance, while the *unorganised drugs* are of plant, animal or mineral origin without any defined cellular structure prepared by intermediate physical processes like incision, drying or extraction with a solvent and cannot be easily identified by their morphology. The merits of this type of classification is that identification becomes easier so also the detection of any adulteration. At the same time, this is more convenient for the practical study. The main drawback of this classification is that there is no correlation of the chemical constituents with their medicinal action, and also there may be a possibility of drug repetition. Dr. T.E. Wallis, a great exponent of this classification is of the view that the drugs should always be classified according some inherent or intrinsic properties.

The *organised drugs* include:
- Barks of cinchona, cinnamon, quaillaia and wild cherry
- Leaves of digitalis, senna, eucalyptus and vasaka
- Seeds of nux vomica, isphagul, castor and linseed
- Fruits of fennel, coriander, strychnos, colocynth and bael
- Woods of red sanders, sassafras and sandalwood
- Roots of rauwolfia, boerhavia, ipecac and aconite
- Rhizomes of ginger, turmeric, and podophyllum
- Flowers of saffron, clove, china rose and artemisia
- Entire drugs of ephedra, ergot, centella, catharanthus and belladonna, etc.

The *unorganised drugs* include:
- Gums like acacia, gutty gum, guar gum, and gum tragacanth
- Extracts of agar and pectin, gelatin, honey
- Dried latex of opium, papain
- Resins of myrrh, asafoetida, balsam and benzoin
- Dried juice of kino and aloe
- Dried extracts of catechu, curare, etc.

TAXONOMICAL (BIOLOGICAL) CLASSIFICATION

This classification is purely botanical as it is based on the principles of natural relationship and evolutionary development. The entire plant is not used as a drug and it is only a part of the plant which is used. Hence, this has no significance and does not help in assigning the plants into a specific taxonomic group. This system only helps in the study of evolutionary development. This fails to correlate between the chemical constituents of the drugs and their biological activity. The knowledge of botany and zoology is always necessary to classify the drugs in this way.

The drugs belong to many groups and families of plant kingdom such as algae and fungi (thallophyta), pteridophyta, pinaceae and ephedraceae (gymnosperms), gramineae, liliaceae, zingiberaceae, iridaceae, dioscoriaceae, araceae and orchidaceae (monocotyledons), and over

100 families of dicotyledons. Animal drugs mainly come from many invertebrate and vertebrate groups.

Under this system, crude drugs like liquorice can be classified as:
- Regnum: Vegetabile
- Division: Magnoliophyta
- Class: Magnoliopsida
- Subclass: Rosidae
- Order: Fabales,
- Family: Fabaceae
- Genus: *Glycyrrhiza*
- Species: *glabra*.

This classification may appear to be interesting but it fails to recognise whether the drug is organised or unorganised and it does not give any indication of the part from which the drug is produced. Also it fails to denote the chemical nature of the active principle and its therapeutic significance.

PHARMACOLOGICAL (THERAPEUTIC OR PHYSIOLOGICAL OR PHARMACODYNAMICAL) CLASSIFICATION

In this type of classification, the drugs are grouped in accordance with their action on the body of the organism or their important constituent or therapeutic use. The method is the most widely followed method and appears to be more relevant. Drugs possessing a common therapeutic action are grouped together irrespective of the morphology of the part or their phylogenetic relationship or the nature of their constituents. This becomes useful in suggesting the appropriate substitutes in case of their non-availability. The most important demerit of such a classification is that the drugs with different therapeutic action are classified into more than one group which results in an ambiguity and confusion.

The drugs are grouped under specific headings in this type of classification such as:
- Carminatives (mentha and cardamom)
- Emetics (ipecac)
- Antiamoebics (kurchi and ipecac)
- Laxatives (agar, ispaghul and banana)
- Purgatives (senna, plantago, cascara and castor oil)
- Expectorants (licorice, ipecac and vasaka)
- Antitussives (opium)
- Bronchodilators (ephedra and tea)
- Astringents (black catechu, tannic acid, myrobalan and ashoka bark)
- Cardiotonics (digitalis and squill)

- Cardiac depressants (cinchona and veratrum)
- Peripheral vasoconstrictors (ergot and ephedra)
- Antihypertensives (rauwolfia)
- anticholinergics (belladonna and *Datura*)
- Central nervous system stimulants (coffee)
- Central nervous system depressants (hyoscyamus, belladonna and opium)
- Analeptics (nux vomica, camphor and lobelia)
- Hallucinogenics (latex of cannabis and poppy)
- Antispasmodics (opium and curare)
- Anticancerous (vinca, podophyllum and taxus)
- Antirheumatics (aconite, colchicum and guggul)
- Anthelmintics (quassia and male fern)
- Antimalarials (cinchona and artemisia)
- Local anaesthetics (cocoa)
- Immunizing agents (vaccines, sera, toxoids and antitoxins)
- Immune-modulatory agents (aswagandha, ginseng, asparagus and picrorhiza), etc.

CHEMICAL CLASSIFICATION

As the pharmacological activity and the therapeutic significance of the crude drugs are based on the nature of the chemical constituents, the drugs are divided into different groups in accordance with their chemical nature in this method. This system is mainly dependant on creation of the groups with identical chemical constituents. This system is useful in the phytochemical studies of the constituents. But, this may result in an ambiguity when a particular drug possesses many compounds that belong to different groups. The drugs belonging to different morphological or taxonomic categories may be brought together provided there is some similarity in the chemical nature of the active principles. Some of the important chemical substances are alkaloids, glycosides, tannins, resins, volatile oils, fixed oils, etc.

This system can be exemplified by:

- Glycosides (digitalis, senna, licorice, aloe, cascara, scilla, dioscroea, ginseng, senega, tobacco, glycyrrhiza and rhubarb)
- Alkaloids (ergot, cinchona, *Datura*, rauwolfia, nicotiana, piper, belladonna, hyoscyamus, withania, calumba, nux vomica, catharanthus, vasaka, aconite, holarrhena, punarnava, shankhpushpi and opium)
- Tannins (myrobalan, ashoka, pale catechu, black catechu, *Behera* and *Amla*)

- Volatile oils (turpentine oil, peppermint oil, mentha oil, lemongrass oil, clove oil and Eucalyptus oil)
- Lipids represented by fixed oils, fats and waxes (castor oil, sesame oil, chalmoogra oil, almond oil, corn oil, coconut oil, palm oil, mustard oil, soya oil, safflower oil, sunflower oil, chenopodium oil, lanolin, bees wax, kokum butter, shark liver oil and cod liver oil)
- Ccarbohydrates (starch, sodium alginate, cellulose, pectin)
- Triterpenoids (rasna, pluchea and vanda)
- Esters (pyrethrum)
- Soluble carbohydrates (honey)
- Organic acids (tamarind)
- Gums (gum acacia, guar gum, gum tragacanth and sterculia gum)
- Mucilages (isphagul seed and bark, linseed, and agar)
- Resins (jalap, colophony, balsam of peru, storax, vidang, myrrh, asafoetida, and ginger)
- Minerals (kaolin and tar)
- Vitamins and hormones (yeast, shark liver oil, oxytocin and insulin),
- Proteins (gelatin and yeast)
- Enzymes (casein, trypsin and papaian), etc.

CHEMOTAXONOMIC CLASSIFICATION

This classification mostly relies on the chemical similarity of a taxon and is based on the relationship between the constituents in different plants. Specific classes of plants show specific chemical constituents as such an entirely new concept of chemotaxonomy that utilises the chemical characters in understanding the taxonomical status of the individual, its relationship with other plants and the evolution arises. This system gives a much wider scope in understanding the interrelationship between the chemical constituents, biosynthesis and possible action. The chemical constituents of certain type are the characteristic of certain groups of plants like tropane alkaloids in majority of the members of solanaceae and volatile oils in the members of umbelliferae show that there is some definite relationship between the chemical constituents and the taxonomical status of the plants. The characters often studied in chemotaxonomy are the secondary metabolites of medical significance like alkaloids, glycosides, flavonoids, etc. The alkaloids in *Hydrastis*, *Berberis* and *Argemone*, and distribution of the alkaloids in ranunculaceae and flavonoids in higher plants are of significance in chemotaxonomy. Hybridisation of DNA, sequencing of amino acids in proteins and serotaxonomy are gaining greater significance in chemotaxonomic classification.

In addition to these, biochemical classification and geographical classification are also being followed. The biochemical classification appears to be more natural in modern pharmacognosy as it takes into account the biogenetic relationship of the natural orders. The geographical classification is based on the availability of the drugs in different parts of the world, as all the drugs do not grow everywhere. Prof. E. Schratz of Germany, a strong supporter of the geographical, commercial and political roles of drugs, taught pharmacognosy through this classification under a caption 'Wirtsschaftliche Geograsphie'.

SEROTAXONOMICAL CLASSIFICATION

Serology is defined as the unit of biology which is concerned with the nature and interactions of the antigenic material and antibodies (the study of the antigen-antibody reaction). It is defined as the study of origins and properties of antisera (Smith, 1976). When the foreign cells (or particles–antigens) are introduced into an organism, the antibodies are produced in the blood (antiserum). The substance that is capable of stimulating the formation of an antibody is called the antigen, and a specific protein molecule produced by plasma cells in the immune system in response to an antigen is called an antibody. The antibodies combine chemically with specific antigens and such a combination elevates an immune response. The application of serology in solving the problems in taxonomy is called serotaxonomy. Nuttal (1901) was the first biologist to compare the immunochemical specificity of the serum proteins for systematic purposes. Later, Dunbar (1910) showed that theta-proteins from the pollen, seeds and the leaves were serologically distinct. Gholke (1914) established serology school in Germany and later Germany became the centre of serological studies in the world.

Phytoserology deals with the immunological reactions between the serum antibodies and the antigens, has established itself as a valid method in taxonomy because it helps to detect the homologous proteins. It uses the specific properties of the antisera produced by the animals against proteins as characters to assess the plant relationships. This branch of systematics (serotaxonomy) developed and became popular first in Germany since the beginning of this century.

According to Serotaxonomy, the classification of very similar plants by means of the differences in the proteins they contain. The technique is based on the highly specific relationship between the antigens and the antibodies produced in response to them. The protein extracted from a plant is injected into the blood of an animal, where it behaves as an antigen. After an interval for the production of the antibodies, a blood sample is taken, and this can be used to compare the first plant protein (antigen) with extracts taken from other plants.

The process of serotaxonomy involves the following steps: The antigen (the protein extract of the plant origin) is extracted. This is injected into the bloodstream of an experimental animal to generate the antibodies. The experimental animal produces the specific antibodies in response to the antigen. The serum with the antibodies is called the antiserum. This is made to react *in vitro* with the antigenic protein as well as the proteins of other taxa whose affinities are to be determined. The amount of precipitation shows the degree of homology. For example, to know the closeness of the taxon A with taxons B, C, D and E, the proteins from taxon A are extracted and are injected into the experimental animal (such as rabbit or mice). The animal in return, produces the antibodies, which are extracted from the blood of the animal as antiserum. When this is allowed to react with the original protein extract from taxon A, complete coagulation takes place. When this antiserum is allowed to react with the protein extracts from the other taxa (B, C, D and E), the degree of coagulation varies. These degrees of coagulation are compared to know the closeness of the taxa, e.g. more the degree of coagulation, more is the closeness of the taxa.

The initiation of an immunological reaction in plants occurs as follows: The antiserum gives a precipitation reaction with the plant extract (antigen-antibody reaction), and the similarity of other species to the first one can be assessed by measuring the amount of coagulation it causes.

The quantitative precipitation in solution is frequently replaced by the more convenient methods like gel diffusion method, immuno-electrophoresis, radioimmunoassay and ELISA. The absorption protein mixtures of different plants often contain some common proteins. The removal of the antibodies for the common proteins from the antiserum is carried out, and the logical comparisons can be drawn from the precipitation reactions, as the antiserum at this juncture contains only those antibodies which can react with the specific proteins. Immuno-electrophoresis is a combination of serological and electrophoretic procedures. Primarily, the antigens are separated by electrophoresis on a gel and then allowed to diffuse towards the antiserum. This method is more specific as better antigenic separations occur during the process. In Radioimmunoassay, the antigens or the antibodies are labelled with radioactivity which facilitates their identification, even though they are in small concentrations. In ELISA (Enzyme-Linked-Immunosorbent Assay), the enzymes couple their catalytic activity with a specific immunoglobulin, which forms the basis for the estimation. In tests like ELISA which involve the labelling of either the antigens or the antibodies and linking this with enzymes for detecting them even in minute quantities.

The importance of serotaxonomy is as follows: The use of serological techniques to compare the proteins extracted from different plants is an important aid in plant taxonomy. The serological data was used in the classification of the orders and the assignment of the families in Apiales, Fagales, Magnoliales, Juglandales, Rubiales, Ranunculales, etc.

(Fairbrothers, 1983). Six species of *Bromus* were separated on the basis of the serological data (Fairbrothers and Jhonson, 1959). Fairbrothers and Jhonson on the basis of their serotaxonomic studies showed that the genera *Magnolia* and *Michelia* show closest affinity within the family Magnoliaceae. Simon (1971) demonstrated the close relationship between Nymphaeceae and Nelumbonaceae on the basis of serological data. Klos applied serotaxonomic data in the classification of Leguminosae.

REVIEW QUESTIONS

1. **Essay and Short Answer Questions:**
   1. Write an account of systems of classification of crude drugs with examples.
   2. What are the different types of classification of crude drugs that are in practice today? Explain any two methods with examples.
   3. How are the crude drugs classified? Add a note on the merits and demerits of different classification systems.
   4. Write short notes on the chemical and chemotaxonomic systems of classification of crude drugs with examples.
   5. Write short notes on the therapeutic and biological systems of classification of crude drugs with examples.
   6. Write short notes on the alphabetical and morphological systems of classification of crude drugs with examples.
   7. Name the different types of classification of crude drugs. Bring out the differences between the organised and unorganised drugs with examples.
   8. How are the crude drugs classified? Bring out the differences between pharmacodynamical and chemical systems of classification with examples.

2. **Choose the Correct Alternative:**
   1. Alphabetical classification is followed in: [ ]
      a. British herbal compendium
      b. European pharmacopoeia
      c. Indian pharmacopoeia
      d. All these
   2. Pick out an organised drug from the following: [ ]
      a. Wood of Sassafras   b. Gelatin
      c. Juice of aloe   d. Benzoin
   3. Pick out an unorganised drug from the following: [ ]
      a. Rhizome of turmeric   b. Ergot
      c. Guar gum   d. Fruit of bael

4. Which one of the following is used as an emetic?   [ ]
   a. Datura   b. Ephedra
   c. Tannic acid   d. Ipecac
5. Pick out the cardiac depressant: [ ]
   a. Liquorice   b. Cascara
   c. Cinchona   d. Kurchi

3. Fill in the Blanks:

1. Latex of cannabis is used as a ....
2. The drugs from tobacco are alkaloids while those from *Scilla* are
   ....
3. Kaolin and tar are minerals while gelatin is a ....
4. Kokum butter is a lipid while pectin is a ....
5. Asafoetida is a resin while catechu is a ....

4. True or False Statements:

1. The simplest classification for disconnected drugs is alphabetical system.   [True/False]
2. Barks, leaves and the seeds represent unorganised drugs.
                                                              [True/False]
3. The unorganised drugs are not represented by the gums, resins and juices.   [True/False]
4. Taxonomical classification fails to correlate between the chemical constituents and their biological activity.   [True/False]
5. Therapeutic classification is the most widely followed and a more relevant method.   [True/False]
6. Chemical classification is useful in the phytochemical studies of the drug constituents.   [True/False]
7. The secondary metabolites of medical significance are studied in chemotaxonomy.   [True/False]

5. Match the following:

1. Oxytocin   [ ]   a. Honey
2. Papain   [ ]   b. Volatile oil
3. Soluble carbohydrate   [ ]   c. Hormone
4. Tamarind   [ ]   d. Enzyme
5. Turpentine   [ ]   e. Organic acids

Chapter 4

Cultivation, Collection, Processing, Drying and Storage of Medicinal Plants

INTRODUCTION

India is one of the richest countries in the world with regard to the genetic resources of medicinal plants. The land mass of India is only 2% but it has 11% of the total known world flora and is acclaimed as one of the top 12 mega diversity nations in the world. The agroclimatic conditions of India are very conducive for introduction and domestication of new exotic plant varieties. The Indian systems of medicine use over 2000 medicinal plants, about 700 in Ayurveda, about 600 in Siddha medicine and about 700 in Unani system of medicine. At present, the demand and the supply of the medicinal plants is mismatching, and about 90% comes from the forests while only 10% is from cultivation. The tribes and local communities living in and around the forests are allowed to collect the minor forest products. A lot of herbal products go uncollected and lost due to non-identification. The availability of medicinal plants in nature has been depleted over the years due to unscientific, unsustainable and discriminative collection and some of the species have become scarce due to overexploitation. The availability of the valuable medicinal plants has been reduced due to the rapid expansion of the area under the cultivation of food and commercial crops, the rapid conversion of non-forest area for other use and degradation of the forest due to fire and grazing, etc. These practices have led to the extinction of many valuable medicinal plants and some others have become endangered. Hence, sincere efforts are needed for the reintroduction of medicinal plants and eco-restoration for enhancing their availability. The species which are exposed to the threat of their existence should be properly identified and immediate steps should be taken for their conservation by *in situ* and *ex situ* programmes and the development of herbal sanctuaries to safe guard the biological wealth will be very helpful and also useful. The cultivation for the domestication of medicinal plants at present is being dictated by the user industries and they are fixing up the price of the commodity. The essential factor is to go in for quick disposal and for a fair price and this limits the present large scale cultivation of medicinal plants. To overcome all these hurdles, there is an urgent need for the cultivation of medicinal plants.

CULTIVATION

Cultivation is always advantageous over collection from wild habitat, because of the following reasons. Cultivation always ensures the purity and the quality of crude drugs. If all the operations of cultivation are maintained uniformly, one can obtain the drug of the highest quality. Cultivation of medicinal plants with rhizomes requires an adequate quantity of fertilisers and suitable irrigation. Proper cultivation always results in the production of a crop with maximum content of volatile oil and other constituents like ginger, turmeric and licorice. In the absence of the weeds, the crude drug contamination can be avoided. If all the operations are carried out by the skilled and experienced professional personnel, the drugs of higher therapeutic quality in addition to a higher yield can be obtained. Cultivation also helps in a continuous supply of the crude drug to the market so that the industries that depend on the drugs do not face a shortage. Medicinal and aromatic plant cultivation like coffee, tea, opium and cinchona also leads to establishment of many cottage and small scale industries and industrialisation. The higher prices of the crude drugs as well as losses due to environmental imbalance like storms, floods, droughts, etc. are the only disadvantage. Cultivation permits the scientists to apply modern methods of technology like mutation, polyploidy and hybridisation to achieve greater yields and to produce many more new drugs.

Medicinal plants are propagated by the usual methods of propagation which remain applicable to normal crops like sexual method (seed propagation) and asexual method.

In sexual method, the seedlings are raised from healthy seeds of a superior quality. The seeds must possess a high percentage of germination and they must be free from disease and pests. The seeds must be subjected to scarification prior to germination and when not in use they must be properly stored in cool and dry place to retain their power for germination but not for a longer time. Prior to germination they must be exposed to a chemical treatment with substances like gibberellins, cytokinins, ethylene, thiourea, potassium nitrate, sodium hypochlorite. Gibberellic acid relieves dormancy of the seeds and promotes the growth of seedlings. Dormant seeds from a fresh harvest germinate immediately if they are soaked in potassium nitrate solution. Thiourea promotes germination in seeds which fail to do so in dark or at higher temperatures. In some cases, special treatment is given such as soaking in water for a day (castor seeds) or soaking in sulphuric acid (henbane seeds) or subjected to pounding with coarse sand (Indian senna seeds) to partially remove their outer seed coat. This method is advantageous because, the seedlings have a longer life, easy to raise and cheaper. The propagation sometimes also results in the production of plants of superior quality by chance (as in Papaya and Orange). This method has also its own limitations such as: the trees raised from seedlings are not uniform in their growth and yielding potential and require more time to bear the fruit and the cost of harvesting is more.

In asexual method, the vegetative part of a plant (stem or root) is placed in a suitable environment that it develops into a new plant. This has some advantages like: the new plants do not show any variation from which the plant part has been collected, the plants maintain uniformity in their growth and yielding capacity, and in fruit trees, uniformity make harvesting and marketing easy. This method helps to generate the seedless fruits as in grapes, pomegranate and lemon. Plants bear the fruits earlier to those produced sexually. There is a possibility of generating the disease resistant varieties (by budding or grafting). This method has its own disadvantages too. The asexually generated plants are not long lived and do not show vigorous growth unlike the sexually produced ones. There is no possibility of evolving new varieties. Asexual method can be achieved either by vegetative propagation or by aseptic method. Vegetative propagation is carried out by means of underground stems like bulbs (squill and garlic), corms (colchicum and saffron), stem tubers (aconite and potato) and rhizomes (ginger and turmeric). It can also be carried out by means of sub-aerial stems like runners (mentha), suckers (chrysanthemum, pineapple and banana), offsets (aloe and valerian) and stolons (arrow root and licorice). Aseptically, the medicinal plants are micropropagated on an artificial medium under aseptic conditions from cell, tissues, organs, embryos, seeds, pollen and root and shoot apices, etc. They are also supplied with external nutrients, hormones, etc.

The Factors Influencing the Cultivation of Medicinal Plants

The factors that affect cultivation of medicinal plants can be listed as: cultivability, climatic (external) factors, edaphic (soil) factors and others like application of fertilisers and pesticides.

a. **Cultivability:** The medicinal plants do grow in a wild state but the cultivation of the wild varieties involves many factors. Some plants like opium, flax and cocoa have been cultivated since ages. Certain types of plants like Indian hemp, ginger, cardamom, cinchona, linseed, etc. are exclusively cultivated. When the wild plant supply falls short, cultivation is enforced. Such plants may be either growing or being cultivated in distant geographical regions and the transportation of such drug may involve excessive economy or if tried to cultivate in a different geographical region they may fail to acclimatise and establish successfully. The cultivation of medicinal plants is preferred to maintain the natural resources intact and also to improve the quality of the drug. Another reason is that a specific variety or a species may need to be cultivated as it is not freely accessible in nature. The collection is to be done at a precise growing period when the active principle is supposed to exist at its peak. It is not possible to know when the product will be at its peak if the desired plant is allowed to grow in a wild state, in nature. But, some plants such as the rubber plant luxuriant in Amazon basin are unwieldy for cultivation as it never grows in the cleared areas.

b. **Climatic Factors:** The climatic factors that influence the chemical content, growth and yield of a medicinal plant are altitude, temperature, rainfall (irrigation), humidity (moisture content) and light.

1. **Altitude:** Altitude at which the medicinal plants are cultivated is an important factor. Plants like cinnamon are grown from 250–1000 meters, cardamom is grown from 600–1600 meters, cloves are grown up to 900 meters, saffron is grown up to 1250 meters, cinchona and coffee from 1000–2000 meters and camphor from 1500–2000 meters from sea level while senna is cultivated at the sea level.

2. **Temperature:** Temperature is another major factor which regulates the overall growth of the plant. For example, the tropical and sub-tropical plants of the temperate regions of the globe grow well in summer rather than in winter because they are not frost resistant. The higher temperatures in general promote the formation of volatile oils but the hot days may account for the physical loss of the oil. For example, the optimum temperatures required for species like cardamom varies between 50 and 100°F, for coffee between 55 and 70°F, for cinchona between 60 and 75°F and for tea it varies between 70 and 90°F. Some plants like camphor and coffee cannot withstand frost while saffron grows best in a cold climate and dry weather is required for pyrethrum.

3. **Rainfall/Precipitation:** The rain fall or precipitation includes many factors like annual rainfall, its distribution throughout the year, its effect on the humidity and water holding capacity of the soil. For example, continuous rain leads to the loss of water-soluble alkaloids (in solanaceae) from the roots and their leaves get leached, thereby resulting in the low yield of the active constituents in the wet season of the year. Most of the cultivated medicinal plants require proper irrigation or a sufficient amount of rainfall except xerophytes like aloe, acacia, etc.

4. **Light:** The influence of light is not the same in all plants. The plants in the wild usually grow under shade. When these are to be cultivated, the required shade is to be necessarily provided. It is observed that full sunshine promotes the content of alkaloids in belladonna, stramonium and *Cinchona ledgeriana*. The leaves of *mentha* showed menthane, menthol and traces of menthofuran under long day conditions while under short days, showed menthofuran as a major constituent. Specific day length is capable of initiating the flowering in many plants and this should be taken into account during the cultivation of medicinal plants for drugs from their flowers.

c. **Edaphic (Soil) Factors**

1. **Soil factors (nature of soil, soil pH, soil moisture and soil nutrients):** Soil supports the growth of plants by providing the anchorage for their roots and also water and essential mineral nutrients for their growth. The growth of the plants is dependent upon the arrangement of the soil particles, nature and size of the soil particles, the amount of organic matter and soil biota. The porosity of the soil and the pH of the soil solution also determine the growth and development of the plants. The physical and chemical properties of the soil greatly influence the growth of plants. Soil fertility plays a major role in providing the balanced proportions of nutrients to plants. Mucilage used as a water retaining material is produced by *Althaea officinalis* and it has been observed that in Western Europe where the soils are mostly clayey, when grown on the soil with high moisture content, the plant contained lesser amount of mucilage. Similarly, all species cannot tolerate the same soil pH and the limit varies from plant to plant. For example, *Datura stramonium* has a pH tolerance of 6.0–8.2 while *Majorana hortensis* shows a tolerance limit of 5.6–6.4. Normally, the plants that contain the essential oils like *Mentha piperata* and those that contain the alkaloids such as *Datura stramonium* seem not to be influenced by the variations in soil pH. All plants require calcium for their normal nutrition and growth but, *Digitalis purpurea*, *Pinus pinaster*, etc. fail to grow on calcareous soils. Hence, a thorough study on the effect of various mineral nutrients on medicinal plant growth is needed, and with a better understanding of the plant responses, better yield of the crude drugs can be achieved.

2. **Additive factors (fertilisers, pesticides, etc.):** Fertilisers and manures play an important role in plant nutrition as the addition of the same to a soil make it fertile. The addition of chemical fertilisers to the soil in which medicinal plants are cultivated supplies all the necessary primary and secondary nutrients as well as the trace elements to plants. The addition of manures like farm

yard manure (compost), poultry manure, castor and neem seed cake, vermicompost in addition to bone meal, fish meal, biogas slurry, blood meal and press mud makes the soil rich in organic and inorganic nutrients required by the plants. The addition of biofertilisers like *Rhizobium, Azotobacter, Azospirillum, Beijerinckia,* Cyanophytes, *Azolla*, etc. are preferred in place of organic and inorganic manures as they are cost-effective and also harmless to the plants cultivated. A considerable amount of the crude drug may be lost by pests before it reaches the consumer after harvest. Hence, pest control assumes primary importance in the context to cultivation of medicinal and aromatic plants. The common pests like fungi, viruses, insects, weeds, rodents, etc. are to be controlled by the use of specific pesticides, weedicides, rodenticides, insecticides, acaricides, herbicides, antifungal and antiviral substances either by mechanical, chemical or biological control methods to enhance the quality and quantity of the crude drug during cultivation. The use of biopesticides is highly preferable.

COLLECTION AND PROCESSING OF CRUDE DRUGS

The drugs are to be processed prior to marketing after collection. Several methods are adapted in the preparation of the drugs and also to meet the standard pharmacopoeial requirements. These include methods of collection, harvesting, drying, dressing, packing and storage.

1. **Collection:** The crude drugs can be collected either from wild species or cultivated varieties, and the collection can be done either by native labourers without a skill or by scientifically trained skilled workers.

    a. **Time of collection:** The different parts of the plants that contain the crude drugs and drug material are to be collected with some knowledge associated with the time of collection and the nature of the plant parts at which time the components will be at their peak stage of accumulation. The prevailing environmental conditions are taken into consideration while collecting the crude drugs. The drugs from the leaf and flower tops like senna, vinca, belladonna and digitalis should be collected before the flowers open up or just before they reach their maturity. Similarly, the leaves of aloe can be collected when they are fresh and succulent for their mucilage. saffron, unopened flower buds of cloves, chamomile and arnica should be collected prior to pollination before their full expansion during morning in dry weather. The bark is to be collected preferably either in spring or early summer during which period the cambium will be very active which becomes easier for collection by detachment except the bark of wild cherry and the bark of cinnamon which are to be collected in autumn and in rainy season respectively. The fruits for drugs are collected when they are mature and fully grown. For example, the fruits of cardamom are collected before they dehisce, tamarind fruits when they have attained full maturity and the fruits of caraway and coriander when they are fully ripe. The roots for the crude drugs are to be collected in spring season before their vegetative growth comes to a halt. Similarly, the rhizomes are collected when the food reserves are full. The unorganised drugs like resins, gums and latex are collected as soon as they begin to ooze out from the plant parts. Acacia gum is generally collected 2–3 weeks after making the incisions on the bark of the tree and opium, papaya are collected after the latex gets coagulated.

b. **Method of collection/harvesting:** Harvesting is done with efficiency by employing skilled workers. If the crude drugs are underground like roots, tubers, rhizomes, etc. they are to be harvested by mechanical devices like diggers. Drugs which are aerial are to be harvested by binders. The flowers, seeds, fruits are to be harvested by seed strippers. The cloves are collected by beating the plant with bamboos. The cochineal insects are collected by brushing. The seaweeds are harvested by forks. Mint is harvested by mowers while fennel and coriander are uprooted and dried followed by thrashing and winnowing.

In the case of unorganised drugs where the concerned part of the medicinal plant is underground, it should be made free from the soil. The part possessing the crude drug is to be shaken thoroughly and it may be brushed during and after drying which separates the soil particles that are stuck. In the case of valerian, the particles of clay are removed by washing it in the streams where it grows. If the part is diseased, it should be discarded. In case of ginger and marsh mallow, the rootlets are to be peeled off. If the underground organs are large in size as in calumba root, they are cut into slices for drying. The seeds of nux vomica and cocoa are to be carefully extracted from the mucilaginous fruits and thoroughly washed to make it free from the pulp.

2. **Drying:** Drying is an integral part of the drug collection. The plant materials that contain the crude drug after collection need to be dried for storage and transportation. The application of a uniform type of drying procedure is not possible in all medicinal plants since the chemical constituents of the collected material vary in their composition. For example, slow drying preferably at lower temperature is carried out to ensure enzyme action in the seeds of cocoa, roots of gentian and in the rhizomes of *Orris*. The plant materials containing the volatile oils need to be dried immediately lest

they lose their aroma. Immediate drying is taken up as moist drugs tend to develop moulds and if so they are to be discarded.

There is a considerable variation in the type of the drying process. Plants like cardamoms, cloves and cinnamon, etc. are air-dried. As the open air drying depends on the weather, the drying time is to be carefully selected. In countries like West Africa with a high humidity in the atmosphere, artificial rapid drying of the material is desired. In European countries, continuous felt driers are used for drying the bulk of drugs as in digitalis. For the procurement of nutmeg, drying is done by open fire. The process of drying is carried out in drying sheds where trays containing the materials are arranged with a gap of 15 cm to ensure the circulation of free air in between them.

3. **Dressing (garbling):** This includes the removal of sand, dirt and extraneous matter (foreign organic matter) of the same plant that does not constitute the drug. In lobelia and stramonium, extra portions of the stems are removed and in cloves, the stalks are separated. The roots, rootlets and stem bases are carefully removed in the case of rhizomes constituting the drug.

4. **Packing:** While packing the drugs, the nature of the drug and the nature of the climate during transportation and storage should be taken into consideration to retain the quality of the drug until it reaches the consumer. For example, aloe is packed in goat skin, balsam is packed in kerosene tins and asafoetida is stored in well-closed containers. Cod liver oil is stored in dark containers to prevent the effect of sunlight while leaf drugs like senna, vinca are pressed and stored as bales. Colophony is packed in big masses to prevent auto-oxidation and cinnamon is packed in quills. Drugs like roots and seeds are packed in gunny bags as they do not need special attention. Some others are stored in bags internally coated with polythene.

5. **Storage/preservation:** The crude drugs after collection and drying need to be properly stored to maintain their original from intact and also to maintain a high quality over a longer period until they are transported to the market.

The crude drugs are highly susceptible to physical and chemical deterioration if they are not properly stored or preserved. The physical factors like humidity, light, temperature and oxygen bring down and reduce the quality of the drug during storage/preservation.

Drugs are stored usually in containers like sacks, bales, wooden cases, paper bags, cardboard, boxes, etc. The drugs are stored in waterproof, fire-proof and rodent-proof premises. The crude drugs that are stored reabsorb about 10–12% of moisture from the surroundings which may bring about enzyme activation to decompose the active constituent within. If the store house is saturated with moisture of >75%, the material like starch, gentian, squill and gelatin get degraded. Similarly, the soil with which the storage cellars are made of also affects the quality of the drug. The clay soil absorbs atmospheric moisture and hence, such cellars need artificial heating to reduce their humidity, while the sandy soil of the cellar loses its moisture content and keep the drug material dry. The material like digitalis and Indian hemp should never be allowed to air dry as they lose their activity to some extent and such drugs should be kept in sealed containers along with a dehydrating agent. The volatile oils should be stored in sealed and well-filled containers in a cool dark place to retain their quality for a longer time.

Light also affects the crude drugs. For example, rhubarb rapidly changes to a reddish tint from yellow, coloured or white flowers of Rose will turn brown and those of santonin become black. Added to colour change, the glycosides and vitamins too get decomposed at a slower pace. The volatile oils of chamomile flowers, ginger and asafoetida, etc. are affected by changes in temperature.

Direct oxidation by oxygen of the air too brings about changes in the constituents of the crude drugs. For example, linseed oil, cannibal of Indian hemp, etc. develop a thick consistency and get resinified. Sometimes, the form or the shape of the drug also plays an important role in the storage and preservation. For example, colophony in its entire form (as big masses) is well-preserved rather than in its powdered form when it gets oxidized and loses its solubility in ether. Similarly, squill if preserved in its powdered form becomes rubbery on prolonged exposure to air and the fixed oil in powdered ergot becomes rancid on storage.

The preservation of the drug in such a way that they are not exposed to the attack of the insects or molds is also important. Different types of insects, nematode worms, molds and mites may infest the crude drugs during storage. Hence, every precaution is to be taken to retain the quality and quantity of the drug. The common insect pests include the members of coleoptera (*Stegobium* and *Calandrium*), lepidoptera (*Ephestia* and *Tinea*) and arachnida (mites like *Tyroglyphus* and *Glyophagus*). The premises of storage and the cup-boards must be periodically fumigated and kept exposed to open air and away from flame when carbon disulphide is used as a fumigant. Cold storage is also a safe means of storage. The drug material is kept in numerous small sealed containers to avoid exposure of the entire drug to humid atmosphere. They can also be preserved in well-closed opaque containers. The methods of preservation of the drug material vary with the form and nature of the drug preserved. If the crude drugs are not properly preserved keeping their active constituent in form or exposed to partial pathogenic or pest attack, the purpose of drug is lost.

PLANT HORMONES AND THEIR APPLICATIONS

Compared with animals where the nervous system mediates cell to cell regulation, in plants such a function is through the vascular system which transports certain regulators. The hormones are organic substances that act as messengers for such regulation needed in small quantities and their sites of action and biosynthesis are different. Plant hormones (plant growth regulators or plant growth substances) are the naturally occurring organic substances other than the nutrients which control the growth processes (morphological and physiological) in their lower concentrations. These include both exogenous (synthetic) and endogenous (native) substances which can modify growth in plants. Most of the plant hormones exhibit a broad action spectrum and thus a single hormone may influence several processes.

The native plant growth substances include auxins, gibberellins, cytokinins, abscisic acid and ethylene. These regulate cell division, cell enlargement, cell differentiation, organogenesis, senescence and dormancy. These are at present employed in tissue cultures as such it is possible to culture any part of the plant *in vitro*. These are capable of enhancing production of the secondary metabolites which are used as drugs.

1. **Auxins:** Auxin is a general term that indicates all the substances which promote the elongation of the coleoptile tissues. Auxins may be natural (produced by the plants) or synthetic (artificially produced) and they have the same action. IAA (indole 3-acetic acid) is the principal natural auxin and it was F. W. Went (1928) who provided experimental evidence for IAA from the tips of *Avena* coleoptile, which is now popular as went curvature test. Other natural auxins are IAN (indole 3-acetonitrile), 4-chloroindole 3-acetic acid and phenyl acetic acid. The synthetic auxins include IBA (indole 3-butyric acid), NOA (2-naphthoxy acetic acid), NAA (alpha-naphthyl acetic acid), NAD (1-naphthyl acetamide), 2,4-D (2,4-dichlorophenoxy acetic acid), 2,4,5-T (2,4,5-trichlorophenoxy acetic acid), 2,4,6-T and 5-carboxy-methyl-N, N-dimethyl dithiocarbamate.

   Auxins are associated with cell and internodal elongation, apical dominance, leaf growth, initiation of the vascular tissues, increased cambial activity, formation of the fruit without pollination (parthenocarpy), growth of the fruits, inhibition of the root growth and leaf abscission, photo and geotropism, etc. The mechanism of their action is by interaction with one or more components of protein synthesis. It is also suggested that they alter the osmotically active contents of the vacuole during expansion and extension of the cell wall.

   IBA is a promising growth regulator which induces rooting in cinchona, pinus, papaya and coffee. IAA, NAA and 2,4-D when added to cultures of ergot increases the content of indole alkaloids. Seedlings of *Mentha piperita* treated with NAA showed about 40% increase in their content of volatile oil. 2,4-D and 2,4,5-T are potent weedicides in higher concentrations.

2. **Gibberellins:** These are a class of natural plant growth regulators which stimulate cell division or cell elongation or both, promote vegetative growth, growth of the fruits, help in breaking dormancy, initiate the flower formation and induce parthenocarpy in the absence of pollination to result in the seedless fruits. They also promote rapid expansion of plant cells, stimulate seed germination, and break dormancy due to over-wintering, and influence increase in stem elongation and increase in the size of the leaves. The effects are marked in the intact plants rather than excised organs such as auxins. So far 56 gibberellins are known out of which 52 have been positively spotted from *Gibberella fujikuroi* and/or higher plants and others from fungi.

Gibberellins were discovered from a pathogenic fungus, *Gibberella fujikuroi* (formerly *Fusarium heterospermum*) on rice by a Japanese plant physiologist, Kurosawa. Paleg identified that their biological activity was due to the presence of a gibbane skeleton. Extensive research on gibberellins has shown that gibberellin-A (isolated in 1938) is a mixture of 6 gibberellins referred to GA_1, GA_2, GA_3, GA_4, GA_7 and GA_9 out of which GA_3 is the most common gibberellin of universal occurrence and is called gibberellic acid. The different groups of plants contain different types of gibberellins and all of them together will not occur in the same plant.

Gibberellins find their application in medicinal plants. Gibberellins in lower concentrations increase the yield of glycosides in digitalis (digoxin). In case of senna, GA increases the dry weight of the shoot but reduces the content of sennoside in the leaves. Castor plants treated with GA increased their height 5 times more but failed to show any change in the content of the fixed oil. GA reduces the alkaloid content in vinca, *Datura* and hyoscyamus. GA induces the activity of gluconeogenic enzymes in the early stage of germination which ensures a rapid conversion of lipid to sucrose which is rapidly utilised in the development of the root and shoots in the embryo. In monocot seeds, gibberellins induce the synthesis of amylase and other hydrolases during the germination and the formation of the seedling.

3. **Cytokinins (cytokinetins or phytokinins):** Phytokinins are the purine derivatives especially from adenine. Either natural or synthetic cytokinins regulate growth by promotion of cell division and leaf senescence, sometimes promoting the development of lateral buds and inhibiting senescence. They also participate in embryo and seed development and influence the expansion of cells in leaf discs and

cotyledons. They also delay the breakdown of chlorophyll and protein degradation in ageing leaves.

Haberlandt (1913) provided circumstantial evidence for the substances from phloem which induced cell division. Van Overbeek (1941) showed that coconut milk also induced cell division in embryos grown in tissue culture. Skoog (1955) isolated kinetin, an active substance which induced cell division. Cytokinins, Zeatin was isolated from maize (1964) and thereafter several cytokinins were discovered in several species. Kinetin (6-furfuryladenine) was first isolated by Miller from autoclaved Herring sperm DNA and found to be inducing cell division in tobacco cultures. All cytokinins are adenine (amino purine) derivatives and found in embryos, seedlings and apical meristems. The natural cytokinins (amino purines) are zeatin, dihydrozeatin, methylthiozeatin and DMAA while the synthetic cytokinins prepared from urea are celorophenylurea, benzylurea, 6-benzylaminopurine, 6-benzyl adenine, benzimadole and N,N'-diphenylurea. Kinins play an important role in nucleic acid metabolism and protein synthesis and they also influence the enzymes responsible for the formation certain amino acids.

In medicinal plants, cytokinins increase sennoside content in senna leaves in addition to enhancing the weight of the shoots. In opium, they result in the formation of elongated capsules and reduce the content of the alkaloids.

4. **Ethylene:** Ethylene is the only volatile gaseous growth hormone which occurs in ripening fruits, flowers, stems, roots, tubers and seeds and in a very small quantity in the plant (0.1 ppm) which increases in quantity during growth and development. This is produced by an incomplete burning of carbon rich substances like natural gas, coal and petroleum. Yellowing of lemons by stove gas was observed by Denny (1924). It was also observed that illuminating gas damages the plants. Gane (1934) established that ethylene was a natural product of ripening fruits and stimulated ripening of fruits. Later, it was also established that it was produced from flowers, leaves, seeds and even roots. It was only after 1969; ethylene was accepted as a phytohormone. The growth responses of ethylene in plants include ripening of fruits, abscission of the leaf, swelling of the stem, bending of the leaf, discolouration of the flower petals and inhibition of stem and root growth. On a commercial scale, it is employed for the promotion of flowering and fruit ripening, induction of fruit ripening, breaking dormancy and stimulation of latex flow in rubber trees.

5. **Abscisic acid (ABA):** This phytohormone is a sesquiterpene and its synonyms are Dormin and Abscissin II, which is universal in its distribution in plants. Osborne identified a diffusible abscission

accelerating substance in senescent leaves (1955). Cornus and Addicot (1963) isolated this compound from the shedding bolls of cotton. The chemical structure was identified in 1965. Such substances were named as Abscissin I and Abscissin II. It is a natural growth inhibitor which stimulates the shedding of leaves, fruits and flowers, induces dormancy of buds and inhibits seed germination. The natural ABA is found in ferns, spores and different organs of angiosperms.

ABA also interacts with other growth regulators. It inhibits GA-induced synthesis of alpha-amylase and other hydrolytic enzymes. On accumulation in seeds, it helps in dormancy. On application to the leaf, it also helps in the closure of stomata and as such it is a potential anti-transpirant. It is noticed that ABA accumulates in plants during the conditions of stress, mineral deficiency, injury, drought and flooding.

In addition to these five groups of plant growth regulators, many other synthetic growth retardants and inhibitors have been reported but their commercial use is yet to be reported. These include MH (maleic hydrazide), diaminozide, glyphosine, chromequat, S,S,S-tributyl phosphorotrithioate, ancymidol, chlorophonium chloride, piproctanyl bromide, etc. Another group of synthetic substances called morphactins are identified to be inhibitors of auxin transport during tropic responses, reduction of apical dominance and promotion of lateral growth. Examples are: chloroflurecol methyl, flurecol-butyl and TIBA (2,3,5-triiodobenzoic acid).

BREEDING FOR IMPROVEMENT

Breeding of plants and animals is an applied branch of biology. The plants and animals of the present day are the products of natural and artificial breeding. Plant breeding is concerned with the production of improved and new crop varieties which are superior to the existing varieties. The improved varieties can be produced only by a change in the heredity of the existing varieties. This also helps in the introduction of superior qualities found in different plants of a particular crop variety into a single plant. According to Poehlman (1931), plant breeding is 'the art and science of changing and improving the heredity of plants'. It can also be defined as 'a process of selection and crossing of different plant varieties in order to get the varieties with superior qualities'. The main objective of plant breeding is to improve the qualities of plants like: an increase in the yield of grains, fodder, fibres, oils, etc. an increase in the quality with reference to the size, colour, shape, taste, nutrients, etc. of the grains, fruits and flowers; the production of types which are resistant to pests and diseases; a change in the growth habit, maturation time, etc. The improvement of the crops can be achieved through several methods like: introduction, selection, hybridisation, polyploidy breeding and mutation breeding. Polyploidy, mutations and hybridisation are briefly described hereunder.

1. **Polyploidy:** The minimum number of chromosomes, though all are different, that function as a harmonious and integrated unit is called a 'genome' or the basic chromosome number of an organism. This is denoted by the letter 'x' or 'n'. The individuals in which the somatic cells have chromosomes in pairs are called 'diploid' (2n). Several cases are known in which the chromosome number becomes changed in the somatic cell, and this condition is known as 'ploidy'. Ploidy can be either aneuploidy or euploidy. 'Aneuploidy' is a condition in which the nuclei contain the chromosomes whose number is not a true multiple of the genome, such organisms are aneuploids. 'Euploidy' is a condition in which the change in chromosome number involves either addition or elimination of complete genome. The basic chromosome number of euploids is represented by haploid/monoploid (n). The organisms above this number are: diploids (2n), triploids (3n), tetraploids (4n), pentaploids (5n), hexaploids (6n), heptaploids (7n), octaploids (8n) and polyploids. In all these cases, the chromosome numbers are exact multiples of their original haploid number.

Polyploidy is commonly met within the plant world while it is rare in animals. According to Stebbins (1950), about one half of the total species of flowering plants are polyploid. Among certain plant families, the proportion of polyploids to diploids is >50%. About two-thirds of all grasses are polyploids. According to Manton (1950), among all the plant groups, ferns show the highest degree of polyploidy. Polyploidy can be seen in common plants like *Chrysanthemum*, *Solanum*, *Brassica*, *Triticum*, *Rosa* and *Nicotiana*. Polyploids are of two types namely, autopolyploids and allopolyploids. Autopolyploids contain more than two identical genomes which are derived by the self-duplication of the parental genome. This is due to failure of anaphase during meiosis. Examples: *Datura*, rice, apple, pear, grapes, guava, *Chrysanthemum*, orange, pineapple and rose are autotriploids (3n). Allopolyploids are the individuals in which the genomes of a multiple set are not alike. The different genomes are derived from two or more distant species by hybridisation. The best example is *Raphano-brassica* experimentally evolved by the Russian geneticist, G. D. Karpechenko as a result of an intergeneric cross between Radish (*Raphanus sativus*) and Cabbage (*Brassica oleracea*).

Polyploidy can be induced through exposure of vegetative and flower buds to radiation like ultraviolet rays, X-rays and other rays of shorter wavelength which increases the rate of cell division and causes the somatic doubling of chromosomes. This is also possible by enhancing the callus growth at the points of injury of a plant by the use of coumarone which brings about the somatic doubling of the chromosomes. Similarly, a number of chemicals are now known to induce polyploidy in plants. These include colchicines, granosan, chloroform, chloral hydrate, some narcotics and alkaloids, veratrin sulphate, acenaphthane, indoleacetic acid sulphanilamide, ethyl mercury chloride, hexchloro-cyclohexane, etc. out of which colchicine is the best chemical for inducing polyploidy. It is obtained from the roots and corms of *Colchicum autumnale* (family Liliaceae) and was first discovered by Pernice (1889) and was first demonstrated to be a specific and efficient chemical in inducing polyploidy by Levan (1938). In India, this is collected from *Colchicum luteum* and *Gloriosa superba* (family Liliaceae). Colchicine checks the anaphasic movement of the chromosomes to the poles as a result of which mitosis fails to complete and the chromosomal number gets doubled. With the increase in the chromosome number, the adaptability and variability of species increase progressively which tend to help in the evolution.

These chemical substances cause disturbance to mitotic spindle in dividing cells and due to the non-aggregation of the duplicated chromosomes, the diploids are converted to tetraploids. This is of a great significance in drug plants as it causes the formation of new species, adaptability to different habitats and accumulation of vitamins in plants like *Digitalis*, species of *Mentha*, Poppy and *Lobelia*. The most potent chemical capable of causing polyploidy is colchicine, an alkaloid from *Colchicum autumnale*, *C. luteum* and *C. speciosum* which prevents the formation of the mitotic spindle and thereby the sister chromatids fail to form daughter nuclei at the anaphase. When the cells undergo DNA replication many a time it results in polyploidy. It has been observed that colchicine treatment enhanced the content of tropane alkaloids like stramonium where the yields enhanced by 150% in tetraploids. *Lobelia, Cinchona, Belladonna, Acorus*, Squill, *Cannabis* and Poppy also showed increased yield of the constituents in tetraploids. In some cases, e.g. in *Digitalis purpurea* and *D. lanata* total glycosides were reduced due to polyploidy while lanatosides A and B showed enhancement in *D. lanata*.

2. **Mutation:** Offspring resemble their parents in one or several respects but there are differences between the two. Such differences, large or small are called *variations*. Some of these variations may be induced by the environment while others are hereditary. The variations caused by the environment are not permanent and are not inherited. But, the variations that appear due to the changes in the hereditary mechanism are permanent and heritable. The sudden heritable variation in the nature of any organism in ordinary sense is called a *mutation* and the offspring with unusual variability in its characters is called a *mutant*. Many definitions for mutations have been proposed from time to time by different biologists. Charles Darwin referred mutations as 'sports' and defined them as the 'sudden appearance of new hereditary

character in the progenies of plants and animals'. Sinnot and others referred it in the broader sense as a *'macro-mutation'* which is 'any change in the genotype' and in a narrower sense as *'micro-mutation'* to be 'a change in the gene'. Bateson defined mutation as 'a discontinuous variation'. According the Hugo DeVries (1901), mutations are 'sudden and drastic heritable changes not traceable to segregation or recombination'. Stebbins described mutation as 'a discontinuous chromosomal change with a genetic effect'. Such a change refers to chemical change in a small part of chromomere and alteration of its physical structure. Amatto and Otto (1956) defined mutation as 'a change in the hereditary constitution of a given species'.

Mutation is 'a sudden heritable change' in the characters of a species built in the genotype of an individual either due to changes in the environment or hereditary constitution. The phenotypic changes observed in the organisms are temporary and can be restored later (variations) and these are not inherited, e.g. changes which occur due to the changes in the environment which are short-lived. When the changes are withdrawn, the original traits are restored. But, the change in the genotype of the individual remains permanent and is heritable. This is referred to as the 'mutation'. These changes are either qualitative or quantitative.

These may be chromosomal or point (gene) mutations. The *chromosomal mutations/aberrations* lead to changes in the gross morphology of chromosomes or changes in the number of chromosomes. The *point/gene mutations* are the changes associated with a gene or cistron of DNA and occur at molecular level. Mutations may also be spontaneous/natural or induced/artificial. Spontaneous mutations occur in nature and are caused by natural factors. These are governed by internal factors and not by the environment. These may occur in a gene or a chromosome at anytime in the development of the organism. The induced mutations are caused artificially by mutagens. The inducing agents may be radiation, chemicals and age effect.

H . Muller (1927) was the first to demonstrate that mutations can be artificially induced by treating *Drosophila* with X-rays. L.J. Stadler (1928) also demonstrated an increase in the rate of mutations in barley and maize due to X-ray treatment. The mutagenic radiations are of two types namely, ionising radiations like X-rays, gamma rays, alpha rays, beta rays, electrons, neutrons, protons and other fast moving particles; and nonionising radiations like ultraviolet rays and visible light. A variety of chemical substances are known to induce mutations in plants and animals. It was Auerbach (1940) for the first time discovered mutagenic property of mustard gas in *Drosophila*. Urethane and formaldehyde produce the same type of mutations as the ionising radiation in *Drosophila*. DES (diethyl sulphonate) and EMS (ethyl methane sulphonate) are most extensively used for inducing mutations in microbes and higher plants. Recently discovered potent mutagen is the heliotrin found in the common Raywort. Caffeine is also used for inducing mutations. Other important chemical mutagens are: EL (ethyleneimine), nitrogen mustard, sulphur mustard, DMN (dimethyl nitrosamine), NG (nitrosoguanidine), NMU (nitroso methyl urea), EO (ethylene oxide), DEB (diepoxy butane), MMS (methyl methane sulphonate), hydrazine, nitrous acid, MH (maleic hydrazide), 5-bromo uracil, 2-amino purine, urethane, triaizine, manganese chloride, phenols and hydroxylamine. The rate of mutation is also influenced by ageing of the organism. It has been experimentally proved in *Drosophila* that sex-linked mutations may accumulate as a result of ageing.

The induced mutations in drug plants is an important milestone in the cultivation of medicinal plants as the content of medicinal constituents showed an enhancement in many plants. For example, solasodine content increased in *Solanum khasianum* (radiation and chemical mutagens), increased morphine concentration in *Papaver somniferum* (chemical mutagens), increased tuber yield and diosgenin content in *Dioscorea bulbifera* (radiation), *Atropa belladonna* (radiation), harvest index of *Mentha arvensis* var. *piperascens* (gamma rays), species of *Capsicum* (sodium azide), etc. The changes due to mutations may be morphological or anatomical and also the changes in the chemical composition of plants. In medicinal plants, these may result in increased yield of the active constituents, in increasing disease resistance, etc. But, the plant may become susceptible to changes in the climate, susceptible to other diseases or show slower growth and such undesirable characters can be eliminated by breeding and selection.

3. **Hybridisation:** A 'hybrid' is an organism resulting by crossing two species or varieties which differ in at least one set of characters, and the process of their production is 'hybridisation'. Hybridisation is defined as 'the method of producing new crop varieties by crossing two genetically different parents'. The hybrids may be monohybrids (one pair of characters), dihybrids (two pairs of characters) or multi/polyhybrids (more than two pairs of characters). This helps in introduction of favourable and required characters into a species or a variety and sometimes new characters not present in both the parents. According to the nature and relationship of plants this can be inter-varietal (intraspecific), intravarietal, interspecific (intrageneric) and intergeneric hybridisation. If the cross is made between plants of two

different varieties of the same species, it is called intervarietal or intra-specific hybridisation. Many new varieties of cultivated crops have been evolved by this method. If the plants to be crossed possess different genotypes belonging to the same variety, it is called intra-varietal hybridisation. Interspecific/intrageneric hybridisation is a cross made between two different species of the same/single genus. These crosses have been successfully tried in wheat, cotton, tobacco, mustard, *Luffa*, etc. Intergeneric hybridisation involves the cross between two different genera belonging to the same family: *Raphano-brassica*, *Triticale* (wheat-rye), sugarcane-sorghum, sugarcane-bamboo and wheat-*Aegilops* hybrids are the best examples. Hybridisation can be carried out in either self-pollinated or cross-pollinated crops.

Hybridisation has led to the production of new species/varieties in medicinal plants. *Withania somnifera* Israeli chemotype II crossed with *W. somnifera* South African chemotype resulted in a new hybrid containing three new withanolides. Similarly, the hybrids of *Digitalis purpurea* and *D. lanata*, and *D. purpurea* and *D. lutea* showed the presence of lanatoside A, B and E without lanatoside C. A cross between *Solanum incanum* and *S. melongena* resulted in the F_1 hybrid bearing more berries and solasodine (0.5%) while the F_2 hybrids proved to be high-yielding sources of solasodine. In recent times, protoplast fusion and asexual hybridisation is being employed.

REVIEW QUESTIONS

1. **Essay and Short Answer Questions:**
    1. Write short notes on the importance of mutations and hybri-disation in the improvement and cultivation of medicinal plants.
    2. Describe in detail the different factors that influence the cultivation of medicinal plants.
    3. Describe in detail the collection and processing of medicinal plants.
    4. Write short notes on the influence of climatic factors and edaphic factors on cultivation of medicinal plants.
    5. Write short notes on the importance of hybridisation and polyploidy in the improvement and cultivation of medicinal plants.

2. **Choose the Correct Alternative:**
    1. The harvested medicinal plants should be protected from: [ ]
        a. Pests   b. Rodents
        c. Birds   d. All
    2. The cultivation of medicinal plants always ensures: [ ]
        a. Purity and the quality
        b. Uniformity and quality

    c. Maximum yield and contamination

    d. All

3. Vegetative propagation is carried out by means of: [ ]

    a. Bulbs   b. Corms

    c. Stem tubers   d. All

4. The plants can be aseptically micropropagated from: [ ]

    a. Tissues   b. Embryos

    c. Shoot apex   d. All

5. The additive factors include: [ ]

    a. Fertilisers   b. Pesticides

    c. Weedicides   d. All

3. Fill in the Blanks:

1. Fresh plant material can be frozen at .... temperature

2. Prior to germination, the seeds must be subjected to ....

3. .... relieves dormancy of the seeds and promotes the growth of the seedlings.

4. The barks are to be collected either in spring or early summer when the .... will be very active.

5. The roots for the crude drugs are to be collected before their .... growth comes to a halt.

4. True or False Statements:

1. The contamination of the crude drug can be avoided in cultivation.

    [True/False]

2. The cultivation of medicinal and aromatic plants leads to the establishment of industries and industrialisation.   [True/False]

3. The seeds used for germination should not possess a high percentage of germination and must be free from disease.

    [True/False]

4. Asexual method helps to generate the seedless fruits and disease resistant varieties.   [True/False]

5. Higher temperatures promote the formation of volatile oils while hot days account for physical accumulation of the oil.

    [True/False]

5. A. Match the following:

1. Slow drying at low   [ ]   a. Oil becomes resinous
   temperature

2. Immediate drying   [ ]   b. To procure nutmeg

3. Direct oxidation   [ ]   c. Dark containers

4. Fish liver oils   [ ]   d. Enzyme action in seeds

5. Drying by open fire   [ ]   e. To prevent molds

B. Match the following:

1. Indole-3-acetic acid   [ ]   a. Weedicide

2. 2,4,6-T   [ ]   b. Gibberellin

3. Coconut milk   [ ]   c. Synthetic auxin

4. Kurosawa   [ ]   d. F.W. Went

5. 2,4,5-T   [ ]   e. Von Overbeek

C. Match the following:

1. Cornus and Addicot   [ ]   a. Yellowing by stove gas

2. Denny   [ ]   b. Miller

3. Isolation of kinetin   [ ]   c. ABA

4. Herring sperm DNA   [ ]   d. Ethylene

5. Gane   [ ]   e. Skoog

D. Match the following:

1. Induced mutations   [ ]   a. Hugo De Vries

2. Colchicine   [ ]   b. Karpechenko

3. Autotriploid   [ ]   c. Pernice

4. *Raphano-brassica*   [ ]   d. *Chrysanthemum*

5. Mutations   [ ]   e. H.J. Muller

Good Agriculture Practices (GAP) Strategies of Obtaining Improved Cultivation of Medicinal Plants

INTRODUCTION

Over the past two decades the interest in the traditional medicine (herbal medicine) and the cultivation of medicinal plants has received an increased impetus substantially both in the developed and developing countries, due to the revival of interest in herbal medicines necessitating the authoritative information on the cultivation and utilisation of medicinal flora, and the global and national markets for medicinal herbs have been growing rapidly and economic gains have been realised significantly. As such, the safety and quality of the herbal medicines have become increasingly an important concern for the health authorities and public alike. Following the use of certain herbal medicines associated with possible explanations in the inadvertent use of the wrong plant species, the adulteration with other medicines and potent substances, contamination with toxic and hazardous substances, over dosage, inappropriate use and interaction with the other medicines which result in adverse drug reaction have been reported. The poor quality of the finished products results due to the use of raw plant materials that are not of a high quality as the safety and quality of raw plant material and finished products depend on many factors either intrinsic or genetic and extrinsic like environment, methods of collection, methods of cultivation, methods of harvesting, postharvest processing and transport and storage practices. The contamination by microbial or chemical agents during the stages of production can also lead to the deterioration of the quality of the product. The medicinal plants collected from the wild population may get contaminated by other species or plant parts through misidentification, accidental contamination or internal adulteration with unsafe consequences, and can also give rise to concerns related to regional or local overharvesting and protection of the endangered species. Hence, one should consider the impact of cultivation and collection on the environment and ecology as well as the welfare of the local communities. At the same time, intellectual property rights with regard to the source material must also be respected too.

To account for all these issues and overcome the drawbacks if any, the World Health Organisation in cooperation with other specialised agencies of the United Nations and many international organisations to strengthen and update the relevant issues, proposed some technical guidelines under the heading, Good Agricultural Practices (GAP) to be followed all over the world. These problems can be overcome to ensure the safety and quality of a variety of food commodities including the medicinal plant material by the establishment of specific guidelines for good agricultural practice by the concerned. The quality control for the cultivation and collection of medicinal plants as the raw material for herbal medicines is more demanding than that for food plants, and as such some countries like China, the European Union and Japan have recently developed some guidelines on good agricultural practices for the medicinal plants which sometimes may not be applicable universally. Recently, at an informal meeting it was recommended that the World Health Organisation should give high priority to the development of globally applicable guidelines to promote the safety and quality of medicinal plant material through the formulation of codes for good agricultural and good collection practices for the medicinal plants and it was also envisaged that the guidelines would help to ensure the safety and quality at the first stage of the herbal medicine production.

The medicinal plant material is supplied through collection from wild populations and cultivation. For the quality assurance and control of herbal medicines, World Health Organisation developed the *Guidelines on Good Agricultural and Collection Practices* (GACP) for the medicinal plants which are basically intended to provide the general technical guidance on obtaining the medicinal plant materials of a good quality for the sustainable production of herbal products classified as medicines. These guidelines also apply to the cultivation and collection of medicinal plants including the postharvest operations which vary in accordance with the situation of a country, and also work on the protection of medicinal plants thus aiming at the promotion of sustainable use and cultivation of medicinal plants.

OBJECTIVES OF GUIDELINES

The main objectives of these guidelines are:

- To contribute to the quality assurance of medicinal plant materials used as the source for the herbal medicines aiming at improving the quality, safety and efficacy of the finished herbal products, and are to be produced hygienically with care so that the negative impacts can be limited.

- To guide the formulation of the national and/or regional guidelines and monographs for medicinal plants and related standard operating procedures.

- To encourage and support the sustainable cultivation and collection of the medicinal plants of good quality which support the conservation of the medicinal plants and the environment.

Such guidelines should be considered in conjunction with the existing documents, publications related to the quality assurance, the conservation and protection of the natural resources of the medicinal plants for sustainable use as well as the guidelines and codes of practices developed by the Joint FAO/WHO *Codex Alimentarius Commission*. In following these guidelines, every care must be taken and the grower should be conscious of the critical steps, the risks associated with the production of low quality, the risks associated with the residue and contamination and the risks associated with the unsustainable wild collection to ensure constant high quality and standard safety level, the full traceability of the production, keep up of the records and to establish the basic production quality assurance system.

Our country has a rich tradition of healthcare systems based on medicinal plants contained in its ancient classical texts such as *Charaka Samhitha* and *Sushrutha Samhitha*. On the basis of the diverse healthcare practices, our Government has recognised *Ayurveda, Yoga and Naturopathy, Unani, Siddha* and *Homoeopathy* as the alternative systems of medicine under its National Health Policy. The department of AYUSH in the Ministry of Health and Family Welfare has the responsibility for quality assurance and standardisation of production processes of medicines and guidelines for the production of raw material used in these medicines. These guidelines lay down the standards for the production of the raw material that goes into the making of the medicines and standardise the production processes from the farm to the factory. Our subcontinent has 16 agroclimatic zones, about 45,000 different plant species and 15,000 medicinal plants. Indian systems of medicine have identified 1,500 medicinal plants of which 500 species are mostly used in the preparation of drugs catering to 80% of the raw materials used in the drug preparation. In addition, there is also a growing demand for the natural products such as the items of medicinal value, pharmaceuticals, food supplements and cosmetics. The herbal medicines are the natural answer for some ailments, but some reports of the patients experiencing negative health consequences are on the rise which is directly linked to the poor quality of the herbal medicines and to the wrong identification of the plant species used in their preparation. Hence, cultivation, collection and classification are of utmost importance for the quality and safety of the products. In addition, the growing herbal market might pose a great threat to the biodiversity through overharvesting of the raw material and if this is not curbed, such practices may lead to the extinction of the endangered species as well as the destruction of the natural habitats and resources. The guidelines released by World Health Organisation ensure the production of good quality herbal medicines which are safe and sustainable and pose no threat to either people or the environment. These cover the cultivation and collection practices of the medicinal plants and also guide the postharvest operations including the legal complications related to the quality standard, status of the patient and other benefits.

A Good Agricultural Practice (GAP) with reference to medicinal plants is, a programme of cultivation which is designed to ensure optimum yield in terms of both quality and quantity of any crop that is intended for health purposes. The good agricultural practices for medicinal plants mainly include: the identification and proper authentication of the cultivated medicinal plants (selection), botanical identity, specimens, seeds and other propagation material, cultivation, site selection, ecological environment and the social impact, climate, soil, irrigation and drainage, plant maintenance and protection, harvest, primary processing, packaging, storage and transport, personnel and documentation.

IDENTIFICATION OR AUTHENTICATION OF CULTIVATED MEDICINAL PLANTS (SELECTION)

The selected medicinal plant species or the varieties meant for cultivation should be the same as that specified in the national pharmacopoeia or recommended by the national authority. In the absence of the national documents, the documents of other countries should be considered. In the case of newly introduced species or variety, it should be properly identified and documented as the source material used or described in traditional medicine of the country.

Botanical Identity

The scientific name of the medicinal plant under cultivation (identity) should be properly verified and recorded with reference to the genus, the species, the subspecies/variety, the author and the family. The common names in English and local names (in other languages) should be recorded. The information related to the name of the cultivar, ecotype, chemotype, phenotype and the genotype should be provided. For commercial cultivars, the name of the cultivar and the name of the supplier should be provided. The details related to the locally named line, origin and the source of seeds, plants or propagation materials should be recorded for land races collected, propagated and disseminated.

Specimens

In the case of the first registration in a country, the grower should submit a voucher botanical WHO - GACP for the specimen to a regional or national herbarium for identification. If possible, a genetic pattern should be compared to that of an authentic specimen. The documentation of the identity should be included in the registration file.

Seeds and other Propagation Material

The seeding materials are to be identified botanically and it should be 100% traceable. This also applies to the vegetative propagated starting material and the material used in organic production should necessarily be certified to be organically productive. It should meet the standards concerning the purity and germination. The seeds and other propagation materials should be specified with reference to the name as per the pharmacopoeia nomenclature and the trade name, botanical name, cultivar, phenotype, genotype, etc. The suppliers should provide all the information relating to the identity, quality and performance of the product in addition to their breeding history. The material should be free from contamination and diseases in order to promote healthy plant growth. The material should be resistant to tolerant to biotic or abiotic factors. When resistant or tolerant species or origins are available, they should be preferred. The quality of the material including any genetically modified germplasm should comply with regional and/or national regulations and be appropriately labelled and documented. Every care should be taken to exclude extraneous species, botanical varieties and strains of medicinal plants during the production process. The propagation material if found to be counterfeit, substandard or adulterated should be avoided. The important precautions with reference to the selection of the propagation material are as follows: The seeds chosen for cultivation should be free from pests, diseases, foreign and inert matter. If fresh, the seeds must have originated from the recent harvests and the seeds from the wild sources must invariably be from the recently collected lots and only the mature seeds should be collected. The process of transplantation should be carried out only with healthy seedlings. In case of stem cuttings, the source should be well-authenticated for the botanical identity and the quality of the vegetative propagules. The stem cuttings chosen for the root induction should be of uniform dimension in terms of their length and diameter and should give desired rooting. Similarly, the root cuttings chosen should be of uniform size and maturity and must be free from disease and infection.

Cultivation

The cultivation requires intensive care and management. The required conditions and duration vary depending on the quality of the plant material required. If, scientifically documented cultivation data is not available, the traditional methods of cultivation should be followed or a method should be developed through research. The principles of appropriate rotation of plants selected according to environmental suitability should be followed and tillage should be adapted. The techniques of building-up of organic matter and conservation of soil humidity and no-tillage systems should be followed. Such techniques of conservation agriculture aim to conserve, to improve and make efficient use of natural resources through integrated management of the available soil, water and biological resources combined with the external outputs. This also contributes to the environmental conservation as well as to enhanced and sustained agricultural production, and is resource–efficient and/or resource–effective. Every care should be taken to avoid the environmental disturbances. The principles of good crop husbandry must be followed including an appropriate rotation of crops.

Site Selection

The selected site should qualify in terms of overall soil health for the purpose of the cultivation of medicinal plant species. The material derived from the same species can show significant differences in its quality when cultivated at different sites, due to the influence of the soil, climate and other environmental factors. Such differences may be related to the physical appearance or to variations in its constituents. The biosynthesis may get affected by the extrinsic environmental factors which include ecological and geographical variables which are to be taken into consideration. The risk of contamination due to the pollution of the soil, air or water by the hazardous chemicals should be avoided. The impact of past land use on the site including the previous crops and application of products of plant protection should be also evaluated. In general, sites with a high degree of stress factors like salinity, acidity and toxicity, water-logged conditions, industrial wastes and effluents should be avoided. Similarly, the sites nearer to grave yards, crematoria should also be avoided. The selected site must be in close proximity to a reliable source of irrigation water.

ECOLOGICAL ENVIRONMENT AND SOCIAL IMPACT

The grower should identify the best possible environment where the plant can express its full potential in terms of both the quality and quantity during its entire growth period, from germination to maturity. The medicinal plant cultivation in a site may affect the ecological balance and the genetic diversity of the flora and fauna in the surrounding habitats. The quality and growth of the medicinal plants can also be affected by other plants, living organisms and human activities. The introduction of non-indigenous medicinal plant species into the cultivation could result in a detrimental effect on the biological and ecological balance of that particular region, and such activities should be carefully monitored overtime.

One should examine the social impact of the cultivation on the local communities to ensure that negative impacts on local livelihood are avoided. Small-scale cultivation is preferable if the farmers are organised to market their products jointly. If large-scale cultivation has been established, every care should be taken that the local communities benefit directly from fair wages, equal employment opportunity and capital reinvestment.

Climate

The climatic conditions such as the length of the day, precipitation and field temperature influence the physical, chemical and biological qualities of the medicinal plants under cultivation. The duration of the sunlight, average rainfall, average temperature, differences in the temperature of the day and the night also influence the physiological and biochemical activities of plants and these should also be considered.

Soil

The soil where cultivation is to be taken up should contain appropriate amounts of the nutrients, organic matter and other inorganic elements to ensure optimum plant growth and quality. These include the soil type, drainage, soil moisture retention capacity, soil fertility and soil pH which determine the plant species and/or the target part. The medicinal plants cannot be grown in soils that are contaminated by sludge, heavy metals, residues of the plant protection products and other not naturally occurring chemicals. The fertiliser use is often indispensable in order to achieve larger yields of plants. Hence, the correct type and quantity of the fertilisers are to be used by determination through agricultural research. In general practice, organic and chemical fertilisers are used. The manure applied should be void of human faeces and if animal manure is to be used, it should be thoroughly composted to meet the safe sanitary standards of acceptable microbial limits and destroyed by the germination capacity of the weeds, and this should be documented. The chemical fertilisers approved by the country of cultivation should be used. These fertilisers should be used sparingly in accordance with the needs of the particular plant species and the soil supporting capacity. The leaching of the fertilisers should be minimised. The cultivator should follow the practices that mainly contribute to soil conservation and minimise soil erosion such as creation of stream-side buffer zones and planting of cover crops and green manure.

Irrigation and Drainage

The quality of irrigation water in terms of total salt concentration, sodium absorption ratio, bicarbonate and boron concentration should be adequate in terms of the target crop. Soil irrigation and soil drainage should be minimised as far as possible and carried out in accordance with the needs of the individual plant species during the various stages of its growth. The water that is used should invariably comply with local, regional and/or national quality standards and should be free from contaminants such as faeces, heavy metals, pesticides, herbicides and substances which are toxicologically hazardous. Every care should be taken to ensure that the plants under cultivation are neither over-watered nor under-watered. The risks of vector disease transmission through irrigation practices should be taken care of. Water harvesting and water conservation methods should be followed and the impounding of water through heavy rains should be avoided.

PLANT MAINTENANCE AND PROTECTION

Initial flush of weeds must be controlled effectively and all intercultural operations like weeding, topping, bud nipping, pruning, shading and earthing up must be adhered to control the growth and development of the medicinal plant to improve the quality and quantity of the material being produced. Minimum amount of agrochemicals should be used to promote the growth of/or to protect the plants and these should be applied only when no alternative measures are available. Use of organic manure is preferred for growing the medicinal plants. Use of compost, vermicompost, poultry manure, and green leafy manure is desirable. But, the use of sludge, city waste, night soil and any other manure with known toxicities must be avoided. Where appropriate, the integrative pest management should be followed. The application of pesticides and herbicides should be avoided as far as possible. If necessary, the approved pesticides and herbicides should be used at their minimum effective level in accordance with the instructions of the individual product and the regulatory requirements that apply for the cultivator. The application and storage of these products has to be in accordance with the recommendations of the manufacturers and the authorities. The pesticide and herbicide applications should necessarily be carried out by the certified and qualified staff with the approved equipment and all such applications should be documented. It is also obligatory that the buyer be informed of the brand, quantity and the date of pesticide use in a written form. The application should invariably precede the harvest by a period either defined by the buyer or indicated by the producer of the product. The minimum interval between such treatments and the harvest should be consistent with the instructions inserted on the label and/or package of the plant protection product. Growers and the producers should always comply with the maximum pesticide and herbicide residue limits as was stipulated by the local, regional and/or national regulatory authorities of the growers and the end users, countries and/or the regions. International agreements like International Plant Protection Conventions and Codex Alimentarius should be consulted on the use of pesticides and their residues. In general, the crop protection methods should be limited to the use of biocontrol agents and biopesticides.

Harvest

The medicinal plants should be always harvested during the optimal season to ensure the production of the material and finished herbal product of the best possible quality and the time of harvest should depend on the plant part to be used. The concentration of the biologically active compounds varies with the stage of plant growth and development which also applies to the non-targeted toxic or poisonous plant constituents. The best time for the harvest should be determined according to the quality and quantity of biologically active compounds rather than the total yield of the plant parts. At the time of the harvest, every care must be taken to ensure that no foreign material, weeds or toxic plants are mixed up with the harvested plant material. The plants should be harvested when there is no dew, rain or high humidity. If done under wet conditions, the material should be immediately transported to an indoor drying facility to prevent possible deleterious effects due to microbial fermentation and molds. All the devices and the machines should be kept clean to reduce the damage and soil contamination and they should be stored in a dry place free from the insects, rodents, birds, other pests and should be inaccessible for the livestock and other domestic animals. You should avoid contact with the soil to minimise the microbial load by the use of clean muslin interface between the harvested material and the soil. The adhering soil from the underground parts must be removed immediately after harvest. The raw plant material should be transported in a clean and dry condition and placed in clean dry and well-aerated containers like sacks, baskets, trailers, containers, etc. before carried onto the transport process facility. Overfilling of the sacks, stacking up of the sacks, occurrence of heating is to be avoided. In case of the plastic containers, special attention is to be paid to possible moisture retention and when not in use, these should be kept dry protected from the insects, rodents and pests. The mechanical damage should be avoided and the decomposed plant material should be discarded during harvest to avoid microbial contamination and loss of the product quality. The delivery of the harvested material must occur as quickly as possible to the processing facility.

Primary Processing

This includes the steps such as washing, freezing, distilling, drying, etc. These steps must confirm the local, regional and/or national standards. Prior to processing, the material should not be exposed to sunlight or rainfall. The buildings must be clean and well-aerated. Suitable pest control measures are to taken care of. The drying process should be initiated in a continuum. Drying directly on the ground should be avoided unless it is required. Sorting is to be carried out after drying. The material must be inspected to eliminate the substandard and foreign products. Everything is to be documented.

Packaging

The product should be packed in clean, dry new sacks, bags or cases. They are to be labelled and the labels should be clear and permanently fixed and made from nontoxic material. It must be guaranteed that no contamination takes place by the use of the packaging material. If the packaging material is reusable, it should be thoroughly cleaned and perfectly dried prior to its usage and must be guaranteed that no contamination occurs by reusing the containers.

Storage and Transport

The packaged material is to be stored in a dry, well-aerated building with limited daily temperature fluctuations and good aeration. The windows and doors must be wire-netted so as to protect it from pests, birds, rodents and domestic animals. Storage of packaged dry crop in concrete buildings with easy to clean floors, with a sufficient distance to the wall, separated from other crops to avoid cross-contamination is always recommended. Organic products must be stored separately. In the case of bulk transport, it is advisable to use aerated containers. Fumigation should be carried out in case of necessity during transport with registered chemicals and by qualified personnel which is to be documented.

Personnel

The growers and the producers should necessarily have adequate knowledge of the medicinal plant concerned which includes identification, cultivation methods, environmental requirement, methods of harvest and storage. The field workers and other personnel associated with the propagation, cultivation, harvest and postharvest processing should invariably maintain personal hygiene and they should wear protective clothing like overalls, gloves, helmets, goggles and face masks during the application of agrochemicals. The growers and producers should necessarily receive instructions related to all issues for environmental conservation of the plant species concerned.

Documentation

All the documents related to the entire process should be maintained. These include the meteorological data, reports of soil and water testing, the source, quantity and the time of procurement and collection of seeds or the planting material, the procedures adapted to handling the plant material during the nursery stage, preparation of the soil, transplantation procedure, crop management, weeding cycles, inter-culture practices, photographic records, etc. for a minimum period of 3 to 5 years. All starting materials and different steps of processing have to be documented. Field records should be maintained by all the growers. All the batches of the material should be perfectly labelled. It is also essential to document the type, quantity and the date of the harvest of the crop in addition to the chemicals and other substances used during the production. The application of the fumigation agents must be entered into the documentation. All the processes and the procedures which bear an impact on the quality of the product, all agreements between the producer and the buyer, and special circumstances during the growth period which may influence the chemical composition, etc. must be documented.

The cultivation, collection and harvesting of medicinal plants and the postharvest processing must be carried out in accordance with the legal and environmental requirements and with the ethical codes and norms of the community and the country. The provisions of the Convention on Biological Diversity must be respected. The medicinal plants that are protected by national and international laws may be collected only by relevant permission. The provisions of the CITES (Convention on International Trade in Endangered Species of Wild Fauna and Flora) must be complied with.

SAMPLE RECORD OF DOCUMENTATION FOR CULTIVATED MEDICINAL PLANTS

a. **Identification of the Cultivated Medicinal Plant**

Scientific name: ....

Pharmacopoeia name: ....

Local name(s) and Language(s) for: ....

Common name (in English): ....

Intended plant part for medicinal use and harvested: ....

Crop code number: ....

b. **Identification of Cultivation Site**

Identification of field site: ....

Location of the field: ....

Village/District/Region/State/Country: ....

c. **Identification of Cultivator**

Name of the grower/cultivator: ....

Contact address for communication: ....

Period of cultivation: ....

Cultivation begins on (Date/Month/Year): ....

Cultivation ends on (Date/Month/Year): ....

d. Seeds and other Propagation Materials

Source of the planted material: ....

Physical description of the planted material: ....

Whether commercially available? (Strike off which is not applicable): Yes/No

If YES, name of the cultivator: ....

Name of the supplier: ....

e. Method of Cultivation

Method of establishment of the propagation material (Strike off which is not applicable):

DIRECT SEED SOWING/TRANSPLANTS

Date of first sowing/transplanting (Date/Month/Year): ....

Percentage emergence: ....

Date of re-sowing/re-planting (Date/Month/Year): ....

Percentage of stand establishment: ....

Spacing between the rows (in centimeters): ....

Spacing between the plants (in centimeters): ....

Size of the planted (covered) area (in square-meters): ....

Number of plants per unit area: ....

Crop rotation methods followed: ....

f. Soil and Irrigation

Type of the soil (Strike off which is not applicable):

CLAYEY/SANDY/SILTY/LOAMY

Percentage of clay: ....

Percentage of sand: ....

Percentage of silt: ....

Percentage of organic matter: ....

Percentage of others (if any describe): ....

Soil pH: ....

Soil fertility (strike off which is not applicable): Good/Poor

Soil moisture retention (strike off which is not applicable): Good/Poor

Soil drainage (strike off which is not applicable): Good/Poor

Irrigation (strike off which is not applicable): Yes/No

Land (topography) [strike off which is not applicable]: Even/Sloping

Type of irrigation system (strike off which is not applicable):

FLOOD/FURROW/SPRINKLER/DRIP

Source of water (strike off which is not applicable):

MUNICIPAL OR CORPORATION SUPPLY/LAKE/
RIVER/WELL/OTHERS

If other, please specify the water source: ....

Water quality (strike off which is not applicable): Good/Bad

Description of the quality of water: ....

Salt concentration in water (strike off which is not applicable): High/Low

Name(s) of the adjacent plants (scientific/local names): ,....................

Types of insects on the adjacent plants:

APHIDS/SCALE INSECTS/CATERPILLARS/LOCUSTS/OTHERS

If others, please specify: ....

g. **Agrochemicals Applied**

   1. **Fertilisers applied before planting** (strike off which is not applicable)

      Organic (composted animal manure)/Chemical

      Name: ....

      Method of application: ....

      Time (Date/Month/Year): ....

      Rate of application: ....

   2. **Fertilisers applied after planting (top dressing)** (strike off which is not applicable)

      Organic (composted animal manure)/Chemical

      Name: ....

      Method of application: ....

Time (Date/Month/Year): ....

Rate of application: ....

3. **Herbicides applied before planting** (if any)

   Name: ....

   Method of application: ....

   Time (Date/Month/Year): ....

   Rate of application: ....

4. **Herbicides applied after planting** (if any)

   Name: ....

   Method of application: ....

   Time (Date/Month/Year): ....

   Rate of application: ....

5. **Pesticides applied** (if any)

   Name: ....

   Method of application: ....

   Time (Date/Month/Year): ....

   Rate of application: ....

6. **Special operations done** (if any)

   Name: ....

   Method of application: ....

   Time (Date/Month/Year): ....

   Rate of application: ....

7. **Plant protection chemicals applied** (if any)

   Name: ....

   Method of application: ....

   Time (Date/Month/Year): ....

   Rate of application: ....

h. **Harvest/Collection**

   Date/Month/Year of harvest: ....

   Time of the day: ....

   Conditions of the day at the time of harvest (specify): ....

   Method of harvest: ....

   Amount of yield per unit area: ....

i. **Drying Practice Adapted**

Drying method: Strike off which is not applicable

SUN DRYING/SHADE DRYING/MECHANICAL DRYING

Duration of drying (in days): ....

Moisture content after drying (percentage): ....

j. **Unusual Circumstances which may influence the quality** (strike off which is not applicable):

EXPOSURE TO EXTREME WEATHER CONDITIONS/EXPOSURE TO HAZARDOUS SUBSTANCES/OUTBREAK OF THE PESTS, etc.

Please specify and describe the circumstances and reasons thereof, if any: ....

....

....

REVIEW QUESTIONS

1. **Essay and Short Answer Questions:**
   1. Briefly describe the good agricultural practices employed in the cultivation of medicinal plants.
   2. Write an account of various good practices employed for obtaining better quality drugs with examples.
   3. Briefly discuss the strategies for obtaining the improved varieties of medicinal plants.
   4. Write an account of good agricultural practices which aim at the improvement of medicinal plants.

2. **Choose the Correct Alternative:**
   1. General agricultural practices are the technical guidelines proposed by: [ ]
      a. UNESCO   b. FAO
      c. WHO   d. UNICEF

   2. These guidelines ensure: [ ]
      a. Medicines of good quality
      b. Safe and sustainable medicines
      c. Postharvest operations
      d. All

   3. *Codex Alimentarius Commission* is a joint venture of: [ ]
      a. UNICEF/FAO   b. UNESCO/UNICEF
      c. FAO/WHO   d. FAO/FDA

4. The alternate systems under National Health Policy of India are: [ ]
   a. Unani   b. Siddha
   c. Ayurveda   d. All

5. Botanical identity of selected medicinal plant refers to: [ ]
   a. Scientific name   b. Common name
   c. Cultivar name   d. All

3. Fill in the Blanks:

1. Expand the term GCP ....

2. Expand the term GHP ....

3. Expand the term GAP ....

4. Expand the term GACP ....

5. Expand the term AYUSH ....

6. Expand the term CITES ....

4. True or False Statements:

1. For cultivation of plants, the sites nearer to grave yards and crematoria should be avoided. [True/False]

2. The stem cuttings chosen for root induction should be of uniform dimension, in terms of length and diameter. [True/False]

3. The seed material free from contamination and diseases should be used for cultivation. [True/False]

4. The introduction of non-indigenous plant species into the cultivation may have a detrimental effect on the biological and ecological balance of the region. [True/False]

5. For commercial cultivars of medicinal plants, the name of the cultivar and the name of the supplier should be necessarily recorded. [True/False]

5. Match the following:

1. Packing labels   [ ]   a. Misidentification
2. Naturopathy and Yoga   [ ]   b. WHO-GACP voucher specimen
3. Contamination of drug   [ ]   c. Non-toxic material
4. First registration   [ ]   d. Protective clothing
5. Agrochemicals   [ ]   e. Alternate system of medicine

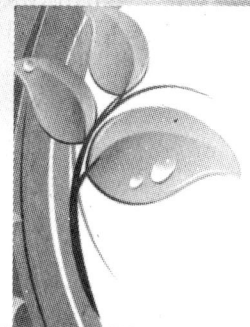

Chapter 6

Systematic Pharmacognostic Study of Carbohydrates and Derived Products

CARBOHYDRATES

The carbohydrates are one of the three main classes of food materials in addition to proteins and fats and one of the most important groups of natural products. These are the primary products of metabolism and are utilised by the plants when required. These help in the production of the secondary metabolites which are deposited in the cells. Carbohydrates are organic compounds which contain carbon, hydrogen and oxygen in the ratio of $1:2:1$ and these are a less efficient source of energy than fats and oils. These are regarded as hydrates of carbon. The final source of carbohydrates in plants is photosynthesis. Widely distributed in plants and animals, they serve as the main source of energy (represented by the sugars) and also store energy (as starch and glycogen). Some carbohydrates give the required support for the plant tissues (as chitin) while some are associated with the shells of crabs and other animals. Other important uses are: they produce alcohol on fermentation; cellulose materials supply various raw materials and are the components of nucleic acids determining the heredity. Thus, carbohydrates find a universal application in medicine, pharmaceuticals and biochemicals.

Carbohydrates are classified into two broad groups namely, sugars and non-sugars.

1. **Sugars (saccharides):** Sugars are sweet and soluble in water and their molecular weights are fixed. These are subdivided into mono-saccharides and oligosaccharides.

   a. **Monosaccharides:** Monosaccharides are the simple carbohydrates with 3 to 9 carbons represented by a general formula $C_nH_{2n}O_n$ and cannot be further hydrolysed into simple sugars and are the building blocks of major carbohydrates like oligosaccharides and polysaccharides. Chemically, a monosaccharide is either an aldehyde or a ketone and a substitution product of a polyhydroxy alcohol. These are grouped according to the number of carbon atoms present in them as trioses (3C such as glyceraldehyde), tetroses (4C which do not occur in a free state like erythroses), pentoses (5C like arabinose, rhamnose, thevetose, xylose and ribose), hexoses (6C like glucose, galactose and fructose) and heptoses (7C such as sedoheptulose) out of which glucose and fructose are the most common hexoses.

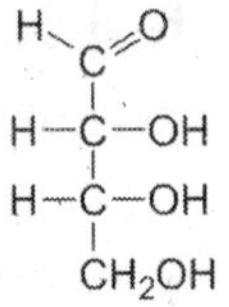

Erythrose (4C)

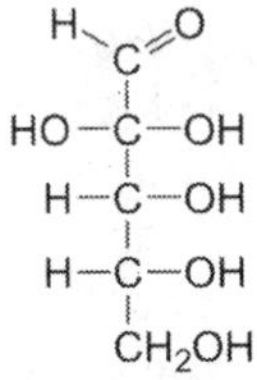

Arabinose (5C)

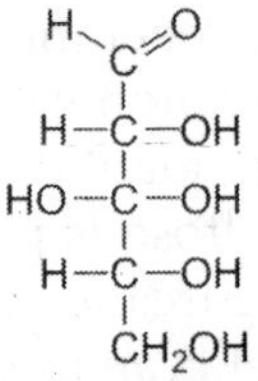

Xylose (5C)

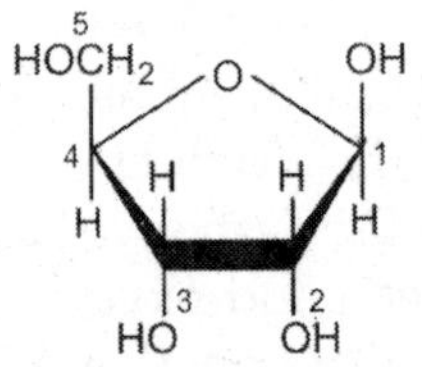

Ribose (5C)

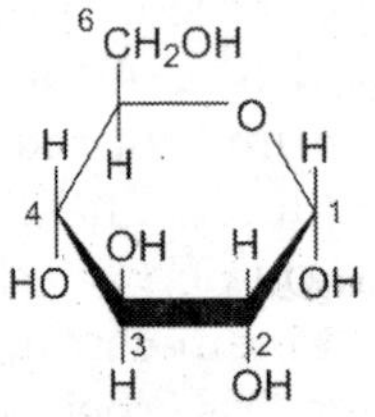

Glucose (6C)

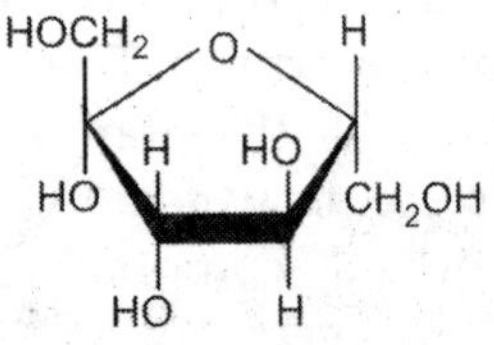

Fructose (6C)

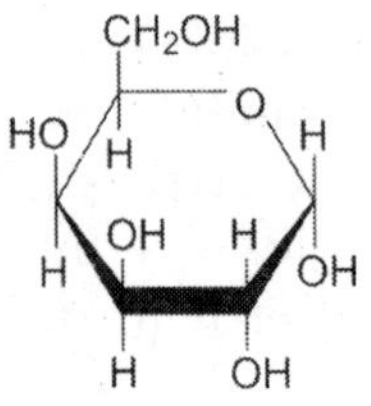

Galactose (6C)

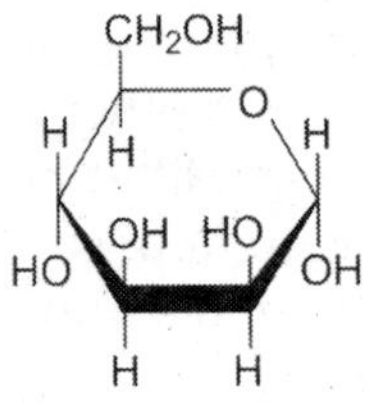

Mannose (6C)

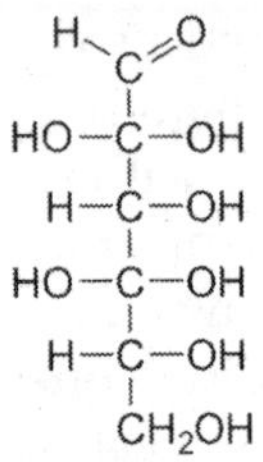

Idose (6C)

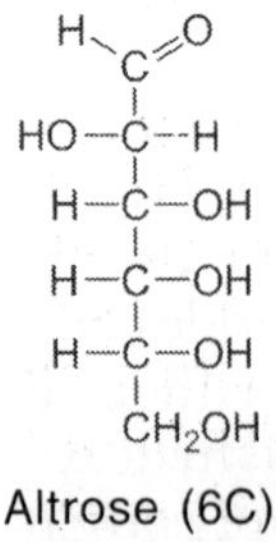

Altrose (6C)

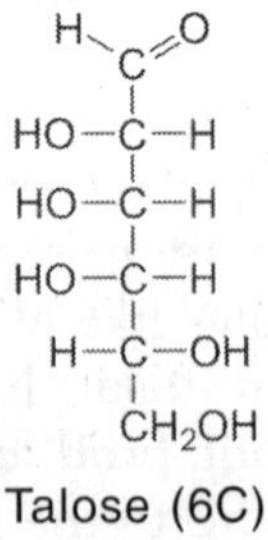

Talose (6C)

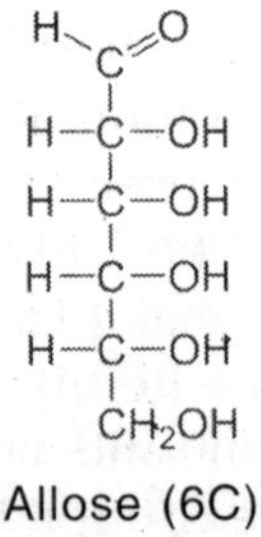

Allose (6C)

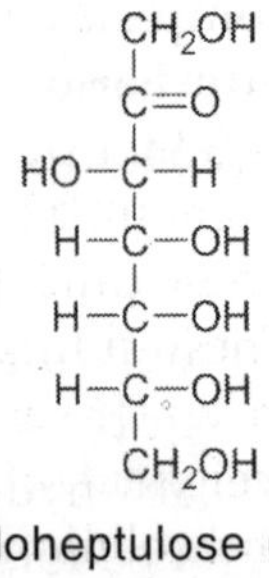

Sedoheptulose (7C)

b. **Oligosaccharides:** Oligosaccharides are composed of two to ten monosaccharide molecules joined together by glycosidic linkages and on hydrolysis yield simple sugars. On the basis of the monosaccharide units present, they are called disaccharides (2) producing 2 monosaccharides of same or different composition on hydrolysis; trisaccharides (3) resulting in the formation of 3 monosaccharides upon hydrolysis and tetrasaccharides (4) generating 4 monosaccharide molecules during hydrolysis. The common examples are sucrose and maltose. Sucrose is the only abundant disaccharide occurring in a free state in the plants while maltose is present in the cell sap. Sucrose occurs in the juices of sugarcane and sugar beet and also the sap of certain plants and yields an invert sugar consisting of glucose and fructose.

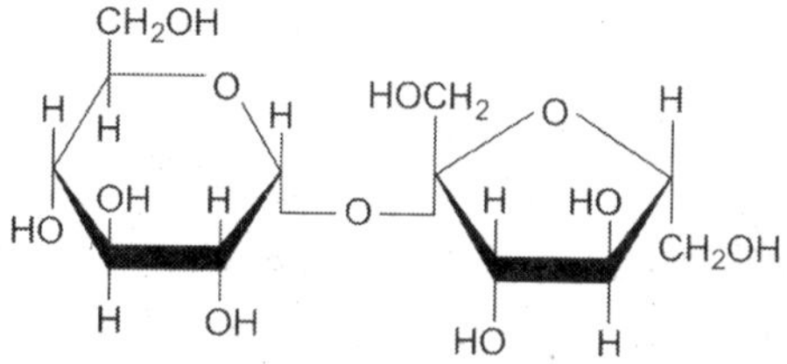

Sucrose

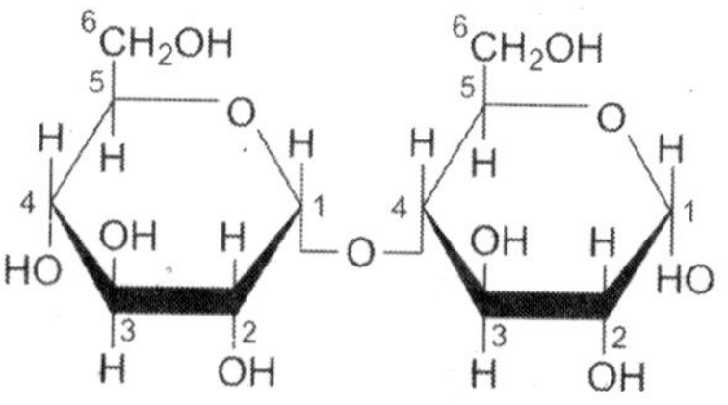

Maltose

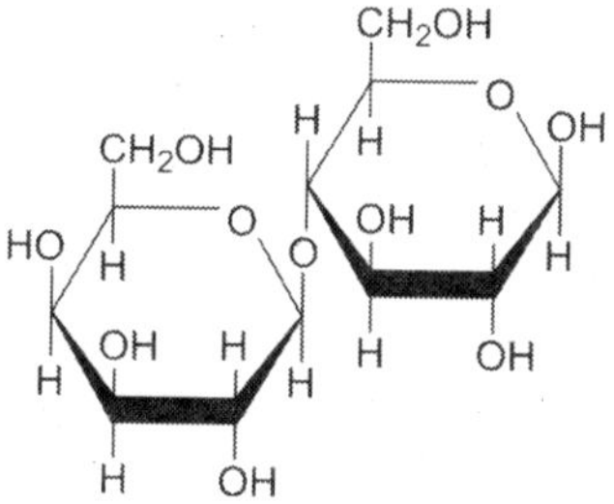

Lactose

2. **Non-sugars (polysaccharides):** Non-sugars or polysaccharides are the complex molecules with a high molecular weight made of a large number of repeating monosaccharide units (more than 10) held together by glycosidic linkages and do not possess the properties of sugars. They are represented by the general formula $(C_nH_{2n-2}O_{n-1})$ n. These can be broken down into their constituent sugars by hydrolysis. These are usually amorphous, solid without a taste and are insoluble in water or form a colloidal suspension, with a higher molecular weight. The two most abundant polysaccharides in plants are starch and cellulose.

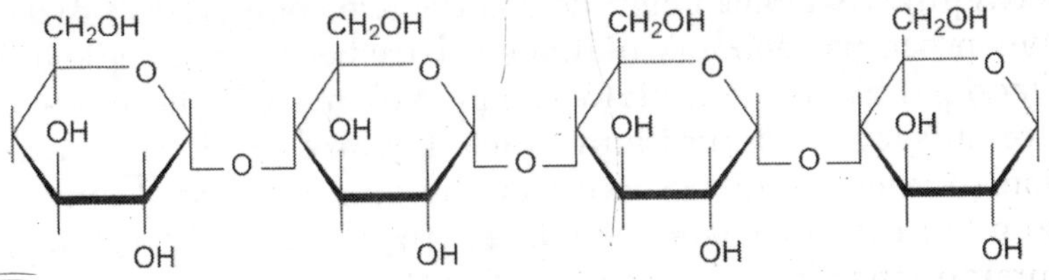

Starch

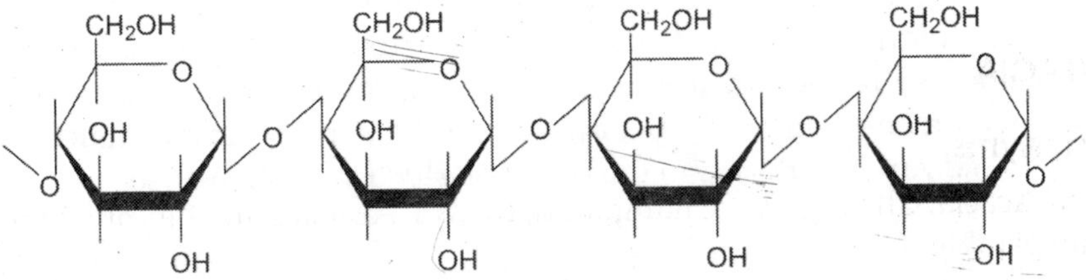

Cellulose

The drugs containing the different categories of carbohydrates are classified as: sugars and sugar containing drugs (sucrose in sugarcane, lactose in cow milk, xylose or wood sugar and honey), drugs with the compounds which are metabolically related to sugars (cherry juice, raspberry juice, citric acid, lactic acid and ethanol), drugs containing the products of reductive metabolism (mannitol and sorbitol), polysaccharides used in coating drugs (starch, inulin, dextran and cellulose) and gums and mucilages (acacia, tragacanth, karaya gum, guar gum and agar).

Carbohydrates make-up the bulk of the dry weight of the plant of which sugars, starches and cellulose predominate. The sugars and starches are digested by humans while cellulose which is insoluble in water cannot be digested but can be easily decomposed by the microbes.

CARBOHYDRATE DERIVATIVES

Hexoses contain the terminal alcoholic groups attached to a pyrane ring and these are easily oxidised. The reaction products are called the uronic acids which occur as constituents of a large number of complex carbohydrates in plants and animals. The aldehyde group on oxidation forms a carboxyl group as a result of which onic acid is produced (gluconic acid) and as a result of reduction of the aldehyde or ketonic group, a corresponding polyalcohol is produced. In some sugars, the terminal alcoholic groups and occasionally, the hydroxyl groups on second carbon are selectively reduced. The hexoses without a hydroxyl group at sixth carbon are referred to as methyl pentoses. In a monosaccharide, when the hydroxyl group gets replaced by a hydrogen atom, the resulting compound is a deoxy sugar and such compounds are the characteristic components of some cardiac glycosides. Variations also occur due to esterification with acids (acetate). Such esters serve as important metabolites and occur in some products of polymerisation such as mucus and nucleic acids. In addition, sugar ethers are the important constituents of some natural drugs. Amino groups also replace the hydroxyl groups of sugars to generate structural variation in some drugs. Acacia gum, gum tragacanth, guar gum, starch, agar, pectin, isabgol and honey are discussed below.

ACACIA

Synonyms

Gum Acacia, Chaar gund, Char goond, Meska, Acacia gum, Egyptian thorn, Gum Arabic, Indian gum, Gum Senegal, Galam gum, Gomme Arabique, Gomme de Senegal, Gomme Mimosae, Gummi Africanum, Khadir, Kher (English), Kumatia, Turkey gum, Meska harra (Moraccan Arabic), Driehaakdoring (Afrikaans), Gummic arabique, Acacia a gomme arabique (French), Gummiarabikumbaum, Senegal-Akazie, Arabisches gummi (German), Arap zamki (Turkish), Khor (Sindhi), Kumta, Kumat (Hindi and Rajasthani), Somali gum, Sudan gum Arabic, Yellow thorn.

Biological Source

Gum Acacia (Gum Arabic) is a natural gum made of hardened sap (dried gum) obtained from the stem and branches of two species of *Acacia, Acacia senegal* Willd. (= *A. verek* Guill. et Perr.) and *Acacia (Vachellia) seyal* belonging to family Mimosaceae or Leguminosae. The taxon, *Senegalia senegal* (L.) Britton is recognised by some authors as the correct name for the gum Arabic tree. However, the name, *Acacia senegal* (L.) Willd. remains widely in use. *A. senegal* is native to semi-desert regions of sub-Saharan Africa as well as Oman, Pakistan and North-Western India. In India, the gum is collected from *Acacia nilotica* (=*Mimosa nilotica*), *Acacia arabica* Willd. and some other species of *Acacia* and though inferior is used as a substitute for the official Gum Acacia. This is sweeter in taste than other varieties. Botanical variations are represented by *Acacia senegal* var. *leiorhachis*, *A. senegal* var.

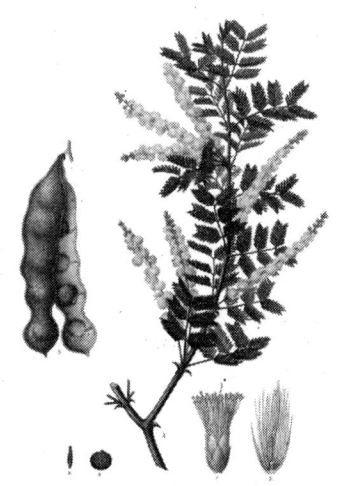

Acacia senegal (L.) Willd.

rostrata and *A. senegal* var. *senegal*. About 500 species of *Acacia* are distributed over tropical and sub-tropical areas of Africa, India, Australia, Central

America and South – West North America but only a few are commercially important.

Geographical Source

The oldest and best known of all the natural gums is gum arabic. The tree *Acacia senegal* grows wild in Sudan, Central and West Africa. Gum acacia originally belongs to Senegal gum, Sudan gum, Kordofan gum or Egyptian gum which is superior and always preferred to any other known gum. The plants are grown in Senegambia in West Africa, the upper Nile region in Eastern Africa and Central Africa. The trees grow wild throughout Sahel from Senegal to Sudan to Somalia. Today the gum is harvested in Mauritania, Senegal, Masli, Burkina Faso, Niger, Nigeria, Chad, Cameroon, Sudan, Eritrea, Somalia, Ethiopia, Kenya and Tanzania. The plant has been historically cultivated in Arabia and West Asia. *Acacia nilotica* (= *Acacia arabica*) (Babul tree) grows wild in India in the states of Punjab, Rajasthan, Andhra Pradesh and Tamil Nadu.

Collection and Preparation

The gum has been harvested in Arabia, Egypt and West Asia since antiquity, and sub-Saharan Africa has a long history as a prized export. The gum flows naturally from the cracks on the bark of the tree under difficult conditions like heat, dryness, wounds and diseases. This flows naturally in the form of a thick and frothy liquid and concretes in the sun into tears. The gum is traditionally harvested by the semi-nomadic desert tribes while on their travels. The hardened exudations are collected in the middle of the rainy season (harvesting begins in July) and exported at the start of the dry season (November). *Acacia senegal* is tapped for the gum by cutting holes or incisions (60 × 5 cm) in the bark from which a product called Senegal gum (*kordofan*) is exuded. Seyal gum from *Acacia seyal* (the species more prevalent in South Africa) is collected from naturally occurring exudations on the bark.

The gum is produced as result of injury to the plant. After the rainy season the bark of the trees is tapped and transverse cuts are made on the stem and branches to expose cambium. As a result of injury, tears of gum are collected on the cambium and newly formed phloem. The gum droplets are about 0.75–3 cm which gradually dry and harden which are manually collected. Within 20–30 days the tears of gum which have formed on the surface may be picked up, made free of bark pieces and foreign organic matter. The material thus collected may be dried in the sun which helps in the removal of moisture. During the process of sun drying numerous cracks appear on the surface of lumps of tears and the gum is bleached. In general, higher the temperature, the higher is the yield. Damaged trees give larger yield of the gum. The yield is improved by natural factors that lessen the vitality of the trees like hot weather, poor soil and lack of moisture. The gum is further processed into the final products. These include 'kibbling' (making the uniform pieces of pebble size), granulating, powdering and spray drying. During kibbling, the large lumps of gum are passed through a hammer mill and it is screened to produce smaller granules of more uniform size. The dissolved gum (in water) is filtered for the removal of contamination, and is sprayed into a stream of hot air to promote the evaporation of water and the powder is screened to assure the uniformity of the size of the particles. The crude gum is stored and exported in jute sacks while the graded gum is packed in heavy duty bags. The semi-processed and processed granules are exported in drums, polyethylene – lined, multi-wall paper bags or cardboard boxes. When stored in cool (21–24°C) in a dry place the gum has an unlimited shelf-life.

Characters

Gum Arabic is colourless (somewhat yellowish), tasteless (bland taste), non-toxic, odourless, acidic (neutral or slightly acidic salt), white powder. It is insoluble in oils and in most organic solvents, but usually dissolves completely in hot or cold water forming a clear, mucilaginous solution. The gum is available in tears, crystals, granules, powder, and spray- and roller-dried powder. It is a multifunctional and a complicated mixture of long and short chains of sugars (arabinogalactan of arabinose and galactose monosaccharides, oligosaccharides and polysaccharides) and glycoproteins of a very high molecular weight. This is a major component of many plant gums including gum arabic. 8–5' non-cyclic diferulic acid has been identified as covalently linked to carbohydrate moieties of the arabionoglactan-protein fraction. The hydrolysis of gum yields L-arabinose, L-rhamnose, D-galactose and D-glucuronic acid. This is very unique among the naturally occurring hydrocolloids because of its high

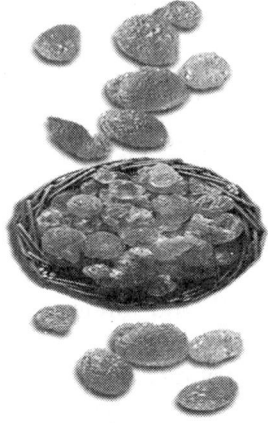

Gum acacia tears

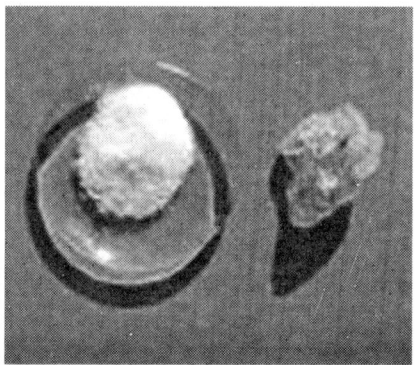

Gum powder and lump

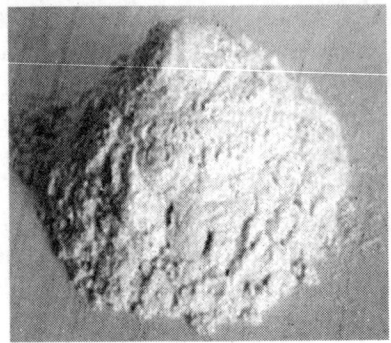

Gum acacia powder

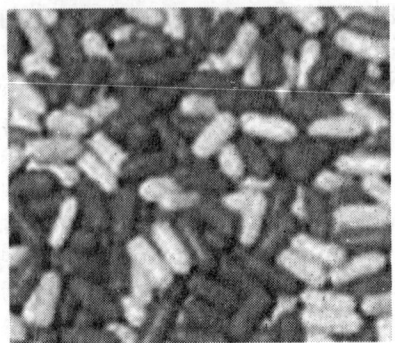

Gum acacia salt

solubility in cold water. It forms sticky glue when mixed with water. It has a low viscosity and adhesive properties. This is insoluble in oils and most organic solvents. It is soluble in aqueous 60% ethanol. With glycerol and ethylene glycol it has a limited solubility.

Chemical Constituents

Gum Arabic is a complex mixture of saccharides and glycoproteins which give it the properties of glue and binder. Acacia gum consists mainly of arabin, the calcium salt of Arabic acid along with varying amounts of magnesium and potassium salts of the same acid in addition to smaller amounts of other salts of these bases. The gum (arabino-galactan-$C_{20}H_{36}O_{14}$) is built upon a backbone of D-galactose units with side chains of D-glucuronic acid with L-rhamnose or L-arabinose ($C_{12}H_{22}O_{11}$) terminal units. The molecular weight is large in the range of 200,000 to 600,000 daltons. It is soluble in water but does not dissolve in alcohol. Arabic acid on hydrolysis gives L-arabinose, L-rhamnose, D-galactose and

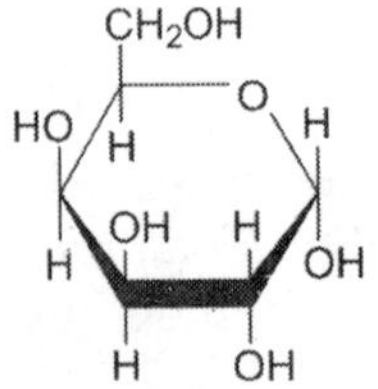

D-galactose ($C_6H_{12}O_6$)

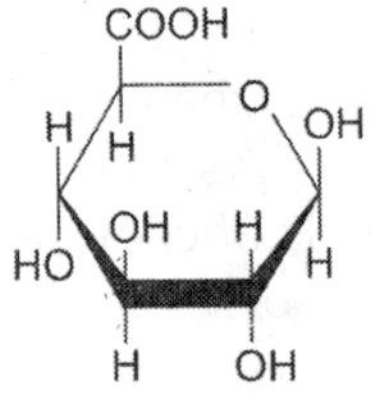

D-lucuronic acid ($C_6H_{12}O_7$)

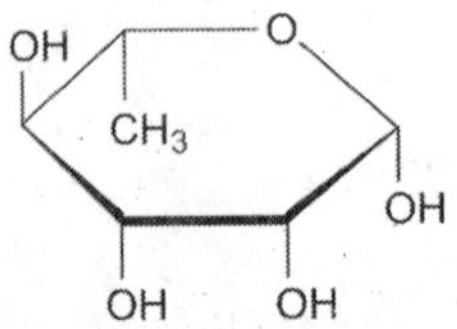

L-rhamnose ($C_6H_{12}O_5$)

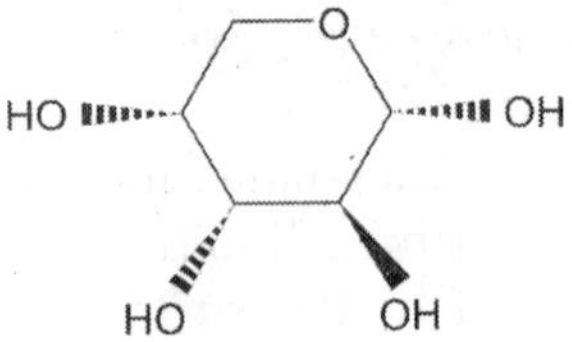

L-arabinose ($C_5H_{10}O_5$)

D-glucuronic acid. Acacia also contains an oxidase enzyme and about 14% (12 to 17%) of water and a trace of sugar. It yields about 2.7–4.0 % of ash entirely of calcium, magnesium and potassium carbonates.

History of Gum Arabic

Gum Arabic was an important article of commerce as early as the 12th century BC. Herodotus in his writings (5th century BC) mentions its use in embalming in Egypt. In the 9th century, the Arab physician, Abu Zayd Hunayn ibn Ishaq al-Ibadi in his 'Ten Treatises on the Eye' described gum arabic as an ingredient in poultices for the eye. In Turkey, the gum was used in the application of gold to manuscripts and they mixed 24-carat gold leaf with melted gum arabic to make gold paste. It was known that the Turkish scribes made lampblack ink with this gum and water. In ancient times, it was used for mummification and inks for hieroglyphics.

Medicinal Uses

Gum Arabic is a demulcent. Its demulcent properties are employed in various cough mixtures, diarrhoea and throat preparations. As it is capable of soothing the irritated mucous membranes, it is used in the preparation of cough drops and lozenges. It is also administered intravenously in haemolysis. In the form of mucilage, it is used as a suspending agent, specifically in mixtures with resinous substance. Gum Arabic is a good emulsifying agent for fixed oils, volatile oils and also for liquid paraffin. It is a good binding agent and is used in the preparation of lozenges, pastilles and compressed tablets. It is a gum of choice, as it is compatible with other plant hydrocolloids, as well as starches and carbohydrates. In combination with gelatin, it is used to form coacervates for microencapsulation of drugs. It is used in intestinal dialysis and cosmetics. Pharmaceutically, it is used in the manufacture of capsules, for coating the pills, in the manufacture of vitamins, mascara and other cosmetics. This is used to treat bleeding, bronchitis, gonorrhea, typhoid fever and infections of the upper respiratory tract because of its astringent properties. Sometimes, this is also used to lower the levels of cholesterol, which is not validated. The gum slows the rate of absorption of some drugs like amoxycillin from the gut.

Non-medical Uses

a. **Culinary and dietary uses:** Gum acacia is highly nutritious and about 6 ounces of the gum supports an adult desert animal like Moor for 24 hours. It is an important ingredient of soft drink syrups, gummy candies, chocolate candies, etc. This has an ability to reduce the surface tension of the liquids leading to increased fizzing and as such it can be used in the production of diet cokes. In the preparation of beverages, it helps oil-based flavours to remain evenly suspended in water. In confectionery, it keeps the oil flavor and a fat uniformly distributed, prevent crystallisation of sugar and thickens chewing gums and jellies. It is used to enhance the shelf-life of flavours in dry packaged products like instant drinks, dessert mixes and soup bases. It is capable of smoothing the creams, fixatives and lotions in cosmetics. It is used in sweeteners and as an additive in foods and beverages, as a thickener in liquids like soft drinks and food flavours. It has a low viscosity and high adhesive properties that make it an excellent ingredient for coating cereals, confectionaries and snack foods. In bakery products, it is used in icings and frostings. In food, the gum is used as a stabiliser. It is edible. The Arab populations use the natural gum to make a chilled, sweetened and flavoured gelato-like dessert. New foliage is used as forage while the dried seeds are consumed by the humans. It is an excellent source of soluble dietary fibre.

b. **Use in artistry, lithography and photography:** It is also used as a permanent binder to fix the pigments onto the surface of the paper by the artists in water colour paints. It is used for gum printing in photography to bind the pigments and to create coloured photographic emulsions which are sensitive to ultraviolet light. Nowadays, it is used in lithography as it helps as an antioxidant coating for photosensitive plates. This has been used since ancient times as part of the black ink. The ancient Egyptian ink was made of carbon soot form the lamps or burnt plant material apart from water and gum arabic. Written on paper or papyrus, this ink has survived for over 3000 years. Because the gum dissolves easily in water, it is used as a binder for water colour printing.

c. **Other uses:** The gum is used as a water-soluble binder in fireworks. It is an important constituent of shoe polish and used in home-made incense cones. It is used as an adhesive on postage stamps and cigarette papers. It can also be used as a flocculating agent in refining the ores, in microencapsulation to produce carbonless copy paper, scratch-and–sniff perfume advertisements, laundry detergents, baking mixes, etc. It also finds it use in sizing and finishing the textiles and for inhibition of metal corrosion. Non-culinary uses include the production of fireworks, paints, inks, glues, ceramic glazes, textiles, cosmetics and more. The roots of the plant nearer to the ground as well as the bark of the tree are used in making strong ropes and cords. The bark of the tree is rich in tannin and is used in tanning and in the production of dyes and inks. Caution is to be taken as very rarely, the gum may cause gas, bloating and loose stools when used as a supplement in addition to some allergic reactions.

Harmful Effects

In particular when used in larger amounts, the gum may cause digestive issues for some people. The potential side effects are: flatulence/gas, bloating, unfavourable viscous sensation in the mouth, early morning nausea, mild diarrhoea and other types of ingestion. To limit these side effects, it is always better to keep the intake well below the maximum daily dose of about 30 grams/day.

Adulteration

The crude gum is often adulterated by adding similar and inferior quality gums which cannot be normally detected. For example, Mesquite gum obtained from *Prosopis juliflora* and artificial gums made from starch or dextrin and in the form of a fine powder, it is adulterated with starch and white dextrin.

TRAGACANTH

Synonyms

Gum Tragacanth (English), Traganth (German), Gomme adragant (French), Tragacantha, Angira (Hindi), Katila (Bengali), Shiraz gum, Gum elect, Gum dragon, Syrian tragacanth, Hog gum, Goat's thorn, Green dragon, Gummi tragacanthae.

Biological Source

It is the dried gummy exudation (sap) obtained by incision from the bark of stems and branches of several species of Middle Eastern legumes of the genus *Astragalus* which include *Astragalus gummifer* Labill. and other Asiatic species like *A. tragacanthus*, *A. kurdicus*, *A. microcephalus*, *A. verus*,

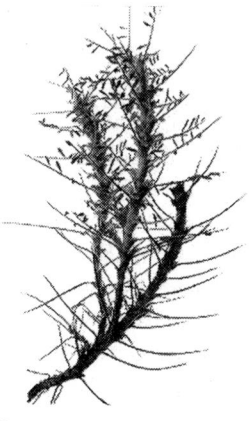

Gum tragacanth plant

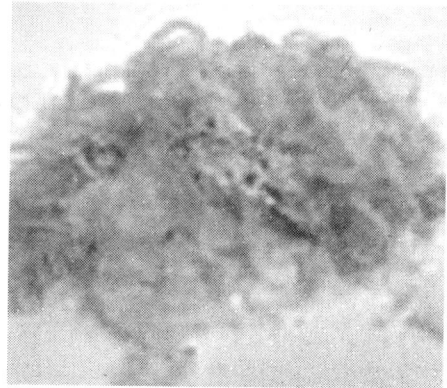

Gum extract

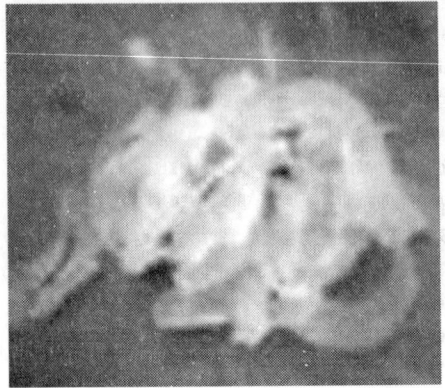

Tragacanth gum

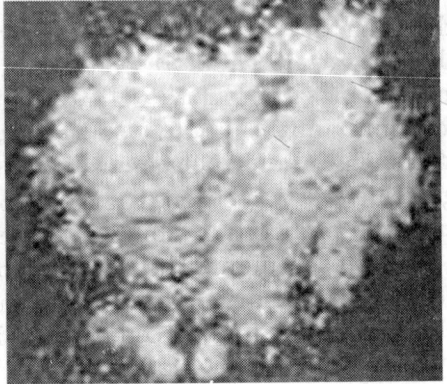

As powder

A. adscendens and *A. strobilifer* (Family: Leguminosae–Fabaceae). The words, *tragos* and *akantha* in Greek mean 'goat' and 'thorn' respectively. Hence, the name 'Goat's thorn' for the plant. Indian tragacanth (Sterculia gum, Karaya gum) is obtained from *Sterculia urens* Roxb. and other species. This was described by Theophrastus several centuries before Christ. The gum has been officially recognised in the U. S. Pharmacopoeia since 1820.

Geographical Source

Tragacanth grows wild in the dry deserts, highlands and mountains of Turkey, Iran, Greece, Iraq, Syria and Russia. In India *Astragalus* species grow in wild state in Kumaon and Garhwal regions of Himalayas. Iran is the biggest producer of the best quality gum. The primary source is the desert highlands of Northern and Western Iran, particularly, the Zagros mountain region.

Collection and Preparation

The plant is a small, low, bushy, perennial shrub having a large tap root which along with the branches is tapped for the gum. The plants require abundance of water during the growing season, but need a dry climate during the time of collection, which extends from April to September (for ribbons) and from August to November (for flakes). The plants are tapped by making careful longitudinal incisions in the tap root and the bark of the branches. When the plant is injured, the gum exudes readily from these cuts in the form of ribbons or flakes. The cell walls of the pith and then the medullary rays are gradually transformed into gum. The gum absorbs water and creates internal pressure within the stem, thus forcing it to the surface through the incision that caused the injury. When the gum strikes the air, it gradually hardens owing to the evaporation of the water and becomes brittle. The nature of the incision governs the shape of the final product. The better grade comes from transverse incisions made with a knife in the main stem and older branches. The gum from such incisions is known as ribbon gum and flake gum, depending on the shape of the solidified exudates. The gum usually shows longitudinal striations caused by small irregularities in the incision. The metamorphosis occurs only at night, and the tragacanth ribbons exhibit transverse striations that show the amount that exudes each night. The whiter and more transluscent ribbons are collected when the drying time is of shorter duration. The collections are first brought to the trading centers and then to wholesale markets where they are sorted by hand, graded, packed and shipped.

Characters

The gum is viscous, odourless and tasteless and is obtained during hot season from the root of the plant and dried. The gum comes out of the plant from natural injuries as white to pale-yellow, flattened, straight, spirally twisted or coiled ribbons or worm-like flakes which can be powdered (white to pale-yellow or pinkish brown). Sometimes, it will be shaped like irregular tears of yellowish or brownish colour. Sometimes, the pieces appear with a red tinge and horny in their structure.

The gum exudate varies in its quality from long, thin, white ribbon to a coarse, yellow-tan ribbon. The powder made from the ribbon is white to light yellow in its colour, odourless, and has an insipid, mucilaginous taste. The flakes vary from yellow tan to brown to give yellowish white to tan powders. This swells rapidly in either cold or hot water to a viscous, colloidal sol or semi-gel which acts as a protective colloid and stabiliser. It is insoluble in alcohol and other organic solvents. The gum can tolerate small amounts of alcohol of glycols. The gum solutions are acidic in the pH range of 5–6. It is fairly stable over a wide range of pH down to extremely acidic conditions of about pH 2.0.

The viscosity is the most important factor in the evaluation of the gum and is regarded as a measure of its quality as well as its behaviour (as a suspending agent, stabiliser or emulsifier). The viscosity of 1% solution may range from about 100–3500 centipose depending on the grade. The viscosity reaches a maximum in 24 hours at 25°C, 8 hours at 40°C, and 2 hours at 50°C. The maximum initial viscosity is at pH 8.0, but maximum stable viscosity is about pH 5.0. The viscosity of the gum solution is quite stable over a wide pH range.

Chemical Constituents

It is a water-soluble carbohydrate gum with a molecular weight of approximately 840,000, which contains the polysaccharides tragacanthin (30–40% water-soluble) and bassorin (60–70% water-insoluble). Tragacanth contains bassorin, a complex mixture of high molecular weight polysaccharides (polymethoxylated acids, galactoarabans) which upon hydrolysis yield D-galacturonic acid, D-galactose, geddic acid ($C_{34}H_{68}O_2$), L-arabinose, D-xylose and L-fucose, in addition to small amounts of rhamnose and glucose as well as traces of starch and/or cellulose. Mannose and glucuronic acid are absent. The gum is soluble in water and swells up to form smooth, stiff, opalescent mucilage. In solution, it is acidic with a pH of 5.0–6.0, and its maximum viscosity is at pH 8.0 but maximum stable viscosity was found to be near pH 5.0 and stability decreases below 4.0 or above 6.0. The portion soluble in water is chiefly polyarabinan-trigalaetangeddic acid while the insoluble part is bassorin. Bassorin on hydrolysis yields tragacanthose, xylose and bassoric acid. It is insoluble in ethanol and does not swell in aqueous ethanol. Bassorin has an elongated molecular shape and forms a viscous solution. The gum also contains water, traces of starch, cellulose and nitrogenous substances yielding about 3% ash. Tragacanthin, which is probably demethoxylated bassorin, composes about 30% of the gum and is the more water-soluble component. The aqueous suspension on microscopic examination shows many angular fragments with either circular or irregular lamellae along with starch grains and stratified cellular membranes.

L-Arap-, →2)β-L-Araf-, α-L-Araf-, →2)-α-L-Araf-, →3)-α-L-Araf-, →4)-α-D-Galp-, →6)-α-D-Galp-, α-L-Araf-(1→2)-α-L-Araf-(1→4)-L-Ara, α-L-Araf-(1→2)-α-L-Araf-(1→5)-L-Ara, β-D-Galp-(1→4)-[β-D-Galp-(1→4)]₂-D-Gal, β-D-Galp-(1→4)-β-D-Galp-(1→4)-D-Gal, β-D-Glcp-(1→4)-[β-D-Galp-(1→4)]₂-D-Galp, α-D-Glcp-(1→4)-[α-D-Glcp-(1→4)]₀.₃-D-Glc.

(The gum contains free α-Araf-(1→2)-α-Araf-(1→4)-Arap and α-Araf-(1→2)-α-Araf-(1→5)-Araf, which correspond to side-chain structures with α-Araf and Arap in the arabinogalactan. β-Galp-(1→4)-[β-Galp-(1→4)]₂-Galp, β-Galp-(1→4)-β-Galp-(1→4)-Galp, β-Glcp-(1→4)-[β-Galp-(1→4)]₂-Galp probably correspond to tragacanthic acid, and α-Glcp-(1→4)-[α-Glcp-(1→4)]₀₋₃-Glc to starch).

Graphical structure of Gum tragacanth

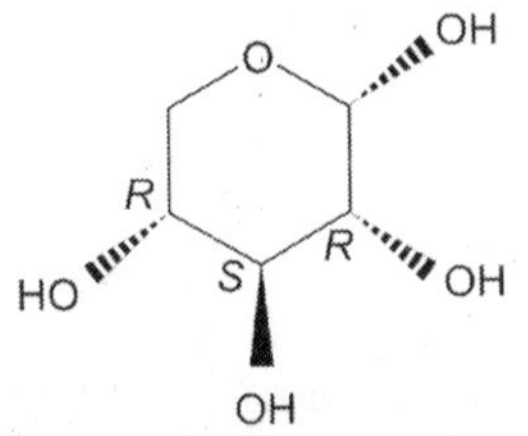

D-xylose ($C_5H_{10}O_5$)

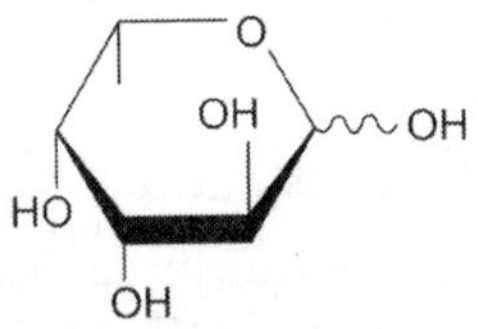

L-fucose ($C_6H_{12}O_5$)

CH₂OH

HO

OH H

H OH

H OH

D-galactose
(C₆H₁₂O₆)

CH₂OH

OH

OH

OH

OH

D-galacturonic
acid (C₆H₁₀O₇)

HO

HO OH

L-arabinose
(C₅H₁₀O₅)

History of Tragacanth

Gum tragacanth is one of the oldest drugs known and has been in commercial use for well over 2000 years, widely used in pharmacy and industry down through the ages. It was described by Theophrastus three centuries before Christian era. Dioscorides and Arabian writers gave it due attention. In ancient times, it has been used as an emulsifier, thickening agent and also a suspending agent. It was officially recognised in the US Pharmacopoeia since 1820. In folk medicine, it has been used as a laxative, and for the treatment of persistent cough, diarrhoea, and as an aphrodisiac. It has been used for centuries in Chinese herbal medicine to overcome fatigue, to lower the blood pressure, to treat colds, nephritis and hypoglycaemia. It would be difficult to locate the first use of tragacanth as the first use of wheat. It came into Smyrna form the interior of Asia Minor, and from Persia and Armenia.

Medicinal Uses

The uses of Tragacanth are dependent on its high viscosity at low concentration, suspending action, stability to heat and acidity, effective emulsifying properties, and an extremely longer shelf-life. Gum Tragacanth is used extensively in pharmaceutical products because of its thickening power and stabilising action in suspended matter. It has no known therapeutic action and is solely used as an excipient for tablets, as a component of medicinal jellies and as laxative and in making emulsions. It is used in the preparation of lozenges and styptic powder. It is very useful in cases of irritation of the mucous membranes of the pulmonary and genitourinary organs. It is also used as a vehicle for active medicines. Gum is having demulcent, emollient and spermicidal properties. It is used to treat coughs and diarrhoea. It is also employed in spermicidal jellies and creams, which immobilise spermatozoa on contact. It is reported that tragacanth gum exerts a strong inhibitory action on cancer cells. The alkaloid within it is used as a remedy for cough and diarrhoea. As a paste it is used as a topical treatment for burns. The mucilage of Tragacanth has been used as an application to burns. The gum is used in the cod liver oil emulsions to facilitate the absorption of poorly soluble substances like steroid glycosides and fat-soluble vitamins. It is also used in low-calorie elixirs and syrups. It also acts as a suspending agent in toothpastes to form a creamy, brilliant product. The longer shelf-life and film-forming properties make it useful in hair lotions, hand lotions and vaginal creams as well as denture adhesives. In folk medicine, it is used as an aphrodisiac.

Non-medical Uses

The gum is used in veg-tanning of the leather and also as a stiffener in textiles. It has been used in textile print paste and sizes for high quality silks and crepes. It has good release properties and gives added body to the fabrics. It is used in dressing leather and in the preparation of leather polishes. It is also used in furniture, floor and auto polishes. It has been used as an adhesive for reconstituted cigar wrapper leaves. It is also used in the artist's pastels as a binder and does not adhere as other gums. It can be used as a paste in floral handicraft to produce life-like flowers on wires used in decoration. It also finds its use in the preparation of incense sticks. This has many industrial uses namely, cloth finishing, calico printing and water proofing of the fabrics.

It is used as an emulsifier, thickener and a stabiliser in pourable dressings of the regular and low calorie types. It is used in relish sauces, condiment bases, sweet pickles, liquors, and mayonnaise. It also finds its use in everyday commercial products like cosmetics and toothpastes to jellies and salad dressings. It is also used in syrups, candies and ice creams. It is useful in the preparation of processed cheese, cream cheese, cottage cheese, etc. Caution is to be taken as at times it may cause allergic reactions.

Side Effects

The excessive intake of gum may cause constipation, diarrhoea, abdominal pain, gas, hay fever, and skin rash. It may also produce allergic symptoms like asthma or contact dermatitis. The gum may also block the intestines if one do not drink a plenty of water with it. It may also cause breathing problems.

Adulteration

The important adulterants of tragacanth gum are the Indian gum (karaya or kadaya), a product of *Coplospermum gossypium*, gum kuteera from *Sterculia urens*, powdered acacia, dextrin, and wheat and corn starch.

AGAR

Synonyms

Agar-Agar (English, Malay and Cingalese), Red sea weed, China grass, Japanese Isinglass, Vegetable (Vegan) gelatin, Ceylon mass or Jaffna moss,

Japanese or Chinese gelatin, (English), Mousse-de-Chine (French), Thav (German), Thao (Japanese), Yang-tsai or Haizaoqiongzhi or Dongfen (Chinese), Chinai ghas (Hindi-Bombay), Darya ki gas (Dukkhini), Samudrapu pachi (Telugu), China grass, Kanten (Japanese), Ceylon agar (agal-agal), Haicai (Mandarin Chinese), Chhai-ian (Taiwanese Hokkien), Hancheon (Korean), Gulaman (Tagalog of Philippines), Apayao (Bikol and Pangasinan of Philippines), Guraman (Ilokano of Philippines) or Gurguraman (Sambali of Philippines), Woon (Thai), Paal kasuv (Tamil and Telugu).

Biological Source

The word, 'agar' comes from the Malay word, *'agar-agar'* meaning 'jelly'. In Japanese, it is called *kanten* meaning 'cold weather' as it is harvested during winter. It is called in Mandarin Chinese as *haicai* meaning 'ocean vegetable' and in Taiwanese Hokkien it is referred to as *chhai-ian* meaning 'vegetable swiftlet'. Agar-agar is the dried hydrophilic colloidal concentrate (gelatin) obtained from a decoction of various red algae (sea weeds) of the

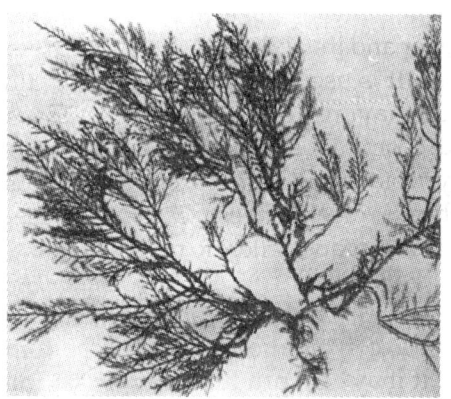

Gelidium amansii

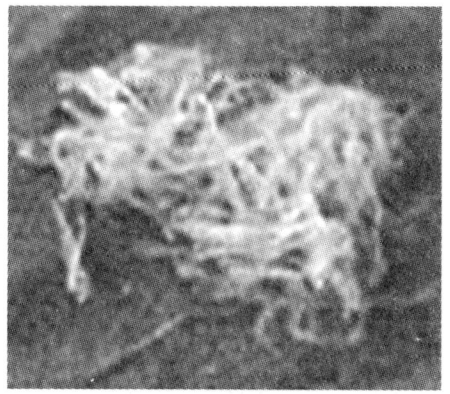

Extracted agar

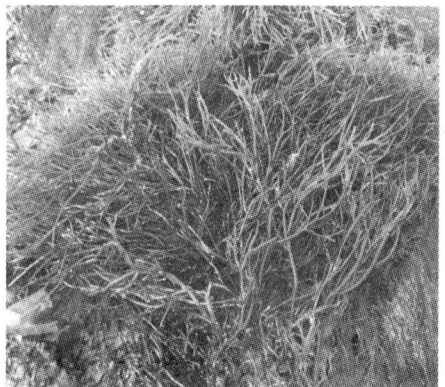

Gracilaria species

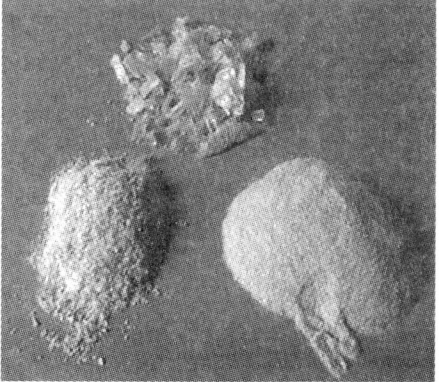

Agar flakes and powder

back waters of Ceylon and the Indian Ocean region, primarily from the genera *Gelidium* and *Gracilaria*. *Gelidium amansii* is the chief source in addition to *G. cartilagineum* (= *G.corneum* Lam.), *G. conferoides*, *Pterocladia lucida*, *P. capillacea* (Family: Gelidaceae) and several other species of *Gracilaria* like *G. lichenioides* (L.) Harv.

Geographical Source

Historically and also in the modern context, it is a chief ingredient in desserts in Japan. Agar is obtained from Japan, Korea, South Africa, both Atlantic and Pacific coasts of USA, Chile, Spain and Portugal.

Collection and Preparation

The production of agar by modern techniques of industrial freezing was initiated in California by Matsuoka who registered his patents (1921 and 1922 in the USA). The present modern manufacturing method by freezing is the classic method and derives from H. H. Selby and C. K. Tseng (1954, 1946) on the basis of the American method developed in California during the years prior to World War II.

Gracilaria is mainly cultivated by three main methods:

1. *Open cultivation in estuaries and bays* (as the sandy soils are required to place the algae to take roots and develop into new plants).

2. *On ropes or nets* (the algae are attached to thrive under water or placed into the bottom of the sea with poles of bamboos).

3. *On ponds or pools* (an artificial pond is created to grow the algae in it).

Algae are largely cultivated in special areas, poles being planted in the sea to form supports on which they develop.

The production of agar-agar from algae is as follows:

1. *Drying of algae:* After collection, the algae are dried in the sun.

2. *Alkalinisation:* After drying, the algae are placed in a container with very hot water in which an alkali (like caustic soda) has been poured.

3. *Washing and bleaching:* The algae are washed with cold water to remove all the impurities. Then, sulphuric acid is added to dealkalinise the algae and sodium hypochlorite for bleaching it. Finally, the algae are cleaned with cold water.

4. *Extraction by cooking:* The product is extracted by subjecting the washed and bleached algae to cooking for about 2 hours.

5. *Filtering:* This separates the product from other waste material like rocks, shells, dirt, etc. Filtering is accomplished by passing water with algae through different filtering tanks.

6. *Gelling:* This process is intended to bring the product to the texture of the gel. The algae are cooled by different processes from 80 to 25°C.

7. *Pressing and drying:* After gelling, the product is compacted by a press and dried with hot air.

8. *Grinding, sieving and packaging:* Finally algae are ground and sieved before they are packed.

The first step is preservation through dehydration, to avoid fermentation which destroys the agar and then the seaweed. The second step is pressing the weed with a hydraulic press in bales (about 60 kg) to reduce the volume. The time for collection of the algae is summer and autumn when the bleaching and drying can take place, but the final preparation of agar-agar is carried out in winter from November to February. The seaweed after collection is spread out on the shore until bleached, and then dried; it is afterwards boiled in water and the mucilaginous solution strained, the filtrate being allowed to harden, and then it is dried in the sun. During the months of May to October these poles are taken ashore and the algae is scrapped off. The algae thus obtained is dried and shaken to remove sand and shells. The dried seaweeds are washed with water to remove salt and dried again by exposing to sun (to reduce the moisture content to about 20%) which also helps in bleaching. They are then boiled with acidified water for 5–6 hours and the mucilaginous decoction is strained through cloth while still hot. On cooling, a jelly is produced, which is cut into bars, these being afterwards forced through wire netting to form strips. The moisture is removed by freezing and drying at about 35°C. The Japanese variety is derived from several kinds of algae and comes into European commerce in two forms: (1) In transparent pieces 2 feet long, the thickness of a straw, prepared in Singapore by treating it in hot water. (2) In yellowish white masses about 1 inch wide and 1 foot long. The latter is the form considered the more suitable for the culture of bacteria.

Characters

Agar is found in the form of strips, flakes or coarse powder which may be white or pale yellow in colour. Agar is tough when damp but brittle when dry having a mucilaginous taste. Agar is insoluble in cold water but when one part of it is boiled for 10 minutes with 65 times its weight of water it forms a clear solution which on cooling yields a firm jelly. The powder is soluble in boiling water. Agar exhibits hysteresis, melting at 85°C (358 K, 185°F) and solidifying from 32–40°C (305–313 K, 90–104°F), and this property lends a suitable balance between easy melting and good gel stability at relatively high temperatures. As many scientific applications require incubation at temperatures close to that of the human body (37°C) and this is more appropriate than other solidifying agents that melt at this temperature (like gelatin).

Chemical Constituents

The gel is an unbranched polysaccharide from the cell walls of red algae. Chemically, this is a polymer of the sugar galactose. The polysaccharides are the primary structural support for the algal cell walls. Agar (gelatin) contains gelose, a gelatinous principle without nitrogen, mannite, starch and albumen. It consists of two different polysaccharides named as agarose and agaropectin. Primarily agar is the calcium salt of a sulphuric acid ester of the complex polysaccharide agarose-agaropectin. Agarose is a neutral galactose linear polymer (made up of D-galactose and a 3,6-anhydro-L-galactopyranose) of molecular weight about 120,000 free from sulphate and is primarily responsible for the gel strength of agar. Agaropectin is a heterogeneous mixture of smaller molecules (that occur in smaller amounts) and a sulphonated polysaccharide having galactose and uronic acid units partly esterified with sulphuric acid. Agaropectin is responsible for the viscosity of agar solution. Acids (acetic acid, hydrochloric acid and oxalic acid) prevent gelatinisation of agar.

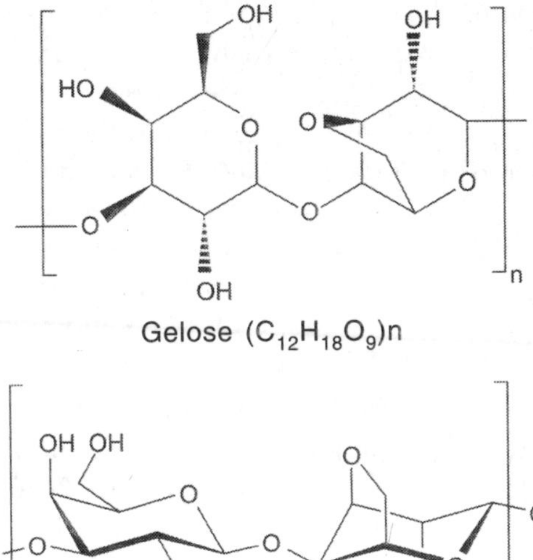

Gelose $(C_{12}H_{18}O_9)n$

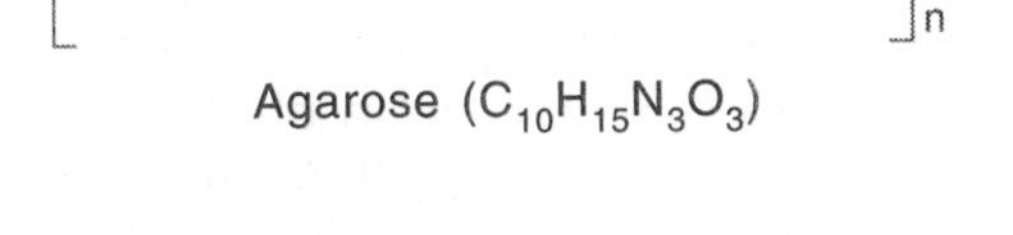

Agarose $(C_{10}H_{15}N_3O_3)$

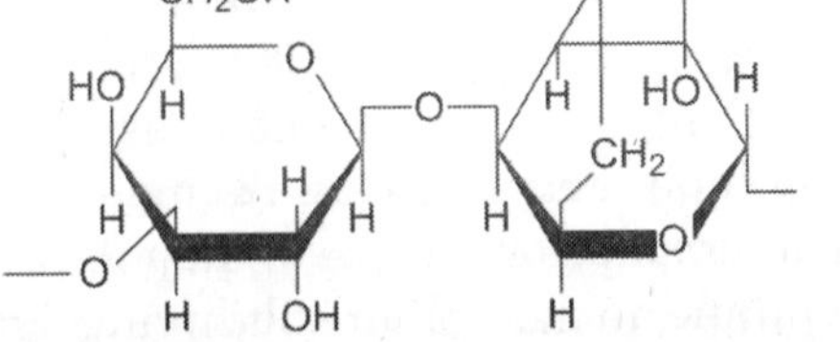

Agarobiose-repeating unit of disaccharide in agar

History of Agar

Agar was the first phyco-colloid to be discovered and prepared as a purified extract and was considered to have been discovered in Japan presumably in 1658 by Mino Tarozaemon and a monument *Shimizu-mura* commemorates its manufacture for the first time. The product was then known as *tokoroten* literally meaning 'frozen sky'. The industrialisation of agar started at the beginning of the 18th century and it has been called *kanten* literally meaning the 'cold weather'. There is a Japanese legend related to the first preparation of agar which runs as: *'A Japanese Emperor and his Royal party were lost in the mountains in the winter of 1658 during a snow storm. When they arrived at a small inn, the inn keeper, Mino Tarozaemon received them ceremoniously and offered them a traditional dish made of the seaweed as dinner, prepared by cooking the species of Gelidium with water. After the dinner, the inn keeper threw away the surplus jelly outdoor—understandably, in the absence of refrigerators back then. The jelly was frozen during the night followed by thawing and draining in the sun to finally leave a cracked substance of a low density after some days. The inn keeper upon finding this soft paper-like substance collected the residue and boiled this in water. To his surprise he found that the jelly could be remade'.* From this was developed 'kantan' which is our modern day agar-agar. Thus, the method of agar manufacture was accidentally discovered. The production of agar by the technique of industrial freezing was initiated in California in 1921 by Matsuoka. The present method of manufacture of agar by freezing is a classic one that was developed in California by H. H. Selby and C. K. Tseng prior to World War II. The shortage of agar during World War II acted as an incentive for its preparation from the coastal resources of the species of *Gelidium*. Payen (1859) described and referred to it as gelose. Robert Koch (1882) was the first to utilise agar in microbiology during his attempts to obtain axenic cultures of *Mycobacterium tuberculosis*. It was Walter Hesse, a country doctor from Saxony who introduced Koch to the powerful gelling agent when he first succeeded in using the agar as the culture medium in cultivating gelatin, which has become a universal component of the solid culture media for the cultivation of the microbes later. The doctor had learnt about agar from his wife, Fanny Hesse, nee Eilshemius. Robert Koch developed the use of agar as a medium for bacterial cultures on the advice of Angelina Fannie, his assistant, who noticed that the jellies and puddings did not melt in the hot summer weather when they contained agar.

Medicinal Uses

Agar is a nutrient and a demulcent and the nutritional properties are due to gelose. The jelly formed with water is a good diet. Agar is used as an emulsifying agent and in the treatment of chronic constipation. It is also used as bulk laxative. The jelly mixed with a little sugar and wine flavoured with a lemon peel and cinnamon leaf is used as a restorative to the invalids. The decoction made of it is an emollient and demulcent and is given in pectoral infections, dysentery and diarrhoea. The jelly is a medicine in leukorrhoea, profuse menstrual flow and irritation of the urinary passages. As it contains iodine, it is also useful in goitre and scrofula. As it is about 80% fibre, it serves as an intestinal regulator which has shown promising results in obesity. In dentistry, agar is used as an impression material.

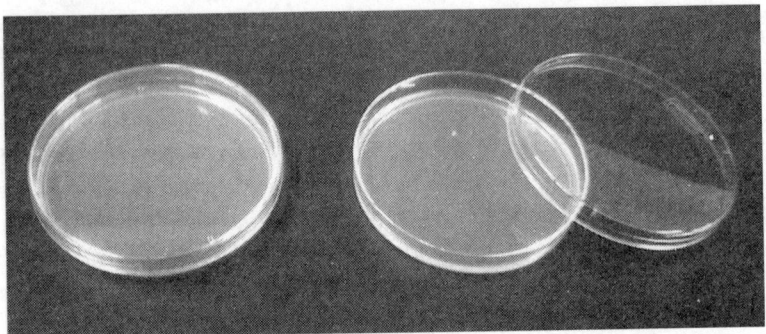

Petri dishes with agar as the culture medium

Non-medical Uses

It is used in the preparation of jellies and confectionary items. It is also a very good culture medium for the cultivation of microbes (bacteria and fungi) for bacteriological investigation. It is used as a solidifying agent in desserts, soups, sauces, etc. In the past century, this has found extensive use as a solid substrate in the culture media for microbiological work. As a vegetarian gelatin substitute it is used as a thickener in soups, jellies, ice creams, Japanese desserts like *anmitsu*, as a clarifying agent in brewing and for paper sizing fabrics. In the form of a gel, agarose medium is porous and can be used to measure microbe motility and mobility. Agarose can also be used for electrophoretic separation in agarose gel electrophoresis and column-based gel filtration chromatography. Research grade agar is used extensively in plant biology for seedling germination in Petri dishes under sterile conditions supplemented with a nutrient and vitamin mixture. Agar is eaten in Japan as a natural gelatin counterpart. It can also be used to make jellies, puddings, desserts, cakes and custards. Japanese cuisine, *anmitsu*, Indian cuisine, *China grass*, Burmese cuisine, *kyauk* and a popular Japanese food, *mizuyokan*, are all made from agar. It is used to prepare salt bridges used in electrochemistry. As a substitute for sand and a soy rice of nutrition, agar is used in the preparation of formicariums. In humans, agar promotes fecal bulk and influences the absorption of the dietary minerals, proteins and fat. In animals, agar decreases the protein digestion and reduces the retention of nitrogen. Agar sometimes is used as an adulterant in jams and jellies. It is used in canning meat, fish and poultry, as a clarifying agent in brewing industry and wine making. It can also be used as a preservative in foods, as a thickener in confectioneries, dairy products, meat products, etc.

Other Uses

Agar is used as an impression material in dentistry; as a medium to orient the tissue specimen and secure it by agar pre-embedding (useful in small endoscopy biopsy specimens) for histopathology processing. It is also used to make salt bridges and gel plugs in electrochemistry; and as a transparent substitute for sand in formicariums and a source of nutrition. It is used as a natural ingredient to form the modeling clay for children to play with; as an allowed biofertiliser in organic farming; and as a substrate to precipitin reactions in immunology. Gelidium agar is used for bacteriological plates, while, Gracilaria agar is used in food applications.

Side Effects

Agar is safe for adults when taken by mouth with at least one 8-ounce glass of water. Without enough water, it can swell and block oesophagus or bowel. Immediate medical attention is necessary if chest pain, vomiting or difficulty in swallowing or breathing occurs after taking it. Agar may also raise cholesterol in some people.

STARCH

Synonyms

The word 'Starch' is derived from Middle English, 'Sterchen' meaning 'to Stiffen'. In Latin, it is 'Amylum' and in Greek, it is 'Amulon' meaning not ground at a mill. In biochemistry, the root 'Amyl' is used for several starch related compounds. The word 'Starch' may come from the Old English 'Stearc' ('Stark, strong rough') which in turn might have a Germanic origin, 'Starchi' meaning 'Strong'. Amylum (= Corn starch, rice starch, wheat starch, potato starch).

Starch is a white, granular, organic chemical that is produced by all green plants. Pure starch is a soft, white, tasteless and odourless powder that is insoluble in cold water or alcohol or other solvents. The basic chemical formula of the starch molecule is $(C_6H_{10}O_5)_n$ where 'n' denotes the number of molecules linked together. Starch is a polysaccharide comprising glucose monomers joined in α-1,4 linkages (glycosidic bonds). The simplest form of starch is the linear polymer amylase; and amylopectin is the branched form. Starch is manufactured in the green leaves of plants from the excess glucose produced during photosynthesis and serves the plant as a reserve food supply. This is stored in the chloroplasts in the form of granules and in such organs as the roots of the tapioca plant; the tuber of potato; the stem pith of sago; and the seeds of corn, wheat, maize, and rice. When required, this is broken down, in the presence of certain enzymes and water, into its constituent monomer glucose units, which diffuse from the cell to nourish the plant tissues. In humans and other animals, the starch is broken down into its constituent sugar molecules which then supply the energy to the tissues.

Biological Source

Starch is a polysaccharide consisting of a large number of glucose units joined together by glycosidic bonds. This is produced by all green plants as an energy store. This is the most important carbohydrate in human diet and is present in staple foods such as rice, wheat, maize, potato and cassava, etc. The glucose is mainly stored in the form of starch granules in chloroplasts (amyloplasts). At the end of the growing season it accumulates in the twigs near the buds, fruits, seeds, rhizomes and tubers to be used in the next growing season. Starch of pharmaceutical use comprises mostly of polysaccharide granules usually separated from the grains of maize or corn (*Zea mays* L.), rice (*Oryza sativa* L.) and wheat (*Triticum aestivum* L.) belonging to Family Poaceae or Gramineae and also from the tubers of potato (*Solanum tuberosum* L.) of Family Solanaceae. Other sources of starch used as food include arrowroot, buckwheat, barley, oat, millet, rye, banana, canna, colacasia, sago, sorghum, sweet potato, yam, edible beans like mung bean and peas.

Synonyms for Maize

Maize, Indian corn (English), Yavanala (Sanskrit), Makka (Hindi), Bhuththe (Bengali), Pysungboo (Burmese), Makaibonda (Maharashtrian), Mukka-cholam (Tamil), Mokka jonna (Telugu), Jagung (Malayalam), Bottah (Kannada), Munwairingu (Sinhalese).

Synonyms for Rice

Rice (English), Vrihi or Thandula (Sanskrit), Chaval (Hindi and Punjabi), Chaul or Dhan (Bengali), Thomul (Kashmiri), Chokha (Gujarathi), Tandul or Bhat (Maharashtrian), Arruz (Arabic), Biranj (Persian), Vari or Vadlu or Biyyam (Telugu), Arshi or Nelli (Tamil), Akki or Bhatta (Kannada), Ari (Malayalam), Hal (Sinhalese), Chan (Burmese).

Synonyms for Wheat

Wheat (English), Yava or Godhuma (Sanskrit), Hintah (Arabic), Ghehun (Hindi), Gam (Bengali), Gahun (Maharashtrian), Godhumalu (Telugu), Godumei (Tamil), Godi (Kannada), Gavu (Konkani).

Synonyms for Potato

Potato (English), Alu (Hindi), Golalu (Bengali) Pomme de terre (French), Kartappe (German), Batata (Kannada and Maharashtrian), Papeta (Gujarathi), Urla-kalanger (Tamil), Urla-gadda (Telugu).

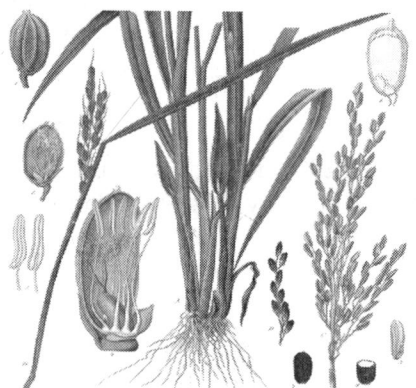

Rice: *Oryza sativa*

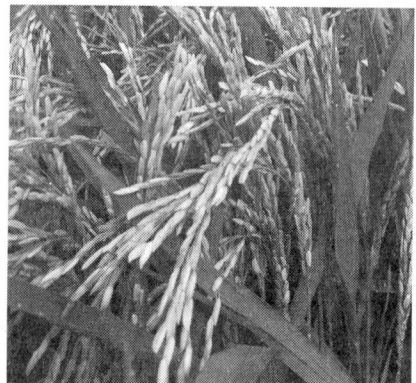

Plant with panicles

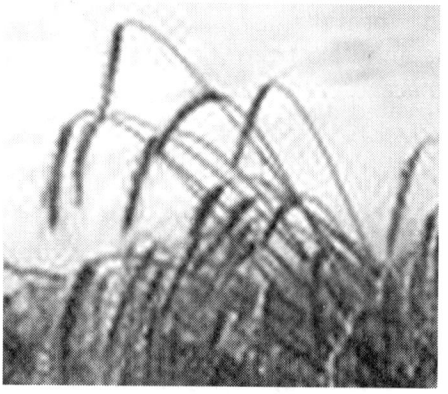

Wheat: *Triticum aestivum*

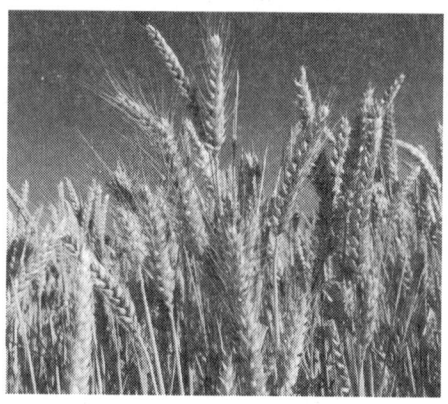

At the time of harvest

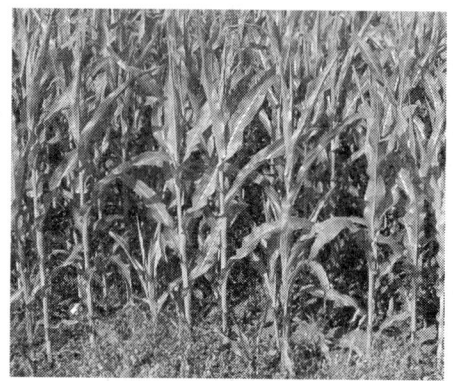

Maize: *Zea mays*

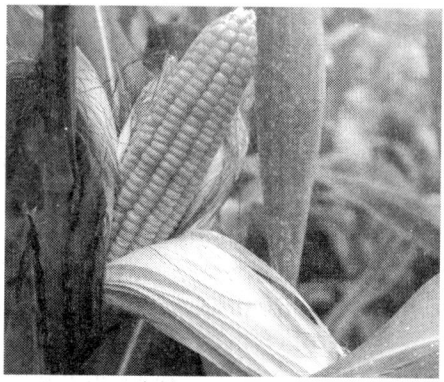

Mature cob

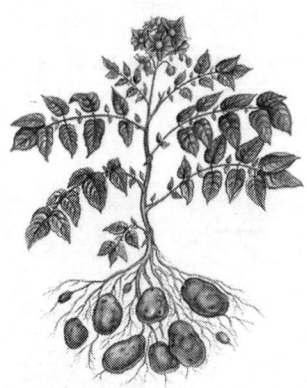

Solanum tuberosum

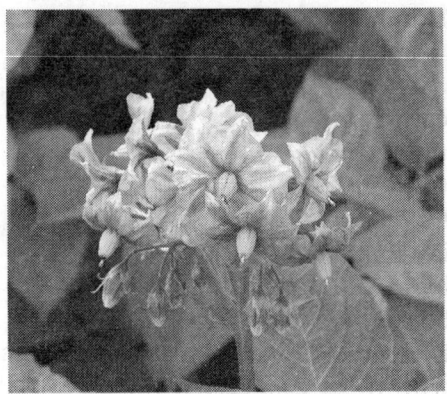

Potato: Flower

Geographical Source

Starch is commercially produced in tropical and subtropical countries. USA, Canada, Australia, China, India, Russia, Thailand, Vietnam, Pakistan are the major producers of starch in the world. Rice is produced in India, China, Japan and other countries. Wheat is cultivated in many temperate countries of the world. Maize is produced in USA, Argentina, India and other tropical and subtropical countries. Potato is cultivated in many countries.

Collection and Preparation

In general, the cereal grains (corn, rice and wheat) mostly comprise of starch bundles, oil, soluble protein, and the insoluble protein termed 'gluten' while potato contains starch, mineral salts (inorganic), soluble proteins and vegetable tissues. The various specific methods are normally employed to separate the starch either from the grains of cereals or from potato.

The method of preparation of starch depends upon the nature of the raw material used and the purity of starch desired. Cereal starches have to be freed from cell debris, oil, soluble protein matter and the abundant insoluble proteins (glutelins and prolamins) known as 'gluten'. Potato starch, on the other hand, is associated with vegetable tissue, mineral salts and soluble proteins.

Collection and Preparation of Maize (Corn) Starch

The grains of corn (maize) are first washed with running water to remove the dust particles and organic matter. Later, the grains are softened by soaking them in warm water at 40–60°C for 48–72 hours along with a solution of sulphur dioxide (0.2–0.3%) to check the fermentation. The grains that are swollen are passed through attrition mill to split and crush them partly to separate the endosperm. The embryos (germs) are isolated by the addition of water as a result of which they float and are segregated by skimming off. The corn oil (germ oil, a source of vitamin E) is recovered from the embryos by expression method. The water that is used to soften the grains dissolves most of the minerals, soluble proteins and carbohydrates from the grains. This can be used as a culture medium for the production of antibiotics such as penicillin. Following the germ removal, the liquid mass is freed from the cell debris and gluten (insoluble protein) by passing through fine sieves and washing. The slurry (milky) obtained is a mixture of starch and particles of gluten are subjected to centrifugation by starch purification centrifuge. The starch being heavier settles at the bottom and the particles of gluten being lighter floats on the surface (this is removed by a jet of water). Finally, the starch is washed thoroughly with fresh water, centrifuged many times and/or filtered, pressed and finally dried either on a moving belt dryer or flash dryer, and finally packed.

Collection and Preparation of Rice Starch

The broken pieces of rice grains are adequately soaked in an aqueous solution of sodium hydroxide (0.4–0.5% w/v) which softens the grains and the dissolution of the insoluble protein, gluten. The grains are then wet-milled and taken up with water. The resulting suspension is purified by passing through the sieves and the starch is recovered by a process of centrifugation. The starch is washed finally, dried, powdered and stored in bags.

Collection and Preparation of Wheat Starch

Wheat being the common staple food, its utility for making the starch is restricted. The wheat flour is first made into a stiff ball of dough which is kept aside for a short duration. During this process, gluten swells up and the balls are shifted to grooved-rollers which move forward and backward slowly. The water is constantly sprinkled to carry off the starch along with it while gluten remains as a soft elastic mass. The slurry is purified by centrifugation, washed, dried, powdered and packed in bags.

Collection and Preparation of Potato Starch

The potato tubers are thoroughly washed to remove the soil, and are chopped (reduced) into small pieces and made into a pulp by crushing in a rasping machine (or in a disintegrator of the hammer-mill type). The resulting slurry is filtered through metallic sieves to remove the cellular matter (vegetable tissues). The milky slurry is purified by centrifugation, and the residue is washed with water, dried and stored in bags.

General Description of Starch

Starch generally occurs in nature as irregular, angular, white masses that may easily be reduced to powder. Starch of rice and maize appears white; wheat starch appears creamy white; while the starch of potato appears pale yellow in colour. The starch is odourless and the taste is bland and mucilaginous. All the four types of starch possess a definite shape and characteristic features.

Maize (Corn) Starch

Synonyms

Corn flour (Commonwealth countries except in Canada), Maize starch (Europe), Corn starch or Corn flour (UK and Australia), Maisstarke (German), Fecule de Maize (French).

Characters

Corn starch is a fine white powder with irregular white masses. There is no distinct odour. It tastes starchy first and later sweet. The aqueous mixture is neutral. The grains are simple, polygonal to round, 5 to 35 microns in diameter with hilum either circular or 2 to 5 -rayed. The lamellae are indistinct and with iodine it becomes deep blue.

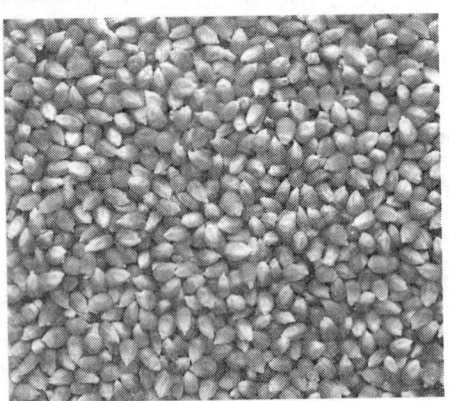

Maize grains

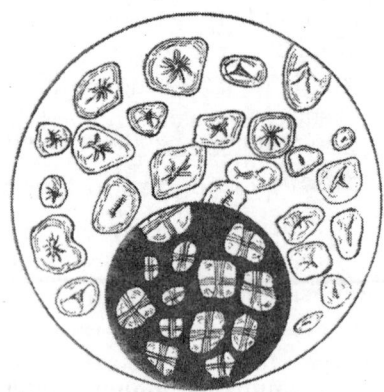

Starch grains: maize

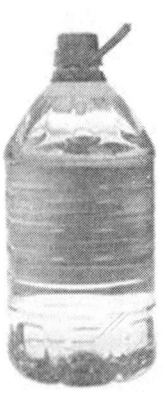

Refined corn oil

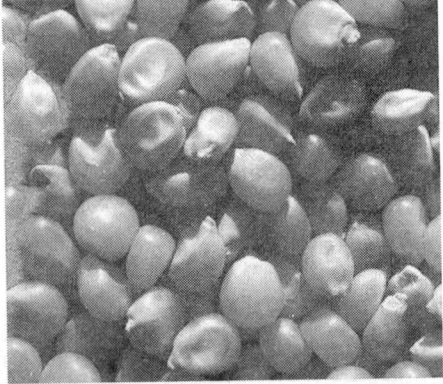

Quality corn

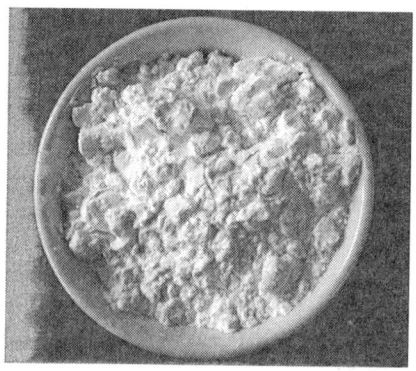

Corn starch

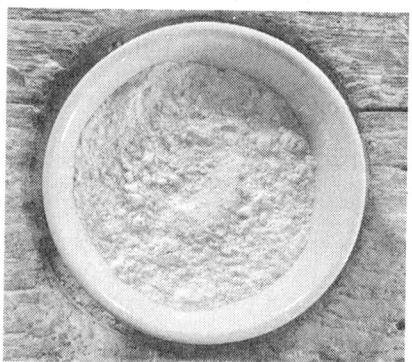

Corn flour

Rice Starch

Characters

The granules are simple or compound. The simple granules are polygonal and 2 to 12 microns in diameter, while the compound granules are oval

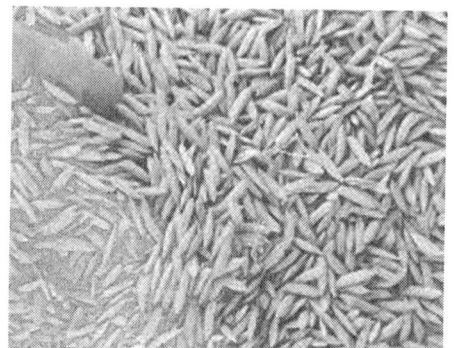

Paddy – Source of starch

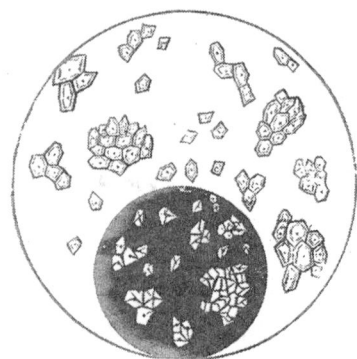

Starch grains of Rice

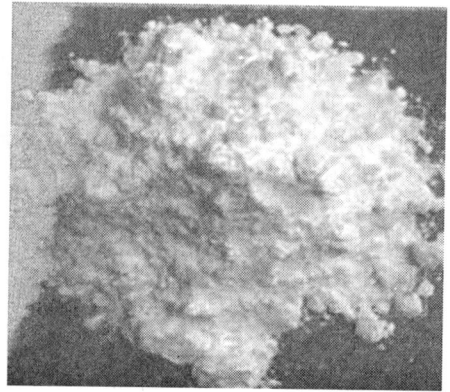

Rice starch

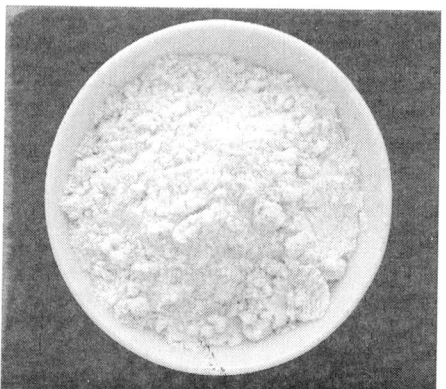

Rice flour

and 12 to 30 microns × 7 to 12 microns in size. The hilum is usually indistinct with indistinct lamellae.

Wheat Starch

Characters

Dough prepared from wheat flour is kept for some time to allow the insoluble proteins, gluten to swell. The mass is shaken constantly with water on rollers. The suspension coming out is dried. The starch grains are simple, circular and large about 28 to 45 microns in diameter. The hilum is central which appears as a dot. The lamellae are indistinct. Starch occurs in irregular, angular masss or as a white powder. It is insoluble in cold water but forms a colloidal solution on boiling with about 15 times its weight of water, the solution forming a transluscent jelly on cooling. Wheat starch is highly refined and closely resembles flour. The starch grains vary in shape and size depending upon the source.

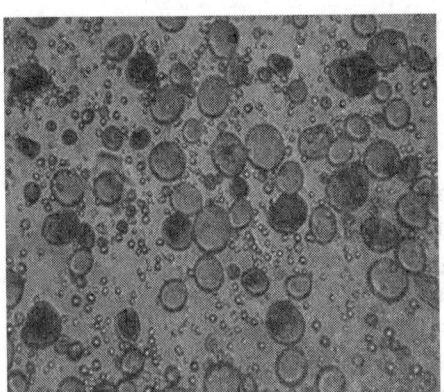

Wheat-starch grains

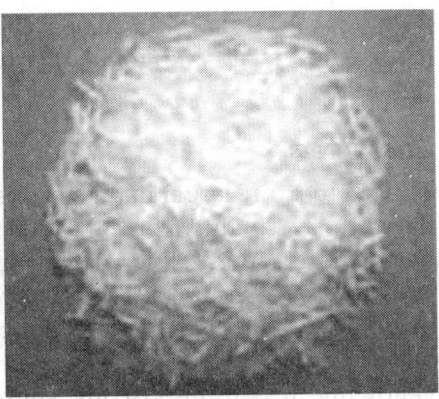

Wheat-sugar

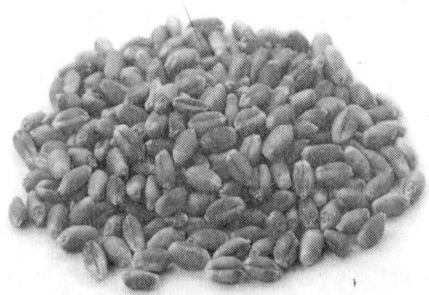

Wheat grains

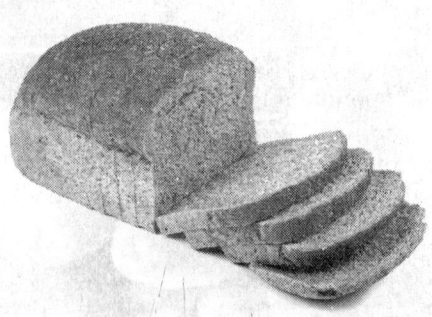

Wheat product—bread

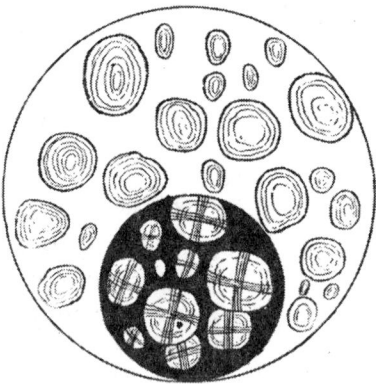

Starch grains of wheat

Potato Starch

Synonyms

Potato starch flour, *Perunajauho* (Finnish), *Potatismjol* (Swedish), *Potetmel* (Norwegian), *Kartoffelmel* (Danish), *Kartoflusterkja* or *Kartoflumjol* (Icelandic).

Characters

The granules are larger in their size, simple, oval to subspherical, somewhat flat, the size ranging from 30 to 100 microns. The hilum is present near the narrower end with clear concentric striations. The starch is very refined and contains minimal amount of protein or fat. The powder is clear white in its colour and exhibits neutral taste after cooking, good clarity, high binding strength, long texture and a minimal tendency of foaming or yellowing. It is more viscous, slightly anionic, with a low gelatinisation temperature and high swelling power.

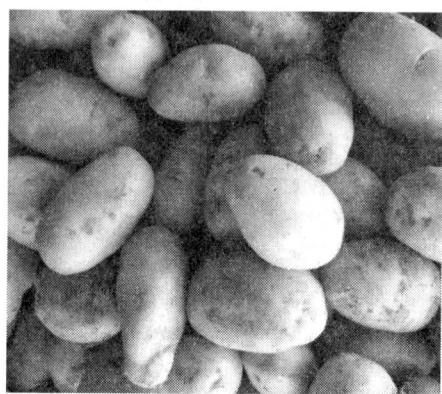

Tubers—source of starch

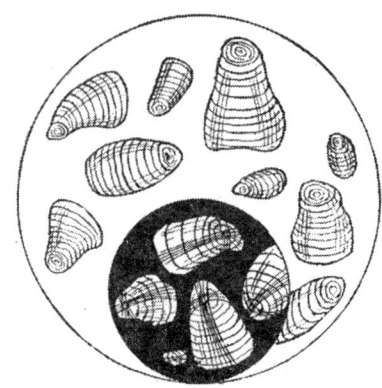

Potato—starch grains

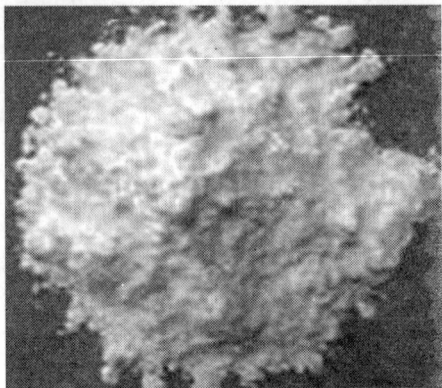

Potato starch

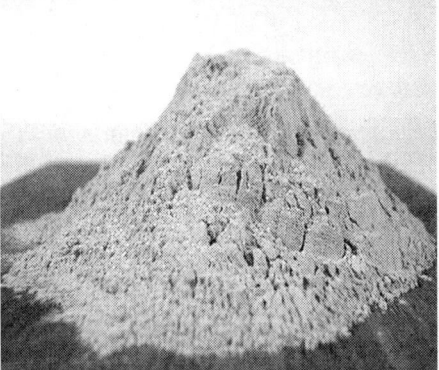

Potato flour

Tests for Starch

Starch taste is mucilaginous. The maize starch is neutral, wheat and potato starch shows acidic reaction and the rice starch is alkaline. Normally, iodine solution (by dissolving iodine in water in the presence of potassium iodide) is used to test for starch and a dark blue colour indicates the prersence of starch. The details of the reaction are not yet fully known. Amylose in the starch is responsible for the formation of a deep blue colour in the presence of iodine. The intensity of the colour depends on the amount of amylose present. If amylose is not present, the colour will be orange or yellow. Waxy starches with little or no amylose will appear red in colour.

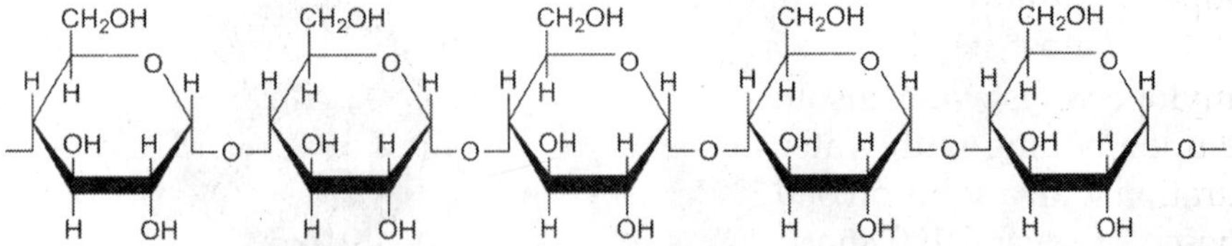

Amylose

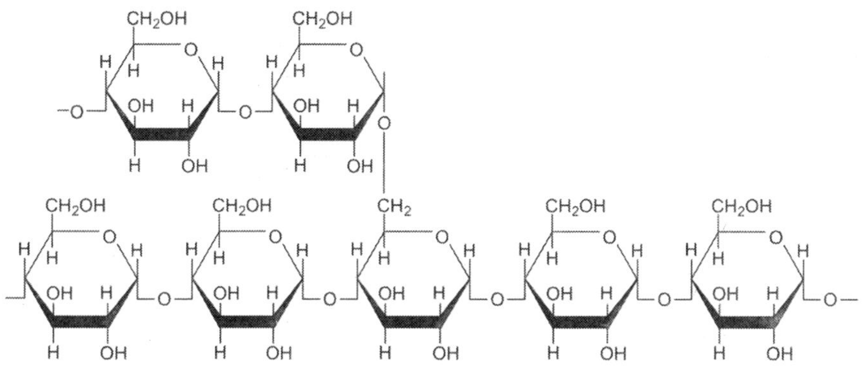

Amylopectin

Chemical Constituents

Pure starch is a soft, white, granular, tasteless and odourless powder that is insoluble in cold water or alcohol or other solvents and can be stored more compactly. The basic chemical formula is $(C_6H_{10}O_5)_n$. Starch is a polysaccharide which comprises of glucose monomers joined in alpha-1,4 linkages. It consists of a linear and helical amylose (20 to 25%) and the branched amylopectin (75 to 80%). In animals, the glucose store is in the form of glycogen which is a more branched amylopectin. The molecules of starch arrange themselves as semi-crystalline granules in plants and each plant species has a unique granular size. The amylose molecules are about 150 times more than amylopectin molecules and smaller in size. When heated, the starch gets dissolved in water and the granules swell and burst and the semi-crystalline structure is lost and the mixture is more viscous. This process is referred to as gelatinisation of starch. It becomes a paste and becomes more viscous during cooking. Upon cooling or prolonged storage, this paste partially recovers and gets thickened by losing water within. This process is called retrogradation. If subjected to dry heat, starch breaks down to form pyrodextrins (brown) and the process is called dextrinisation. Some of the cultivated plant varieties contain pure amylopectin without amylase. These are called waxy starches (maize, rice and potato). Starch is usually adulterated with tapioca starch obtained from *Manihot esculenta*.

Starch granules essentially contain two complex polysaccharides, amylopectin (α-amylose) and amylose (β-amylose); the former constitutes over 80% of most starches.

Amylopectin is water-insoluble swells up in water to give rise to a thick paste upon boiling with water. It produces a distinct violet or bluish-red colouration with a solution of 0.1N iodine. It has highly branched structure composed of several 100 short chains of about 20–25 D-glucose units. One terminal of each of these chains is joined through C-1 to a C-6 with the next chain.

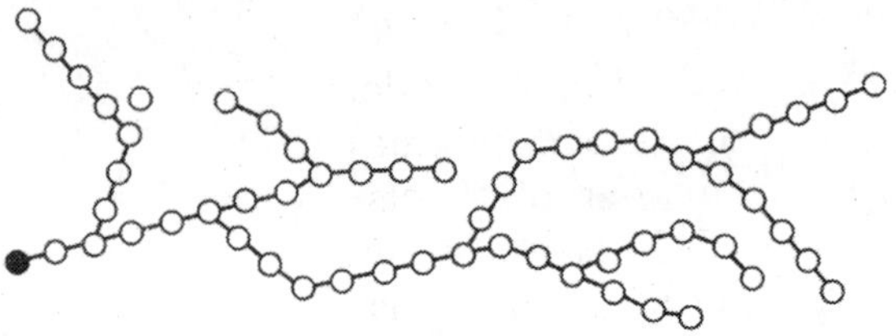

Amylopectin

Amylose is water soluble, and gives an instant bright blue colour with a solution of 0.1N iodine. Upon hydrolysis, this yields a disaccharide (maltose +/−) and the only monosaccharide (D-glucose +), and as such it has been suggested amylase comprises of chains of a number of D-glucose units, and each unit is linked by an alpha-glycoside linkage to C-4 of the next unit. This constitutes up to 25% of the total starch content and the proportion varies with species. This is found to be either absent or present to a very small extent (≤6%) in some glutinous or waxy starches in the plant kingdom.

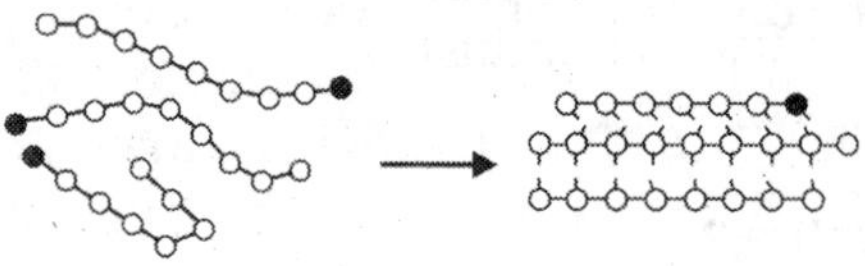

Amylose

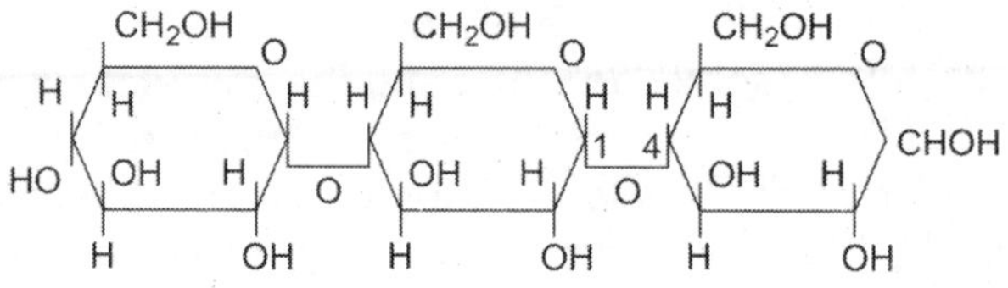

Glucose units

History of Starch

Egyptians used starch paste to stiffen the cloth and also during weaving linen and to glue the papyrus. Romans employed it in the preparation of the cosmetic creams, to powder the hair and to thicken the sauces. It was used to make the dishes similar to *gothumai* wheat halva by the Persians and Indians. The rice starch was used for the surface treatment of paper in China. In 1811, Vauquelin discovered that when starch is heated at higher temperature, it is converted into a substance which is completely soluble in water and resembles gum Arabic in its physical properties. Biot and Persoz (1833) gave the name 'dextrin' to this gum like substance, while Payen and L'ersoz gave the name 'diastase' to the agent in the malted grain which can transform starch.

General Uses of Starch

Starch possesses both absorbent and demulcent properties. It is employed in dusting powder because of its unique protective and absorbent property. It is used in the formulation of tablets and pills as a vital disintegrating agent and a binder. It is also used as a diagnostic aid for the proper identification of the crude drugs. It is used as diluents (or filler) and a lubricant in the preparation of capsules and tablets. It is used as an indicator in iodimetric analyses. It is also used as an antidote of choice for iodine poisoning. The dietetic grades of corn starch are generally marked as 'Maizena' and 'Mondamin'. 'Glycerine of Starch' is used not only as an emollient but also as a base for the suppositories. The starch is the starting material for the large scale production of liquid glucose, glucose syrup, dextrose and dextrin. Starch finds its extensive industrial application for the sizing of paper textiles. Starch also possesses nutrient properties as a food and in cereal-based weaning foods for babies (Farex-R and Cerelac-R of Nestle). The starch can also be used topically and externally to allay itching. It is also used profusely in laundry starching. Starch is used to make foam for packaging. The glucose form starch can be fermented to biofuel ethanol. It is used as industrial alcohol and can also be used as nitro-starch (for explosives).

How Bad Are Starches?

Starches are bad because they are a more concentrated source of carbohydrates and calories than fruits, non-starchy vegetables and dairy products though many of them are excellent sources of fibres, vitamins, minerals and phytonutrients. They are an important part of a healthy, balanced diet when chosen correctly and consumed in reasonable portions. The good starches are potatoes, bread, cereal products, rice and grains and pasta in the diet.

Health Risk of Starches

Too much starch in the diet is associated with dental caries, obesity, and diabetes mellitus. The starch (especially cooked and contained in the processed foods) can cause spikes in blood glucose levels after a meal. Hence, consumption of starch is advised to be in moderation. The individuals with celiac disease and congenital sucrose-isomaltase deficiency may need to avoid the foods rich in starch.

Medicinal Uses

Starch is used as a nutritive, demulcent, protective and as an absorbent. In the manufacture of tablets, it is used as a disintegrant. A starch suspension may be swallowed as an antidote for iodine poisoning. It can be used as an excipient and a binder in the preparation of the tablets.

Culinary Uses

Starch is widely used in the form of prepared foods such as bread, pan cakes, cereals, noodles, pasta, porridge, etc. Commercial refined starches like corn starch, tapioca, and wheat and potato starch are used in industry. Because of its absorbent properties, starch is an important ingredient of all talcum powders. Starch is also the starting material for the commercial manufacture of liquid glucose, dextrose and dextrin. Starch is used as a thickener and a stabiliser in the preparation of puddings, custards, soups, sauces, gravies, pie fillings, salad dressings, noodles and pastas. It is also used as a mold in the preparation of jelly beans and wine gums.

Non-medical Uses

The starch is used in paper manufacturing to increase the strength of the paper and also in surface sizing of the paper and also as a binder for coating the pigments to improve smoothness, hardness, whiteness and gloss. It is used in the preparation of corrugated paper board, paper bags, confections, adhesives and wall boards. Starch is used in the manufacture of different types of glues used for book binding, wall paper adhesives, paper sacks, gummed paper, envelope adhesives, school glues, gummed tape, etc. It is also used in the production of laundry starch (clothing starch), in printing industry, in the production of bioplastics (biodegradable polylactic acid), body powder (beauty products) in the preparation of drilling fluids (oil extraction), biofuel (ethanol) and production of hydrogen.

Other Uses of Different types of Cereals

1. **Rice:** Rice is the most important cereal which forms the basis of the diet of millions of people in South-East Aisa. About 90% is eaten as cooked preparations as plain boiled rice in addition to being mixed with pulses, curd, vegetables, fish or meat. Indian preparations of rice include *kheer* and *pulao*. In South India, fermented preparations like *dosa*, *idli* and *uppma* are prepared from a mixture of rice and blackgram after fermentation for 8 to 12 hours and toasted in a pan or cooked in steam. Rice flour is used in confectionery, ice creams, puddings and pastry. Rice starch is used industrially in cosmetics, as a thickener in calico printing, in finishing the textiles, for making the dextrins, glucose and adhesives. It is used in the preparation of fermented drinks like 'sake' in Japan and 'wang-tsin' in China. Hull is used as a fuel, as bedding for poultry, for packing and insulation. Hull is used also as filler in concrete and bricks, as a source of sodium silicate in making soaps, polishes and cleaning agents. Rice bran oil is edible. The straw is used as a cattle feed, soil mulch, a fertiliser and for making straw boards. The rice straw is also used for the manufacture of a very fine paper in China and Japan. It is also used for thatching, making hats, mats, sacks, ropes and baskets.

2. **Wheat:** Wheat is consumed all over the world in various forms. In advanced countries, it is consumed in the form of leavened bread, but, in India, 85–90% of it is used in the form of chapathies, and other culinary preparations like tandoori roti, nan, paratha and poori. The soft wheat flour is used for making the cakes, biscuits, pastries, crackers, etc. The hard wheats provide excellent flour for bread making. Durum wheat is preferred for the manufacture of macaroni, spaghetti, vermicelli and other products such as noodles. Smaller amounts are converted into breakfast food like wheat flakes, puffed wheat and shredded wheat. Industrial uses include the manufacture of starch, gluten, distilled spirits, malts, pasta, etc. The starch is used for finishing clothes in the laundries while gluten is used in the production of monosodium glutamate for flavouring the food. Wheat bran rich in proteins and vitamins is used as a livestock feed. Wheat straw is used as a livestock feed, for animal bedding and for the production of the compost. The straw is also used in making the corrugated paper and high qualilty insulated building board. Paste made of wheat starch is used as an adhesive for paper mending along with Japanese tissue paper. It is also used in mending flat paper and book hinges. Wheat flour is one of the most important foods in European and North American culture and is an ingredient of breads and pastries. Atta flour is whole-grain wheat flour and is important in Indian and Pakistani cuisine used for a range of foods like roti, naan and chapathi. White wheat flour is the traditional base for wall paper paste and also for papier–mache.

3. **Potato:** At present, potato occupies a prominent position in the food economy of the world. As a vegetable, potato is consumed boiled, steamed, fried, baked or roasted. The processed products of potato include chips, crisps, dehydrated and mashed potatoes, potato flour and canned potatoes. A dehydrated potato product, *'chuno'* is a valued food by the Andean people. Potato is a good substrate for the growth of the microorganisms. The potato broth has long been used as a nutrient medium in microbiology. Potato can also be processed into many commercial products like starch, alcohol, glucose, lactic acid, etc. The starch is used for sizing the cloth and paper, in the laundry industry, and in food preparations. *'Vodka'*, the Russian alcoholic beverage is prepared by the fermentation of cooked potatoes. Potato starch is often a substitute thickener for corn starch in cooking and is considered to be superior for foods that require high temperatures as it is gluten free. In food, it is used to prepare thick gravy or soups or stews instead of wheat or corn flour. The potato starch and its derivatives are used in many recipes like noodles, wine gums, cocktail nuts, chips, sausages, bakery cream, instant soups and sauces, etc. It

is also used as wall paper glue, for finishing and sizing the textiles, and as an adhesive for paper sacks.

4. **Maize** or **corn:** Maize is used as a staple human food, a livestock feed and also as a raw material for many industrial products. Maize was the main food source of ancient civilisations of the Western Hemisphere like the Aztecs, Mayas and Incas. In Mexico, boiled maize is crushed and made into a flat cake called the *'tortilla'*. Corn meal and corn flakes are the products for consumption by the humans. Corn oil is used in cooking. Corn starch is a universal foodstuff. Corn syrup and corn sugar are used in the confectionery, jams and jellies. Maize is the cheapest and most palatable feed for pigs, cattle, sheep and poultry. Corn starch is a substitute for talc in bath powder and as a starching material for clothes. It is also used in the manufacture of asbestos ceramics, dyes, plastics, oil cloth and linoleum. Corn syrup is used in shoe polish, glass paper, rayon and tobacco industry. Corn sugar is used in the preparation of chemicals, leather preparation, dyes and explosives. Furfural, a compound obtained from maize after being cooked under pressure with acids, is used in the production of nylon, in refining diesel, vegetable and lubricating oils, in refining butadiene and in the production of plastics. Zein, a protein from maize, is spun into a soft, durable artificial fibre. This is also used as a foaming agent in fire extinguishers, in the production of linoleum and oil cloth, a sizing material in textiles and as a binding material for cork manufacture and to bind paper, glass, wood, etc. Upon fermentation and distillation, maize produces ethyl alcohol, butyl alcohol, propyl alcohol, acetaldehyde, acetone, glycerol, acetic acid, citric acid and lactic acid. *'Chicha'* is the most common and one of the cheapest beverages of Peru and Bolivia prepared from maize. Corn oil is used in the preparation of soaps, varnishes, paints, etc. The cobs are used for the production of pipes, chemicals, and plastics and also used as livestock feed. The leaves are used as cigarette wrapper. The husks from the cobs are used for making mats, hats and mattresses. The stalks and leaves are sometimes used for production of paper, paper-board and wallboard. The maize cobs which have been pulverised are used extensively as a mild abrasive for the removal of carbon from aeroplane mirrors. Maize flour has been important in Mesoamerican cuisine since ancient times and remains a staple food in Latin American cuisine. Corn (maize) flour is popular in the Southern and South Weestern US, Mexico, South America and Punjab region of India and Pakistan. Corn starch is the refined form of corn flour. Corn starch is used as an anti-caking agent in confectionery. This is also used in the manufacture of environmental friendly products like a biodegradable blue ray compact disc (CD) from Pioneer Company of Japan (2004). It is also used in the production of powders, skin

cleansing milk, deodorants, etc. The starch is a nutrient and a demulcent. Pharmaceutically, it is used as a base for dusting powder for uncoated pills. It is also used as an antidote for iodine and bromine poisoning.

Plant Starch vs Animal Starch

The animal starch is not a starch *per se*, it refers to the constituent of the animal's glycogen owing to the similarity in structure and composition of amylopectin. While the plants store their excess glucose in the form of starch, the animals do so in the form of glycogen. Glycogen is a branched polymer of glucose that is mainly produced in the liver and muscles cells that functions as secondary long-term energy storage the animal cells. Glycogen is also a complex carbohydrate that primarily serves as a storage carbohydrate similar to starch. The main difference between the amylopectin in plants and amylopectin in animals is that the latter has more extensive branching at every 8–12 glucose units.

GUAR GUM

Synonyms

Guar flour, Jaguar gum, Guaran, Guarkernmehl (German), Gomme de Guar, Gomme de Jaguar, Farine de guar (French), Goma Guar, Guaro Dervo (Spanish), Indian Cluster bean.

Biological Source

Guar gum is the powdered endosperm of seeds of *Cyamopsis tetragonaloba* (L.) Taub. (= *C. psoralioides* DC.) (Family: Leguminosae–Fabaceae).

Geographical Source

The plant is probably indigenous to India although it has never been observed in a wild state. It is being grown from hundreds of years in India and Pakistan as a fodder, green manure and vegetable and was introduced into USA in 1900. Now, it is cultivated exclusively in India, Pakistan, Australia, Indonesia, Burma and parts of Central Africa. Quite recently, the cultivation has been undertaken in the arid South-Western United States. In India, two cultivars are recognised, the giant and the dwarf. The plant is commercially cultivated in Gujarat, Punjab, Haryana, Rajasthan, Madhya Pradesh, Tamil Nadu, Maharashtra, Karnataka, Andhra Pradesh and Uttar Pradesh. India and Pakistan are producers of guar seed and guar gum and around 85% guar is produced in India. The major part is consumed by oil and natural gas industry and after that major part goes to food processing industry. India exports guar gum to 145 countries in the world.

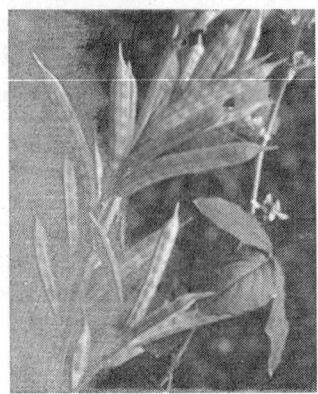

Cyamopsis tetragonaloba

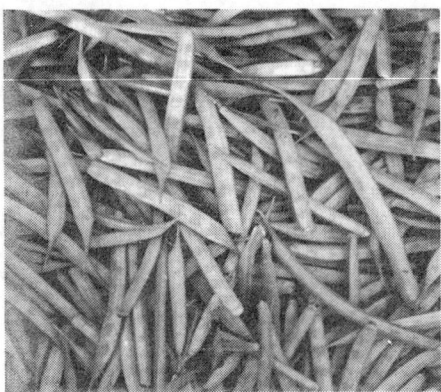

Mature fruits of guar

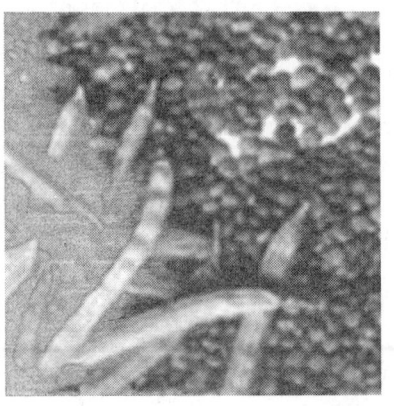

Dry fruits and seeds of guar

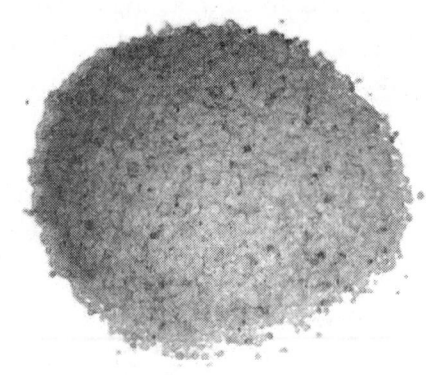

Guar gum

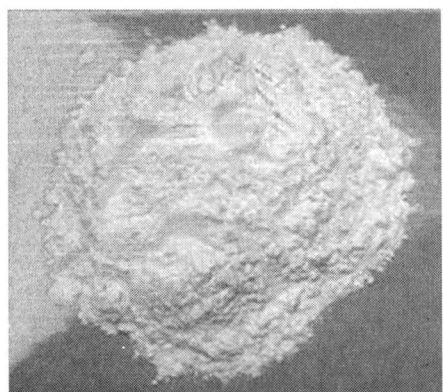

Food grade gum powder

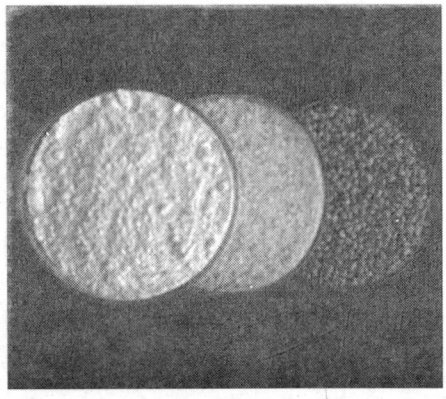

Food grade gum

Collection and Preparation

The guar seeds are mechanically dehusked, hydrated, milled and screened according to the application, and it is generally produced as a free-flowing, off-white powder. Guar gum is industrially prepared from well-developed seeds. The seeds are put into a grinder to bifurcate guar seeds. The seeds are separated into husk and embryo. The husk contains fibrous matter and the gum is located in the endosperm. Guar seeds contain 14–17% of hull, 38–45% of endosperm and 45–50% of germ. Cotyledons are separated from the endosperm by winnowing. The endosperm, i.e. crude guar gum, is pulverised by means of micropulveriser and grinding for 15 minutes. The endosperm being harder is not affected by micropulveriser. Finally, it is sifted through sieves of 4 to 60 mesh to give granular and powdered gum.

Characters

Guar gum is colourless or pale yellowish-white coloured, coarse to finely ground powder, practically odourless with a bland taste. Guar gum disperses and swells rapidly in hot or cold water with a translucent suspension. 0.5% aqueous solution of gum is neutral to litmus. It is insoluble in organic solvents. The viscosity depends on temperature, pH, particle size, etc.

Chemical Constituents

The principal constituent of the gum is a galactomannan (guar gum) or mannogalacton, a complex polysaccharide which consists of 34.5% of D-galactose and 65.4% of D-mannose and readily forms a viscous gel with water. Fatty acids, both free and as esters, have been reported by GLC-NS analysis. The gum is more soluble in water and is a better emulsifier. In water, it is non-ionic and hydro-colloidal. It remains stable in solution over

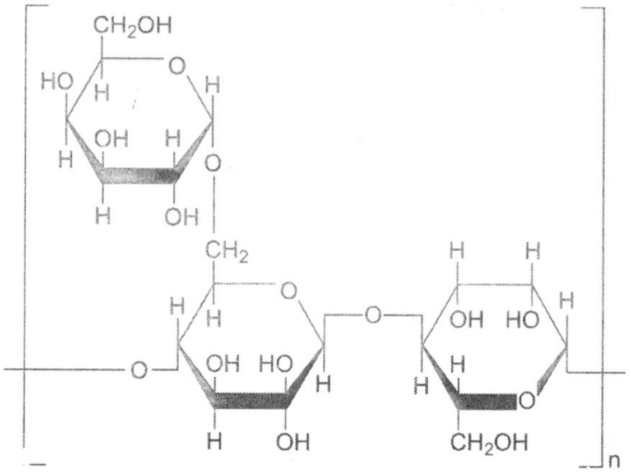

Guaran—the repeating unit in Guar gum

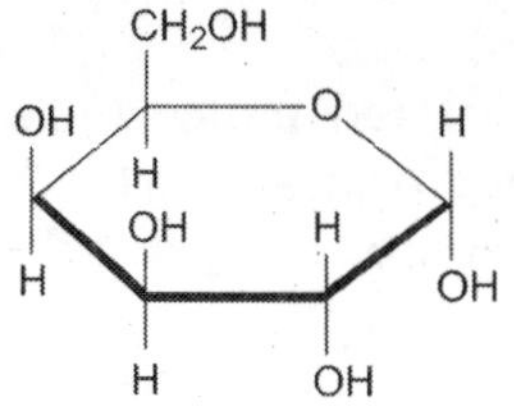

D-galactose ($C_6H_{12}O_6$)

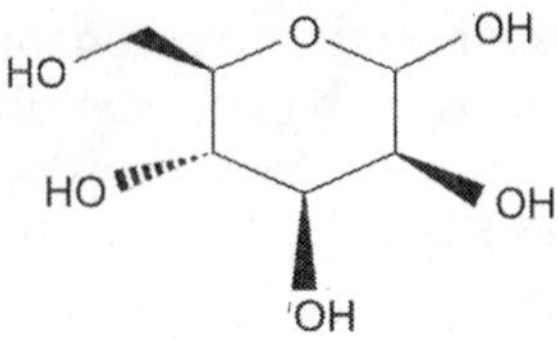

D-mannose ($C_6H_{12}O_6$)

a pH range of 5.0–11.0 but degrades at a pH of 3.0 at 50°C. Strong acids cause hydrolysis and loss of viscosity of the gum. It is insoluble in most of the hydrocarbon solvents.

History of Guar

Guar is a native to the Indian subcontinent and is grown mainly in India, Pakistan, and USA and also in some parts of Africa and Australia. In old times, it was only used as a rich protein food for cattle (the beans and the stems) and also as a green vegetable in India. The plant has been cultivated in India since centuries and India accounts for 80% of the total guar produced in the world. Historically, it has been an important source of nutrition for humans as well as animals. Just after the Second World War, there was a severe locust bean gum shortage which adversely affected the paper and textile industries and guar gum was found to be the most suitable substitute. It was introduced into America in 1903 and the technology of extraction of the gum was commercialised in USA in 1953 and a decade later in India (1960s). In India, when the farmers realised its drought tolerance, they grew it as a forage crop for cattle, which resulted in its name as *guar* meaning 'cattle fodder'. The gum has been used for centuries as a thickening agent for foods and pharmaceuticals and it continues in paper, textile and oil drilling industries.

Medicinal Uses

Guar gum has recently received some attention as a possible oral hypoglycaemic drug. It can produce changes in gastric emptying and in the gastrointestinal transition time, which can delay absorption of sugars and oligosaccharides from the gut. It is used as a binder or a disintegrator in the preparation of tablets pharmaceutically. It is useful as a bulk laxative as it promotes regular bowel movement, relieves constipation, colitis and irritable bowel syndrome. It is also used to treat obesity, diabetes and for preventing atherosclerosis (hardening of the arteries). Following ingestion, it speeds up the removal of the waste and bacteria from colon and also helps absorption of toxic substances and bacteria during infective diarrhoea. Many studies indicated that the gum ingestion decreases significantly, the cholesterol levels in the human serum which may be due to its high soluble fibre content. It also helps as an adjuvant for the diabetic drugs used for the treatment of non-insulin dependent diabetes.

Non-medical Uses

a. **Culinary and dietary uses:** The young tender pods are used as a vegetable and the mature dry seeds as a valuable cattle feed. It is also used as a forage crop and a green manure in India, Pakistan, Indonesia and Eastern countries. The flour is chiefly used as a stabiliser and a thickener in the production of the food products, for sizing the textiles and products of paper. It is also used as an emulsifier in salad dressings, as a flocculent in mining industry in addition to the manufacture of cosmetics. The flour forms excellent films as such it is used for backing the postage stamps. The drought–resistant bean is eaten, fed to cattle and used as a green manure. It is used to increase the dough yield, to give greater resiliency and improve the texture and shelf-life of bakery goods. It is useful in dairy industry as it helps thickening the milk, yoghurt, chewing gums and liquid cheese products, sauces, ketchups, etc. It is used in the preparation of dry soups, sweet desserts, and canned fish in sauce and frozen food items. It is used to stabilise the ice creams in a short time and to slow down the melting of the ice creams. It acts as a lubricant and prevents loss of weight during storage by binding the moisture in meat products. It is used in cosmetics as it thickens the creams and lotions. In foods and beverages the gum is used as a thickening agent, a stabilising agent, as a suspending agent and a binding agent.

b. **Industrial uses:** The guar gum is used in various industries because of its ability to suspend the solids, to bind water by hydrogen bonding, to control the viscosity of the aqueous solutions and to form strong and tough films. It has many industrial applications in paper, textile and oil drilling, mining, explosives and ore floatation. Industrially, the gum is used as a controlling agent in oil wells to facilitate easy drilling and prevent fluid loss, as an emulsifier because it helps to prevent oil droplets from coalescing and also as a stabiliser as it helps to prevent solid particles from settling. It is used primarily as a proppant transport/proppant suspending agent in hydraulic fracturing (in shale oil and gas extraction industries). In textile industry, it is used in sizing, finishing and printing. It is used to improve sheet formation, folding and denser surface for printing in paper industry. It is useful as a waterproofing agent mixed with ammonium nitrate and nitroglycerine in explosives industry. It can be used as a thickener in toothpastes, as a conditioner in shampoos in cosmetic and toiletry industry.

Side Effects

The side effects of consuming guar gum by mouth include increased gas production, diarrhoea and loose stools. These effects usually decrease or disappear after several days of use. Higher doses of guar gum or not drinking enough fluid (water) along with the dose of gum can cause choking or blockage of the oesophagus and the intestines.

PECTIN

Synonyms

Acide pectinique, Acide pectique, Apple pectin, Citrus pectin, Fractionated pectin, Fruit pectin, Grapefruit pectin, lemon pectin, Pectinic acid, Pectina, Pectine d'Agrume, Pectine de Pomme.

Pectin is derived from Greek, *Pektikos* meaning 'congealed' or 'curdled' and is a structural heteropolysaccharide in the primay cell walls of terrestrial plants. It was first isolated and described by Henry Braconnot (1825).

Biological Source

Commerically pectin is produced as a white to light brown powder mainly from citrus fruits. Pectin is the purified carbohydrate product obtained by acid hydrolysis from the inner portion of the rind of *Citrus* peels, i.e. *Citrus limon, Citrus aurantium* (Family: Rutaceae) and the remains of apples after squeezing for juice. Other fruits like apricots, plums, carrots, gooseberries (with much pectin), cherries, grapes, strawberries papaya, guava and mangoes (with less pectin) are also the source of pectin.

Geographical Source

USA, Switzerland and other European countries are producing pectin either from citrus peels or from apple pomace.

Collection and Preparation

The main sources of pectin are pears, apples, guavas, quince, plums, gooseberries and other citrus fruits which contain large amounts of pectin. The soft fruits such as cherries, grapes, and strawberries contain the small amounts. The main raw material for pectin production is the dried peels of citrus or apple pomace, both byproducts of juice production. Pomace from sugar beets is also used to a small extent.

The preserved or fresh peels of citrus are heated with 20 times its weight of water at 90°C for 30 minutes in presence of hot dilute acid (citric acid, lactic acid or tartaric acid) maintaining the pH between 1.5 and 3.5. During the process of extraction, the protopectin loses some of its branching and chain length, and goes into solution. The aqueous extract thus obtained is filtered and the filtrate is concentrated in a vacuum and the pectin is precipitated by the addition of ethanol or isopropanol (alcohol). The precipitated pectin is separated, washed and dried. Following drying and milling, pectin is usually standardised with sugar and sometimes calcium salts or organic acids to have an optimum performance in its application. Pectin is incompatible with calcium, so necessary precaution should be taken to keep it away from its metallic salts throughout the process of extraction.

Characters

Pectin is white to cream coloured, odourless, amorphous, mucilaginous, coarse or fine powder. It is completely soluble in 20 parts of water and the solution is viscous, colloidal and acidic to litmus. Pectin forms a stiff jelly if it is heated with 9 parts of water. It is insoluble in alcohol and other organic solvents. Pectin is more stable in acid media than in alkaline media. It occurs in ripe fruits and certain vegetables. Protopectin, the precursor, present in unripe fruits gets converted to pectin as the fruits ripen. In over-ripe fruits the pectin becomes pectic acid. In plant cells, pectin consists of a complex set of polysaccharides present in most primary cell walls and abundant in the non-woody parts of terrestrial plants. This is present throughout the primary cell wall but also in the middle lamella between the plant cells where it helps to bind the cells together. The amount, structure and chemical composition of the pectin differs from plant to plant and within a plant overtime and in different parts of the plant.

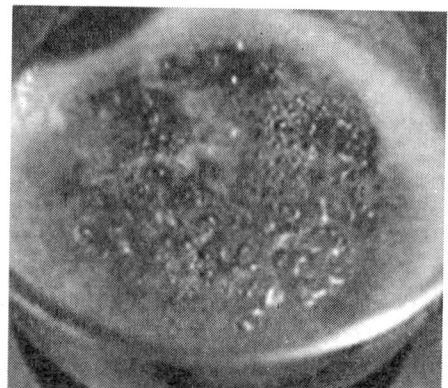

Liquid pectin

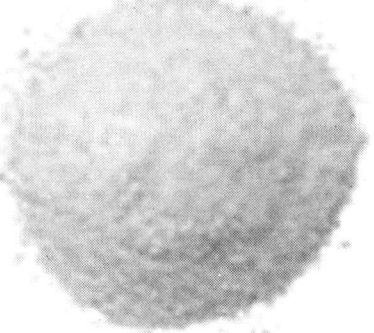

Pectin powder

Forms of Pectin

The different types of pectin behaving differently are: *Dry pectin*—which comes in multiple forms, tailored to the amount of sugar in a recipe; *Liquid pectin*—which is similar to dry pectin but pre-dissolved to avoid clumping; *HM (high methoxyl) pectin*—that comes in fast-set and low-set varieties; *Fast set HM*—that is best for chunky jams and marmalades while *slow-set HM* works well for clear jellies; *Low methoxyl (LM) pectin*—which combines with calcium instead of sugar to create a set that is good for low and no sugar preserves.

Chemical Constituents

Pectin is a linear chain of alpha-(1–4) linked D-galacturonic acid that forms the backbone, a homogalacturonan, with regions where galacturonic acid is replaced by (1–2) linked L-rhamnose. From the rhamnose residues, side chains of various neutral sugars (D-galactose, L-arabinose and D-xylose) branch off. Isolated pectin has a molecular weight of 60–130,000 g/mol varying with the origin. The parent substance protopectin on controlled hydrolysis gets converted into pectinic acids (pectins). These are polygalacturonic acids in which some of the carboxyl groups are present as methyl esters. I.P. specifies that pectin should have not less than 7% of methoxyl groups and not less than 78% of galacturonic acid.

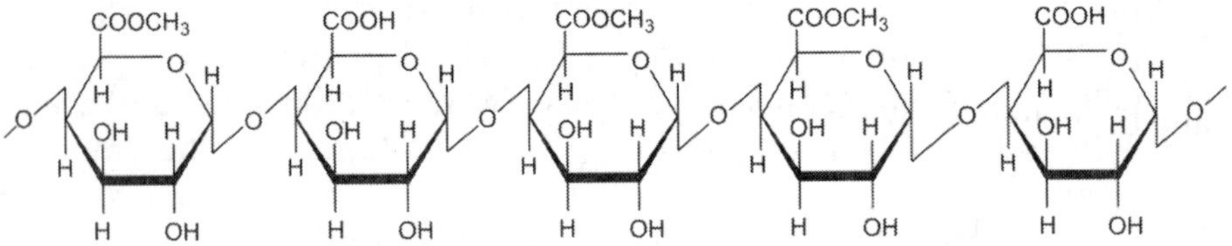

Pectin—a polymer of a-galacturonic acid

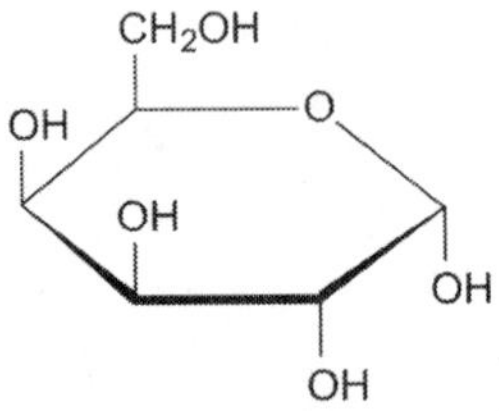

D-galacturonic acid ($C_6H_{10}O_7$) 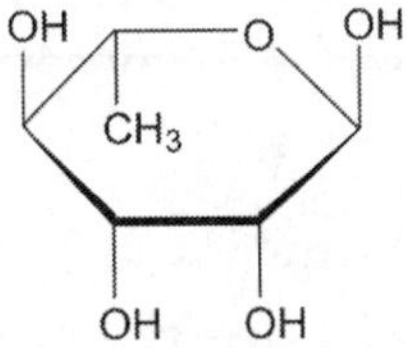   L-rhamnose ($C_6H_{14}O_6$)

History of Pectin

Pectin was first isolated and described by Henri Braconnot (1825) but the action of pectin to make the jams and marmalades was known at least since the 18th century. During industrialisation, apple juice was used to obtain dried apple pomace (waste of crushed apples) which was cooked to extract pectin. The early colonists in New England made their own pectin and extracted it from apple peelings. The actual role of pectin was understood during 1820s at which time, the housewives began using the knowledge of which type of the fruits and what parts of the fruits should be used to make better preservatives in winter. In 1908, the liquid pectin was first sold in Germany as a commercial product. In 1919, the Douglas Pectin Co. of Fairport, New York, made the first pectin plant in the British Empire to manufacture pectin which was later put on the retail market in 1923 under the brand name of Certo. In 1920s and 1930s, factories were built to commercially extract pectin from dried apple pomace and citrus peel. At first, pectin was sold as a liquid extract but later it is used as a dried powder.

Medicinal Uses

Pectin is a protectant having a property of colloidal absorption of toxins and thus used in the treatment of diarrhoea. The efficacy of pectin in the gastrointestinal tract is largely due to its colloidal action. Many antidiarrhoeal formulations contain pectin. Pectin is also used as haemostatic for both internal as well as external haemorrhage. It is also used as an emulsifying agent, gelling agent and as a plasma substitute. It is also used in gentle heavy metal removal from the biological systems. It is also used in throat lozenges as a demulcent. The consumption of pectin has been shown to reduce the blood cholesterol levels. In medicine, it is used against constipation and diarrhoea as pectin increases the viscosity and the volume of the stool. It is also used as a demulcent in throat lozenges, as a stabiliser in cosmetics, medical adhesives and colostomy devices. In humans, it reduces low density lipoprotein (LDL) levels thereby lowering the cholesterol levels. Pectin can also activate cell death pathways in cancer cells.

Non-medical Uses

Pectin is used in many cosmetic preparations and also thickening agent in food industry for the sauces, jams and ketchup. It is used as a gelling agent in jams and jellies. It is also used in fillings, sweets, as a stabiliser in fruit juices and milk drinks and also as a source of soluble dietary fibre. Mainly pectin is used as a gelling agent, thickening agent, food additive and as a stabiliser in food and cosmetic products. It is an ingredient in jam sugar, marmalades, diet products, acidic protein drinks (yogurt) and baked goods. It is an excellent substitute for vegetable glue in cigar industry. It is used as a stabiliser in emulsions.

Side Effects

When pectin is taken by mouth either alone or in combination with guar gum and insoluble fibre, it can cause stomach cramps, diarrhoea, gas and loose stools. The people who are exposed to pectin dust work, may develop asthma.

ISABGOL

Synonyms

Isapghol (Bengali, Persian, Dukhhine, Punjabi, Bombay and Marathi), Uthamujeerun, Umto jeeru (Gujarati), Ispaghula, Isabgol, Indium psyllium, Isphagul or Spongel seeds (Spaghula seeds) (English), Snigdhajeera, Snigdhabijah, Snigdhajirakah, Sat isabgola, Isabgola (Sanskrit), Baje-i-katuna (Persian), Is-mogul (Kashmeeri), Isapagala vittulu (Telugu), Ishappukolvirai, Iskol and Isphiogol (Tamil), Issabagolu (Canarese), Psyllium husk, Psyllium seeds, Fleam, Desert Indian Wheat, Desert plantain, White or blonde psyllium (English), Isabgol or Isabgul, Ishabgula (Hindi), Ashwagol kul (Ayurvedic).

Biological Source

The dried and ripe seeds and the seed coat (husk) of *Plantago ovata* Forssk. (= *P. ispagula*), *P. lanceolata*, *P. arenaria* and *Plantago afra* (= *P. major*, *P. asiatica*, *P. psyllium*) constitute the drug (Family: Plantaginaceae). Isabgol is derived from two Persian words, *'isap'* and *'ghol'* meaning *'horse's ear'* describing the shape of the seed.

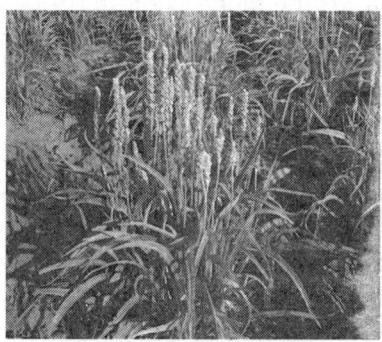

Plantago ovata—isabgol

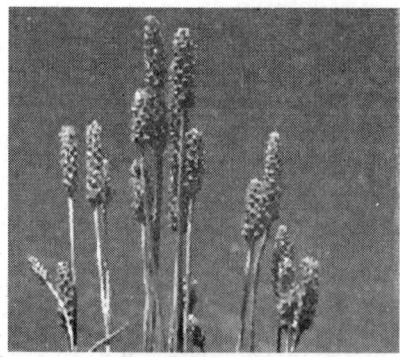

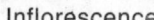
Inflorescence

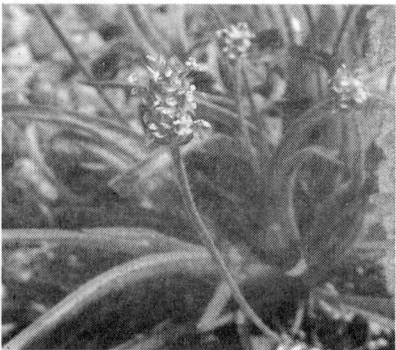
Close-up

Geographical Source

This Persian plant is indigenous to West Asia, North Africa and the Mediterranean countries. It has been introduced into India and the plant is cultivated extensively in North–West India and Punjab and Sind of Pakistan. The species are also found in Australia and New Zealand. About 50,000 hectares of area is under cultivation of isabgol. India is the largest producer and exporter of Isabgol. It has a long history of use throughout the world and has been used in traditional medicine in the US, Europe, China, etc. The mucilage is highest in *P. ovata*, amounting to 25% or more by weight of the total yield of the seed.

Collection and Preparation

Isabgol is predominantly grown as a cold season crop over medium, well drained, loamy soil. It requires cool climate and dry sunny weather. The seed is sown in November to mid December. Seed (4 kg/ha) mixed with 10 times of sand or sieved farm yard manure should be sown in lines 30 cm apart. Irrigation is done 7 to 8 times at an interval of 8 to 10 days. The crop matures during March-April, 110–130 days after sowing. The weather should be dry and sunny at harvesting. Average yield varies between 800–1000 kg/ha.

The plants are cut at the ground level after 10 AM, bundled and transported to thrashing shed. They are allowed to dry for 2–3 days and then thrashed with the help of bullocks or a tractor. The harvested seed must be dried to below 12% moisture to allow for cleaning, milling and storage.

Characters

The seeds are very small, 2–3 mm long and 0.8–1.5 mm wide, pinkish grey to brown in colour. Concave surface contains the hilum covered with thin membrane having two perforations and a red spot in the centre. The seeds have a mucilaginous taste and have no odour. 1 gm accommodates 500–600 seeds. The seeds are transluscent and concavo-convex.

Chemical Constituents

The seeds contain 10–30% of the hydrocolloidal polysaccharide which is localised in the outer seed coat. The mucilage from the seeds of isphagol on hydrolysis yields D-xylose, L-arabinose and aldobiuronic acid. The seeds also contain mucilage, fixed oil, aucubin glycoside, albuminous matter, various bases, sugars, sterols and protein. The mucilage is white, fibrous and hydrophilic. After absorbing water, it forms a gel which is clear, colourless mucilage which increases in volume by 10-fold or more. The viscosity of the mucilage is not affected by variations in temperature and pH. The soluble non-starch polysaccharides result in the production of propionate, butyrate and acetate by fermentation.

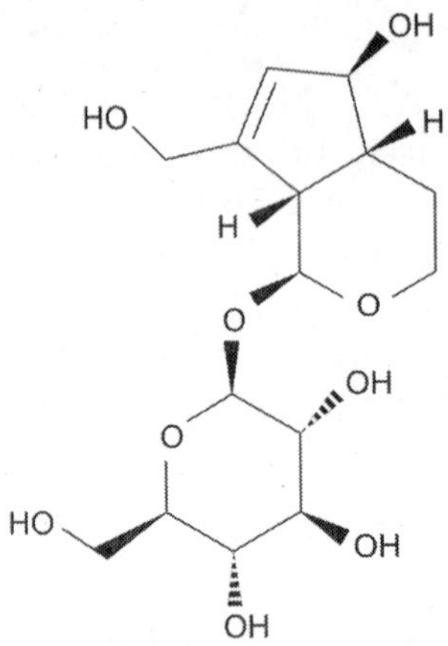

Aucubin ($C_{15}H_{22}O_9$)

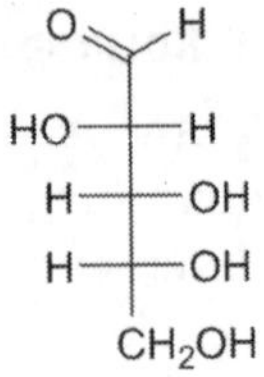

D-arabinose ($C_5H_{10}O_5$)

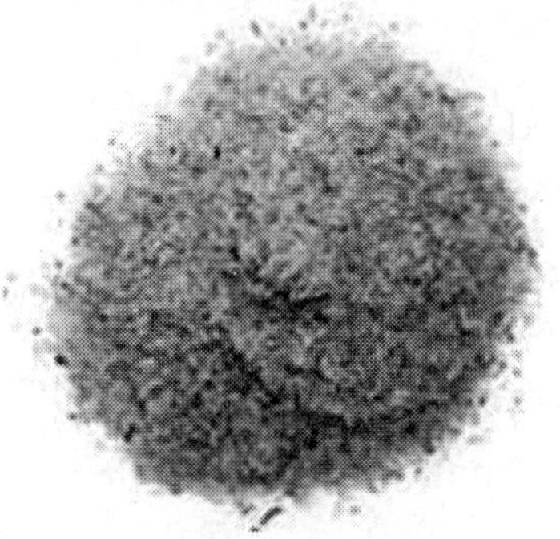

Isabgol—powder

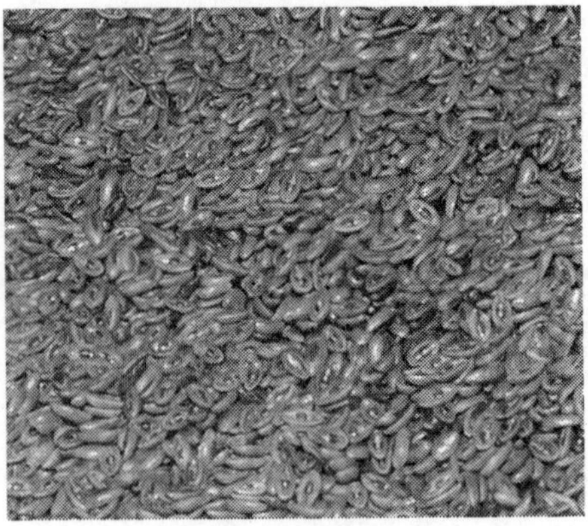

Isabgol—seeds

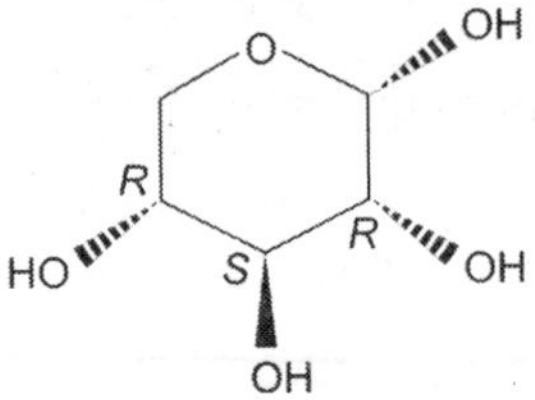

D-xylose ($C_5H_{10}O_5$)

History of Isabgol

Isabgol mainly originated in Persia and from there it is imported to India. The plant has a long history of use throughout the world and has been used in traditional medicine in the USA, Europe, India and China as laxative, emollient, demulcent and diuretic. German authorities approved the use to reduce serum cholesterol levels in 1990s. USFDA in 1998 authorised the use of food and dietary supplements containing sat-isabgol. In India, the use is as old as the Ayurveda (holistic system of medicine) in which the seeds are used as laxative, demulcent and astringent with particular reference to chronic colitis.

Medicinal Uses

Isphagol is centuries old and a prehistoric natural herbal treatment. The seeds are cooling and are useful in several kinds of chronic dysentery, chronic colitis, diarrhoea, catarrah, blenorrhoea, fever, burning sensation, cough, constipation and affections of the kidneys and bladder. It is also aphrodisiac, urinogenetic, antipyretic, antidiarrhoeal, antidysenteric, cooling, demulcent, astringent, emollient, diuretic and expectorant. It is a safe laxative and is beneficial in habitual constipation. It is also used as a remedy for gonorrhoea, urethritis, gastritis, gastric and duodenal ulcers, cystitis, etc. It also relieves bleeding, body heat and syphilitic taints, intestinal irritation, difficulty in passing urine and piles. It is a mild purgative and is used as a remedy for arsenic poisoning. It is used in rheumatic and gouty affections, swellings and in ardent fevers. The powder made from the husk relieves chronic constipation, and reduces the high blood (serum) cholesterol through proper excretion of bile acids. This is an effective remedy for acidity, obesity, diarrhoea, bowel regulation, ulcers, piles, spermatorrhoea, nocturnal emissions, chronic amoebic dysentery and dysuria. The husk (ispghulae testa or *Sat isobgulo*) makes the intestines and the stomach soft and smooth. It is a diuretic and helps in the free flow of urine. It is a mild laxative and helps in the removal of harmful substances out of the stomach and intestines. The husk also absorbs water in the abdomen and the intestine to turn into a jelly which protects the walls from irritation. It helps relieve the pain due to gastric and peptic ulcers due to its inherent anaesthetic property. It is used against the inflammatory conditions of the mucous membranes of the gastrointestinal and genito-urinary tracts. It also reduces the blood glucose levels when ingested along with the food. The natural fibres present decrease the symptoms of fatigue and loss of energy. This can be used as an effective drug in the treatment of gonorrhoea, whitlow of the fingertips, rheumatism and gout. The embryo oil which contains 50% of linoleic acid prevents arteriosclerosis. It is also a drug for gallstones, stool incontinence and psoriasis, etc.

Non-medical Uses

a. **Culinary and dietary uses:** It is a natural food which is cooling, soothing, softening and non-addictive which prevents heart attack. The components of the husk compensate the deficiency of food fibres (true dietary fibre) and also satisfy acute thirst. It is a popular constituent of high-fibre breakfast cereals, breads and ice creams and frozen desserts. The mucilage is used in ice creams and frozen desserts as a thickener. The mucilage of isabgol is a natural dietary fibre for animals too. The dehusked seed is rich in starch and fatty acids and is used as a chicken feed and cattle feed in India. The technical grade isabgol can be used as a hydrocolloidal agent to improve retention of water to improve seed germination and transplanting. The plant is also used as a food plant by the larvae of some species of butterflies and moths.

b. **Other use:** The plant is astringent, antitoxic, antimicrobial, anti-inflammatory and antihistamine and styptic. A poultice of the leaves of the plant relieves suffering from the insect bites, rashes caused due to poison-ivy, minor sores and boils when used externally. In folklore, it is believed to cure even the snake bite. It is taken internally as a tea, tincture or syrup for cough and bronchitis. The varieties with broad leaves are used as a leafy vegetable for salads, green sauce, etc. In India, the seeds and the mucilage from the husk are useful in irritable bowel syndrome, as a dietary fibre supplementation, for mild to moderate hypercholesterolemia, for reducing blood glucose, diverticular disease. It has been used as an indigenous ayurvedic and unani medicine for the whole range of bowel problems.

Adverse Effects

Psyllium can cause bowel obstruction if taken without adequate amount of water. Gas of stomach bloating may also occur. Choking is a hazard if taken without adequate water as it thickens in the throat. This can also cause allergic reactions including anaphylaxis. It may also act as a potent inhalant allergen capable of causing symptoms of asthma. It is also known to cause difficulty in breathing, difficulty in swallowing, pain in the stomach, tightness of the chest, itching, skin rash, nausea and vomiting.

Adulteration

Ispagol is commonly adulterated with the seeds of *Plantago lanceolata* which contain very little mucilage.

HONEY

Synonyms

Madhu, Makshika (Sanskrit), Honey (English), Miel (French), Honig (German), Mel, Shehad, Asal, Injubin, Asatul-nahl (Arabic), Shadad-Angabina (Persian), Saht (Punjabi), Mhach (Kashmiri), Shahad (Dukkhanis), Madha (Hindi, Bengali and Gujarati), Madh (Marathi), Mhou (Konkani), Taen (Tamil and Malayalam), Tayne (Telugu), Jaentuppa (Canarese), Mipanny (Sinhalese), Pya-ya (Burmese), Ayur-mader (Malay).

Biological Source

Honey is a sweet food made by some insects which use the nectar from flowers. The variety produced by the honeybee, *Apis mellifera* (=*Apis mellifica*, Order: Hymenoptera, Family: Apidae) is one of the most commonly referred to which is consumed by humans. Honey produced by other species of *Apis*, other bees and insects have different properties. Honeybees form honey from nectar by regurgitation and store it as a source of food in honeycombs made of wax inside the beehive.

Geographical Source

Honey is produced in India, Russia, West Indies, California, Australia, New Zealand and various parts of Africa.

Collection and Preparation

Honeybees make honey from plant nectar. The honey so made by the bees is stored in the bee hive and used during the cold weather or drought as a food source for the hive. The bees work very hard to make more honey than they need, the excess of which is harvested by the beekeepers. A beekeeper on average can expect to yield about 50 pounds (4.2 gallons) each year from a healthy colony in a fertile area. This can vary from year to year and from location to location.

The removal of bees from the honey is necessary to obtain honey. The easiest way to harvest the honey from a beehive is through the use of a fume board. A fume board looks like a telescoping top (or outer hive cover) the inside of which contains an absorbent material that is sprayed with a nontoxic solution that the bees do not enjoy. The board is placed on the top of the full honey super that one wishes to harvest. After a few minutes, the bees move away from the smell and vacate the honey super, which lets you remove the box of honey with minimal disturbance. The beekeepers often use a smoker to pacify the bee colony.

The worker bees, by means of a long, hollow tube from the maxillae and labium, take nectar from the nectarines of flowers they visit and pass it through the oesophagus into the honey-sac or crop. The final honey is the virgin honey that drains from the comb and collected fresh. In cold weather the bees use their stored honey as their energy source. The nectar, which consists largely of sucrose, is mixed with salivary secretion containing enzyme invertase and while in the honey-sac is hydrolysed into inert sugar. On arrival at the hive the bee brings back the contents of the honey-sac and deposits them in a previously prepared cell of the honeycomb.

Thus, the honey comb is smoked to remove the bees and a hot knife is used to cut the wax cappings of the cells of the honeycomb. These cappings can be used to make candles. Once the cappings have been removed, one can begin to separate the liquid honey from the comb. The honey is separated from the cut comb by drainage or by centrifugation or by expression. The honey extractor, either electric or manual, uses the centrifugal force to separate the liquid honey from the comb without destroying the comb. This allows the beekeeper to reuse the frame of empty comb in the honey super. Alternatively, the honey filled comb can be cut out of the frame, crushed, and strained through cheesecloth. The resulting beeswax can be used for candles. After straining (or extraction), the liquid honey is allowed to settle for a few days in a closed container and is then ready to bottle.

The honey obtained by applying pressure is liable to contamination with the beeswax present in the comb. Honey obtained from the comb is heated to 80°C so that the impurities floating on the surface are removed and the density adjusted between 1.35 and 1.37. After heating and removal of impurities, honey should be cooled rapidly; otherwise the colour darkens on storage.

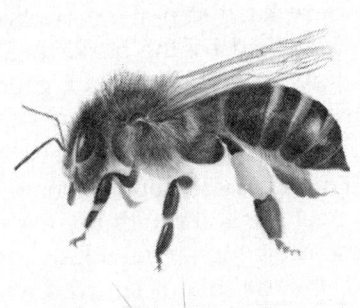

Apis mellifera—honeybee

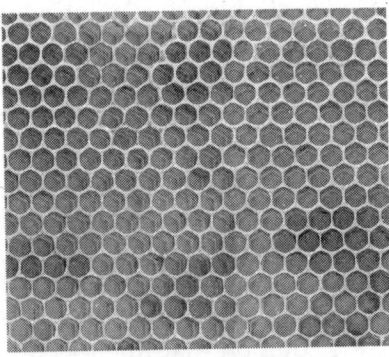

Honeycomb

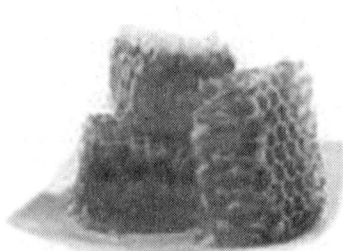

Hive with honey

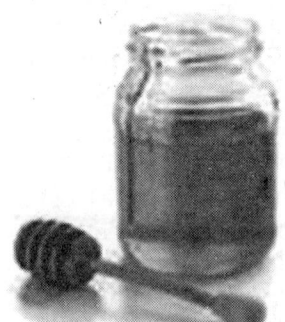

Raw honey

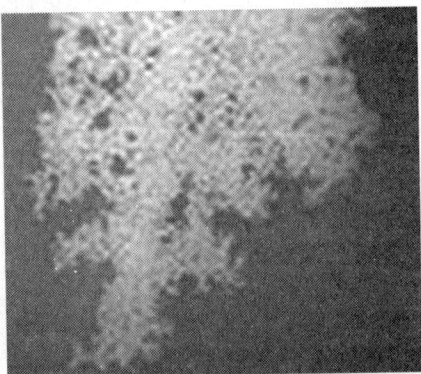

Crystallised honey

How Flower Nectar is turned into Honey?

The sweet, viscous honey is the product of industrious honeybees working as a highly organised colony, collecting the flower nectar and converting it into a high-sugar food store. The production of the honey by the bees involves several chemical processes, including digestion, regurgitation, enzyme activity and evaporation. The bees create honey as a highly efficient food source to sustain themselves all the year-round, including the dormant months of the winter. The bees store honey in wax structures called the honeycombs. Honey is collected from wild bee colonies, or from the hives of domesticated bees, and this practice is called beekeeping. In the honey-gathering industry, the excess honey in the hive is harvested for sale, with enough honey left in the hive to sustain the population of the bees until it becomes active again in the following spring.

Honeybee Colony

The colony generally consists of 3 main types of honeybees namely, one *Queen Bee* (the only fertile female insect), a few 1000 *Drone Bees* (a seasonally variable number of the fertile males to fertilise the new queens), and 20,000–40,000 of *worker bees* (the sterile females). The worker bees take on specialised roles as *foragers* and *house bees* in the production of the honey.

Collecting the Nectar

The actual process of transforming the flower nectar into honey requires team work. First, the older worker bees fly out form the hive in search of nectar-rich flowers. A forager bee using its straw-like *proboscis* sucks up the liquid nectar from the flower and stores it in a special organ called the *honey stomach* or *crop (proventriculus)* which lies just dorsal to its food stomach. This can hold 40 mg of nectar. The nectar begins with a water content of 70–80%. The bee continues to forage until its honey stomach is full (visiting 50–100 flowers per trip from the hive). The moment the nectar reaches the honey stomach, the salivary enzymes and proteins from the bee's hypopharyngeal gland are added to the nectar to begin the breaking down of the sugars (raising the water content slightly). The forager bees return to the hive where they regurgitate and transfer the nectar to the hive bees. The hive bees use their honey stomachs to ingest and regurgitate the nectar forming the bubbles between their mandibles, repeatedly until it is partially digested. The bubbles create a large surface area per volume and a portion of the water is removed through evaporation. The digestive enzymes of the bee hydrolyse the sucrose to a mixture of glucose and fructose that are less prone to crystallisation (this process is called *inversion*), and breakdown other starches and proteins increasing the acidity.

All the hive bees work together as a group with the regurgitation and digestion for as long as 20 minutes, passing the nectar from one bee to the next, until the product reaches the honeycombs in storage quality. The bee ingests the sugary offering and further breaks down the sugars by its own enzymes. The house bees within the hive pass the nectar from one individual to individual until the water content of the nectar is reduced to about 20%. The last house bee at this point regurgitates the fully inverted nectar into a cell of the honeycomb. It is then placed in the honeycomb and left unsealed while it is still high in its water content (about 50–70%). At this point, all the hive bees beat their wings furiously, fanning the nectar to evaporate its remaining water content. The temperature inside a hive being a constant 35°C (93–95°F), helps further evaporation, and as the water gets evaporated (to a content of about 18–20%), the sugars thicken into a substance which is recognisable as honey in the comb. When the individual cells of the comb are full of honey, the house bees cap the cells with beeswax, thus sealing the honey into the comb for late consumption. The bees wax is produced by the glands on the abdomen of the bee. Another source of honey, other than honey bees, is from a number of species of wasps, like *Brachygastra lecheguana* and *B. mellifica* (found in South and Central America). These species are known to feed on the nectar and produce honey. Some other wasps like *Polistes versicolor*, even consume honey themselves, alternating between feeding on the pollen in the middle of their life cycles and feeding on honey, which can provide for their energy needs.

Most of the foraging bees are dedicated to the collection of nectar for honey production, but 15–30% of the foragers collect the pollen on their flights. This is used to make *beebread*, which is the main source of dietary protein to the bee. The pollen also provides the bees with fats, vitamins and minerals. The bees add the enzymes and acids to it from the secretions of their salivary glands to keep the pollen from spoiling. The worker bee lives only a few weeks and during that time produces only 1/12th of tablespoon of honey. But working together, 1000s worker bees of the hive can produce >200 pounds of honey for the colony within a year. Of this amount, a beekeeper can harvest 30–60 pounds.

The production of honey is not possible at all without nectar from the plant flowers. The nectar is a sweet, liquid substance, it is an evolutionary adaptation that attracts the insects to the flowers and offers them nutrition. In return, the insects help pollinate the flowers by transferring the pollen clinging to their bodies from flower to flower during their feeding activity. The relationship is synergetic where both the parties benefit. The nectar in its natural state contains about 80% water along with complex sugars. If the same is left unattended to, it becomes a useless food source due to fermentation. But, by transformation into honey, it is an efficient and usable carbohydrate (14–18% water) which can be stored indefinitely without fermentation or spoilage. The long shelf-life of honey is due to an enzyme found in the stomach of bees. The bees mix glucose oxidase with the expelled nectar they previously consume which creates two by-products, gluconic acid and hydrogen peroxide which are partially responsible for the honey's acidity and its ability to suppress the growth of bacteria.

Characters

Virgin honey is a clear translucent (semi-transparent), syrupy, thick liquid of pale-yellow to yellowish brown colour having a distinctive flavour and a sweet acrid taste. On storage, honey becomes opaque and granules may be formed due to crystallisation of sugar. It is soluble in water and insoluble in alcohol and other organic solvents. Honey is optically active with rotation between + 0.6 and 0.3. Most of the microbes do not grow on honey because of its low water activity of 0.6. But, sometimes, it contains dormant endospores of *Clostridium botulinum* which can be dangerous to infants as they can transform into toxin-producing bacteria in the intestinal tract leading to poisoning (*Botulism*) and death. The flavours vary according to the source of the nectar and as such many types and grades are available in the market. The source can be determined by the study of pollen and spore present in it (*melittopalynology*).

Chemical Constituents

Honey gets its sweetness from its monosaccharides, fructose and glucose and it has the same relative sweetness as that of the normal sugar. Fresh honey is a supersaturated liquid containing more sugar than the water which can typically dissolve at ambient temperatures. At room temperature, this is a super-cooled liquid in which glucose will precipitate into solid granules. At the temperature of 20°C, the density of honey ranges between 1.38 and 1.45 kg/l. The viscosity of honey is affected greatly by both the temperature and water content. As cooling progresses, honey becomes more viscous at a rapid rate. While the honey is very viscous, it has low surface tension. Being hygroscopic, it has the ability to absorb moisture directly from the air, as such it is stored in sealed containers to prevent fermentation. Honey also exhibits varying degrees of electrical conductivity. The average pH of honey is 3.9 but can range from 3.4 to 6.1. It contains many organic and amino acids, and these may be aromatic or aliphatic. The latter contribute greatly to the flavour. The organic acids account for 0.17–1.17%. The gluconic acid is the most prevalent, while the minor organic acids consist of formic acid, acetic acid, butyric acid, citric acid, lactic acid, malic acid, pyroglutamic acid, propionic acid, valeric acid, capronic acid, plamitic acid, and succinic acid.

Honey is an aqueous solution of glucose (31.0%), fructose (38.5%), sucrose (1.0%), water (17.0%), other sugars like maltose and melezitose (9.0%), ash (0.17%), and small quantities of dextran and other complex carbohydrates. The amount of sugars may vary depending upon the source of the nectar and the activity of invertase enzyme responsible for converting nectar into honey. It contains dextrose, levulose, wax, volatile oil, mucilage, formic acid, ash, traces of enzymes, vitamins, proteins and colouring matter. Many compounds which function as the antioxidants such as chrysin, pinobanksin, vitamin C, catalase and pinocembrin occur in honey in tracer quantities. It also contains pollen dust, ethereal oil, many phosphates, lime

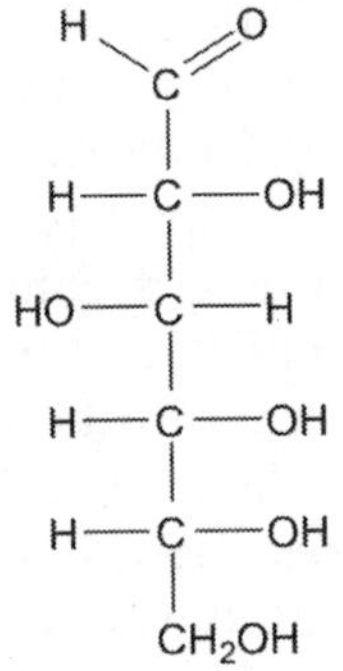

D-glucose ($C_6H_{12}O_6$)

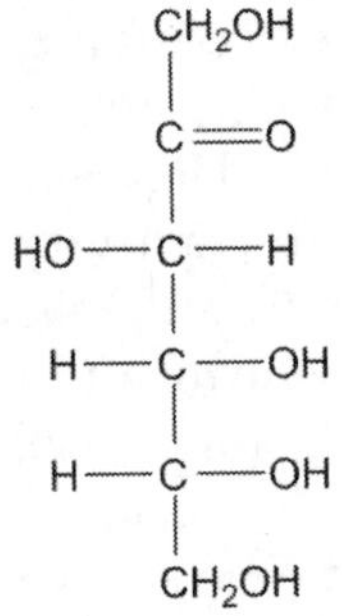

D-fructose ($C_6H_{12}O_6$)

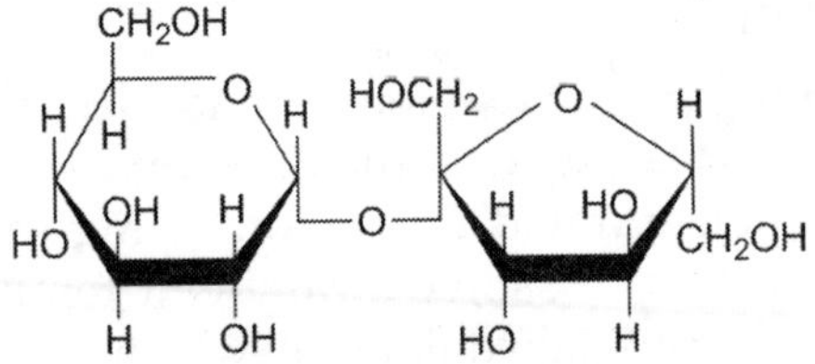

Sucrose ($C_{12}H_{22}O_{11}$)

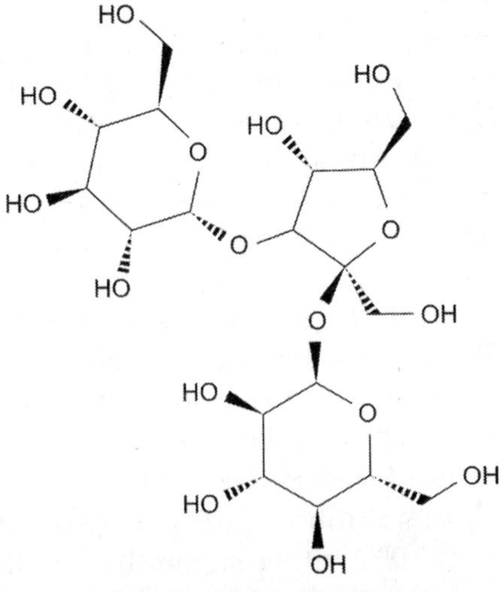

Melizitose ($C_{18}H_{32}O_{16}$)

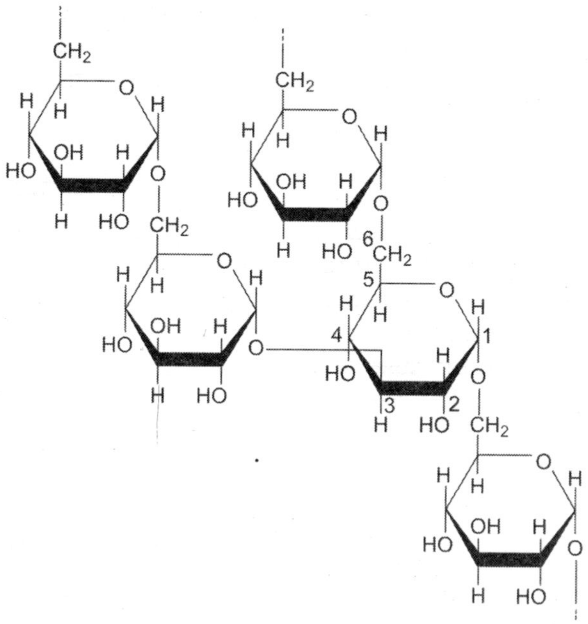

Dextran $C_{18}H_{32}O_{16}$ or $H(C_6H_{10}O_5)_xOH$

and iron in it. Honey contains both water soluble and fat soluble vitamins. It contains a diastatic ferment similar to that of saliva which converts starch into sugar. Honey is 36% denser than water with a specific gravity of 1.36 kg/litre.

Varieties of Honey

Susrutha described about eight different varieties of honey in his compendium, *Susrutha samhitha*. They are: *Mahshika* or the honey collected by the common bee, *Madhumakshika*; *Bhramara*, the honey collected by a large black bee, *Bhramara* which is useful in phlegm, cough, fever and epistaxis; *Kshaudra* or the honey collected by a small bee of tawny colour, *Kshudra* useful in the diseases of the eye; *Pauttika* or the honey collected by a small black bee which resembles a gnat, *Puttika*; *Chhatra* or the honey produced by yellow wasps which make their hives in the form of an umbrella and useful in worms, leucoderma, gonorrhoea, giddiness, hysteria and poisoning; *Argha* or the honey collected by yellow bees, *Bhramara*, beneficial in diseases of the eye, piles, cholera, cough, jaundice and ulcers; *Audalaka*, a bitter and acrid substance in the nests of the white ants; and *Dala* or the unprepared honey on the flowers which is said to be useful in increasing digestion, generation of the bile useful in gonorrhoea and vomiting. Out of all these, the first four are used in medicine.

Types of Honey by the Floral Source

In general, honey is classified by the floral source of the nectar from which it was made. The various types are:

a. **Blended honey:** This is a mixture of two or more honeys differing in floral source, colour, flavour, density or geographical origin. This is the most commercially available honey.

b. **Polyfloral honey:** This is also known as wildflower honey which is derived from the nectar of many types of flowers. The taste may vary from year to year, and the aroma and the flavor can be more or less intense, depending on which blooms are prevalent.

c. **Monofloral honey:** This is made primarily from the nectar of one type of flower. These have distinct flavours and colours because of the differences between the principal nectar sources.

Classification by Processing and Packaging

The different varieties of honey according to their processing and packaging are:

1. **Crystallised honey:** This is also called the 'granulated honey' or 'candied honey'. This occurs when some of the glucose has spontaneously crystallised from solution as the monohydrate. This can be returned to a liquid state by warming.

2. **Pasteurised honey:** This has been created when honey has been heated in a pasteurisation process at temperatures of 72°C (161°F) or higher, to destroy the cells of the yeast. It also liquefies any microcrystals in the honey. Heat also affects the appearance (the natural colour gets darkened), taste and the fragrance.

3. **Raw honey:** This refers to the honey as it exists in the beehive or as obtained by extraction, settling or straining without adding the heat. This contains some pollen and also may contain small particles of wax.

4. **Strained honey:** This type of honey has been passed through a mesh to remove the particulate material (such as pieces of wax, propolis and other defects) without removing the pollen, minerals or the enzymes.

5. **Filtered honey:** This is the honey of any type which has been filtered to the extent that all or most of the fine particles, pollen, air bubbles or other materials normally found in suspension have been removed. This is very clear and will not crystallise quickly and is preferred.

6. **Ultrasonicated honey:** This honey has been processed by ultra-sonication, a non-thermal processing. During this process, most of the cells of the yeast are destroyed. The cells that survive lose their growing ability and fermentation is reduced. This also eliminates the existing crystals and inhibits further crystallisation.

7. **Creamed honey:** This is also called 'whipped honey', 'spun honey', 'churned honey', 'honey fondant' and 'set honey'. The honey has been

processed to control crystallisation. The honey contains a large number of small crystals that prevent the formation of large crystals. The honey is smooth and spreadable in its consistency after processing.

8. **Dried honey:** The moisture has been extracted from the liquid honey to create completely solid, nonstick granules referred to as the dried honey. The process may or may not include drying and anticaking agents. This is used in baked goods and also to garnish the desserts.

9. **Comb honey:** This is also called 'cut-comb honey' and refers to honey that is still in the honeybee's wax and is traditionally collected using standard wooden frames in honey supers. The frames are collected and the comb is cut-out in chunks before packaging. Alternative to this method is the labour-intensive method, in which plastic rings or cartridges can be used that does not require the manual cutting of the comb.

10. **Chunk honey:** This honey is packed in wide-mouthed containers consisting of one or more pieces of comb honey immersed in extracted liquid honey.

11. **Honey decoction:** The decoctions are made from honey or its by-products which are dissolved in water and reduced (by means of boiling). Other ingredients are added to it after boiling (e.g. abbamele from citrus). The final product remains similar to molasses.

12. **Baker's honey:** This type of honey is outside the normal specification, due to a foreign taste or odour or because it has begun to ferment or has been overheated. This is generally used as an ingredient in food processing.

History of Honey

Honey has a long history of its use in foods and beverages as a sweetener and flavouring agent. It has also a role in religion and symbolism where it has been used as a talisman and a symbol of sweetness. The people of ancient Egypt used honey in cakes and biscuits. The people of Middle Eastern countries used honey for embalming the dead. Romans too used honey instead of gold to pay their taxes. The bee, honey and the uses were described in detail in *Naturalis Historia* written by Pliny, the Elder. The Egyptians offered honey to their God of Fertility, *Min*. In some parts of Greece like Rhodes, it was an earlier custom where a bride dipped her fingers in honey and made the sign of a cross before her entry into a new home. The Vedas and ancient literature of India which is thousands of years old mentioned the use of honey as a great medicinal and health food. Jews used honey as a symbol for their new year, Rosh Hashana. The Quran also promotes honey as a nutritious and healthy food and Prophet Mohammad strongly recommended honey for healing. Honey plays an important role in the festival of *Madhu Purnima* celebrated by Buddhists in India and Bangladesh. The Hebrew Bible, the Christian New Testament, the Book of Judges and the Book of Exodus also contain many references to honey.

Medicinal Uses

Honey is used as a demulcent, laxative and a sweetening agent. It is readily assimilated and hence is a good nutrient to infants and patients. Stored honey for more than a year old is said to be a good astringent and demulcent. It is also a detergent, pectoral, emollient and a laxative. It is a common ingredient of several cough mixtures, cough drops and vehicle for ayurvedic formulations. Recently, it is used in preparation of creams, lotions, soft drinks and candies also. Honey possesses nutritive properties too. The fatty acids present stimulate peristalsis, appetite and digestion. It is readily absorbable and most potent to provide the energy for the muscles of the heart. Along with lime, it regulates the secretions of internal glands of both sexes irrespective of the age from infancy to old age. If taken with cold water, it helps in bringing a sound sleep in babies. It has a capacity to decrease flatulence, increase the general metabolism and the amount of urine in children. It stimulates the mucous surfaces and also acts as a styptic. It is much used in the preparation of confections, decoctions, pills and powders. It is a remedy for constipation, indigestion, bronchial affections, asthma, chronic colds, and sore throat. It has a marked effect in severe cases of malnutrition with a weak heart, in cases of pneumonia in reviving the action of the heart and keeping the patient alive. In Western countries, honey is used more extensively in curing rickets, marasmus, malnutrition, scurvy, etc. In older people, it provides the required energy and heat to the body in addition to drying up of the phlegm and clearing the system of mucous. The Hindu, Greek and Arabic practitioners give honey along with their other medicines to diabetics, accountable for the levulose, ferment, special protein and vitamins present in it. The special protein secreted by the honeybee in the honey is capable of producing antibodies in the serum of rabbits. A paste made of honey with flour promotes the maturation of abscesses and buboes. It cures aphthae in the mouth, and on application to sore nipples and swollen mammae, it helps to dry up milk. Along with lime, it can be used as an external application to the temples during headaches, to the abdomen around the navel during colic and other parts of the body during sprains. It helps clean the teeth and the skin.

Clarified honey (*Mel depuratum*), the honey of commerce is a viscid transluscent liquid of light yellowish or brownish yellow colour which gradually becomes partially crystalline and opaque with a characteristic odour and very sweet taste. This is used as a demulcent, laxative and nutritive. It is one of the best medicinal vehicles used to cure cough, asthma, fever, dyspepsia, etc.

In myth and folk medicine, honey has been used both orally and topically to treat various ailments including gastric disturbances, ulcers, wounds on the skin, and skin burns by the ancient Greeks and Egyptians, and in Ayurveda and traditional Chinese medicine.

Non-medical Uses

Dietary Use

Honey is mainly used in cooking, baking, desserts, as a spread on the bread and added to beverages as tea. It is also used as a sweetener in commercial beverages like mead (honey wine or honey beer) and is also used as an adjunct in beer.

Religious Importance of Honey

In ancient Greek religion, the food of Zeus and the 12 Gods of Olympus was honey, in the form of nectar and ambrosia.

In Hinduism, *Madhu* (honey) is one of the 5 elixirs of life (*Panchamrita*). In Hindu temples, honey is poured over the deities in a ritual called *Madhu abhisheka*. The Vedas and other ancient literature mention the use of honey as a great medicinal and healthy food.

In Jewish tradition, honey is a symbol for the New Year, *Rosh Hashanah*. At the traditional meal, apple slices are dipped in honey and are eaten to bring a sweet new year. Sometimes, the greetings also show honey and an apple symbolizing the feast. Small straws of honey are given out in some congregations to usher in the New Year.

The *Hebrew bible* also contains many references to honey. In the *Book of Judges*, Samson found a swarm of bees and honey in the carcass of a lion; and in Old Testament law, offerings were made in the temple to God. The *Book of Leviticus* says that '*Every grain offering you bring to the Lord must be made without yeast, for you are not to burn any yeast or honey in a food offering presented to the Lord*' (2:11). In the *Books of Samuel*, *Jonathan* is forced into a confrontation with his father *King Saul* after eating honey in violation of a rash oath Saul has made. The proverbs 16:24 in the J.P.S. Tanakh 1917 version says: '*Pleasant words are as a honeycomb, Sweet to the soul, and health to the bones*'. The *Book of Exodus* describes the Promised Land as a '*land flowing with milk, and honey*' (33:3). In 2005, an apiary dating from the 10th century B.C. was found in Tel Rehov, Israel, that contained 100 hives and is estimated to produce a half ton of honey annually. Pure honey is considered *kosher*, though it is produced by a flying insect, non-kosher creature, other products of non-kosher animals are not kosher.

In Buddhism, honey plays an important role in the festival of *Madhu Purnima*, celebrated in India and Bangladesh. This day commemorates Buddha's making peace among his disciples by retreating into the wilderness. The legend has it that while he was there, a monkey brought him honey to eat. On *Madhu Purnima*, Buddhists remember this act by giving honey to monks, and monkey's gift is frequently depicted in Buddhist's art also.

In the *Christian New Testament, Matthew 3:4, John the Baptist* is said to have lived for a long period of time in the wilderness on a diet consisting of locusts and wild honey.

In Islam, an entire chapter (*Surah*) in the *Qur'an* is called *an-Nahl* (the bees). In his teachings (*hadith*), *Muhammad* strongly recommended honey for healing purposes. The Holy Book promotes honey as a nutritious and healthy food (Al-Quran 16:68–69).

Health Hazards and Honey

When taken in typical food amounts, honey is generally safe. But, it may have potential adverse effects in combination with excessive consumption, existing diseased conditions, or drugs. According to one study, the mild reactions to higher intake of honey are anxiety, insomnia or hyperactivity in about 10% of children. But, according to another study, no symptoms were detected. The consumption of honey may adversely interact with the existing allergies, levels of high blood sugar (as in diabetes) or anticoagulants used to control bleeding and other clinical conditions. From eating honey, the people who have a weak immune system may be at risk of bacterial or fungal infection though there is no high quality clinical evidence that this commonly occurs.

Adulteration

The most common adulterant of honey is the artificial invert sugar in addition to plant syrups (like maple, birch or sorghum), azo dyes and other foreign colouring substances.

REVIEW QUESTIONS

1. **Essay and Short Answer Questions**
    1. Write short notes on:
        a. Types of carbohydrates
        b. Uses of gum arabic
        c. Constituents of gum tragacanth
        d. Uses of agar
        e. Difference between potato starch and corn starch
        f. Differences between rice starch and wheat starch
        g. Differences between potato starch and wheat starch
        h. Differences between corn starch and rice starch
        i. Pharmaceutical and other uses of starch
        j. Characters and uses of pectin

2. Write an account of the source, macroscopic and microscopic properties, constituents and uses of guar gum.

3. What is the source of Isabgol? Describe the macroscopic characters of the seed. Add a note on its chemical constituents and uses.

4. What is the source of honey? Describe the method of collection, characters, constituents, varieties and pharmaceutical uses of honey.

2. Choose the Correct Alternative

1. Which of the following is a nitrogen containing substance?   [ ]
   a. Agarose   b. Agaropectin
   c. Agar   d. Agar solution

2. Which of the following is used as both a demulcent and a sweetening agent?   [ ]
   a. Starch   b. Pectin
   c. Honey   d. Indian gum

3. Enzyme present in acacia is: [ ]
   a. Oxidase   b. Lipase
   c. Amylase   d. Transferase

4. The following is not a hydrolysis product of tragacanth: [ ]
   a. Galacturonic acid   b. D-galactopyranose
   c. L-arabinose   d. Galactose

5. The best known and the oldest gum of all the natural gums is: [ ]
   a. Tragacanth gum   b. Guar gum
   c. Karaya gum   d. Acacia gum

6. The sugar present in gum arabic is: [ ]
   a. Arabinose   b. Arabinogalactan
   c. Arabinase   d. Agarose

3. Fill in the Blanks

1. Chemically ispagol consists of ....

2. Water insoluble portion of tragacanth is known as ....

3. Guar gum is the powder of the endosperm of the seeds of ....

4. Gum Arabic is the hardened sap from the stem of ....

5. Tragacanth gum of best quality comes from ....

6. The water soluble and insoluble components of tragacanth gum are .... and ....

7. The chief source of China grass is ....

8. The gelatinous principle of agar is ....

9. .... is insoluble in organic solvents.

10. .... is the principal constituent of guar gum.

4. True or False Statements:

1. Agar contains nitrogen containing substance. [True/False]
2. Pectin can be used as a plasma substitute. [True/False]
3. Guar gum is located in the endosperm of seeds. [True/False]
4. Agarose is the water insoluble portion of agar. [True/False]
5. Monosaccharides cannot be further hydrolysed. [True/False]
6. The monosaccharides in oligosaccharide are joined together by glycosidic linkages. [True/False]
7. Polysaccharides have no taste and are insoluble in water. [True/False]
8. Gum Arabic is highly soluble in glycerol. [True/False]
9. Agar powder is not soluble in boiling water. [True/False]
10. Agaropectin determines the viscosity of agar solution. [True/False]

5. A. Match the following:

1. Cod liver oil   [ ]   a. Suppositories
2. Olive oil   [ ]   b. Vitamin A
3. Linseed oil   [ ]   c. High iodine value
4. Shark liver oil   [ ]   d. Used for eczema and psoriasis
5. Kokum butter   [ ]   e. Vitamins A and D

B. Match the following:

1. Dextrin   [ ]   a. Braconnot
2. Pectin   [ ]   b. Biot and Persoz
3. Waxy starch   [ ]   c. Payen and L'ersoz
4. *Mel depuratum*   [ ]   d. Potato starch
5. Diastase   [ ]   e. Clarified honey

Chapter 7

Systematic Pharmacognostic Study of Lipids

LIPIDS

Lipids have a wider distribution in vegetable and animal kingdom and in plants they occur abundantly in fruits and seeds. In animals, lipids of a complex nature occur in brain and liver and play a significant role in the structure of cell membranes. Lipids are esters of long-chained fatty acids and alcohols. These are sparingly soluble in water but dissolve in organic solvents like chloroform, methanol, ether, benzene, hot alcohol and petroleum ether, the first two being the universal lipid solvents. They yield fatty acids on hydrolysis which can be readily utilised.

Lipids are normally grouped under three headings, simple lipids, compound lipids and derived lipids.

Simple Lipids

A simple lipid is a fatty acid ester of different alcohols and it carries no other substance. These belong to a heterogeneous class of nonpolar compounds, mostly insoluble in water, but soluble in nonpolar organic solvents (chloroform and benzene). These are esters of fatty acids with various alcohols. Simple lipids are represented by neutral fats, fats and oils and waxes.

Neutral Fats

Neutral fats are the esters of fatty acids with glycerol. These are also called triglycerides as three molecules of fatty acid undergo condensation with a single molecule of glycerol to form fat (tributyrin). Neutral fats are

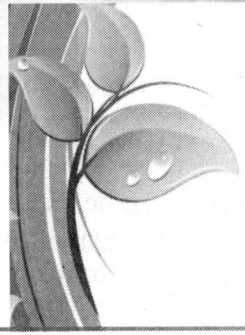

Tributyrin ($C_{15}H_{26}O_6$)
Linear formula ($CH_3CH_2CH_2COOCH_2)_2CHOCOCH_2CH_2CH_3$

composed of mixed glycerides (triglycerides which on hydrolysis yield non-identical fatty acids) which do not possess any free acid or basic group.

Fats and Oils

The fats are esters of fatty acids with glycerol. The fats are also called triglycerides because all the 3-hydroxyl groups of glycerol are esterified. Fats are tasteless, odourless, colourless and neutral in their reaction. They are liquids or solids or semisolids lighter than water and immiscible with water. The fats are insoluble in water, but readily soluble in ether, chloroform, petroleum ether, benzene and carbon tetrachloride. They are readily soluble in hot alcohol but slightly soluble in cold alcohol. They are themselves good solvents for other fats, fatty acids, etc. Several neutral fats are readily crystallised (beef and mutton). They have lower melting points. The specific gravity of the solid fats is about 0.86. They spread uniformly over the surface of water (due to lower surface tension).

Though they are nonvolatile, they decompose on strong heating and readily form emulsions when they are agitated with water in presence of emulsifiers like soap and gelatin. The vegetable fats contain phytosterol while the animal fats contain cholesterol. They have a larger amount of saturated fatty acids and undergo melting at higher temperatures (e.g. Lard). The saturated fatty acids possess higher melting point and are solids at room temperature. They have a maximum number of attached hydrogens and one terminal carbon has 3-hydrogen while the other end has a carboxylic group attached to it. They occur in a large proportion in animal triglycerides like palmitic acid and stearic acid. The fats are found in nature in large quantities, and are the best reserve of the food material in the human body. They act as insulator for the loss of body heat. They also act as a padding material for protecting the internal organs.

The oils are fats in the liquid state. The oils (fixed oils) contain a high proportion of unsaturated fatty acids, melt at a lower temperature and are liquids at room temperature. (e.g. coconut oil, olive oil and cotton seed oil). But, at lower temperatures, these may attain the state of a fat and fats too attain the state of oil at higher temperature. In general, all vegetable lipids are liquids (oils) at ordinary temperature while those from animals are fats, except cocoa butter (solid oil) and cod and shark liver oils (liquid fats). The unsaturated fatty acids have a lower melting point and are liquids at room temperature. They possess one or more double bonds. They occur more in plant glycerides such as oleic acid, linoleic acid and linolenic acid. Oils are grouped into three categories namely, drying oils, nondrying oils and semidrying oils.

$$CH_3(CH_2)_7-C=C-(CH_2)_7-\overset{\overset{\displaystyle O}{\|}}{C}-OH$$

Oleic acid ($C_{18}H_{34}O_2$) or [$CH_3 (CH_2)_7CH=CH(CH_2)_7COOH$]

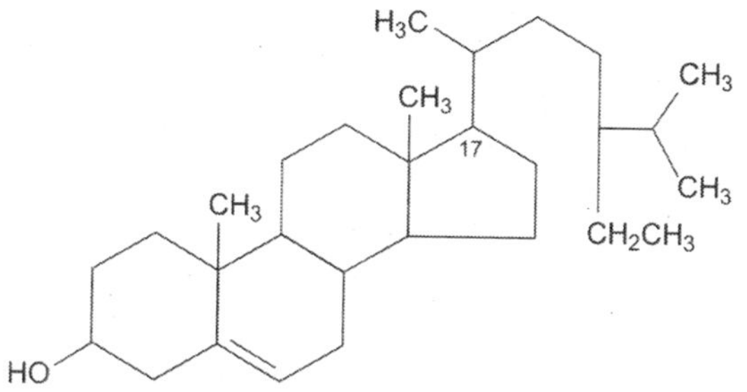

Stigmasterol or Stigmasterin (Phytosterol) $C_{29}H_{48}O$

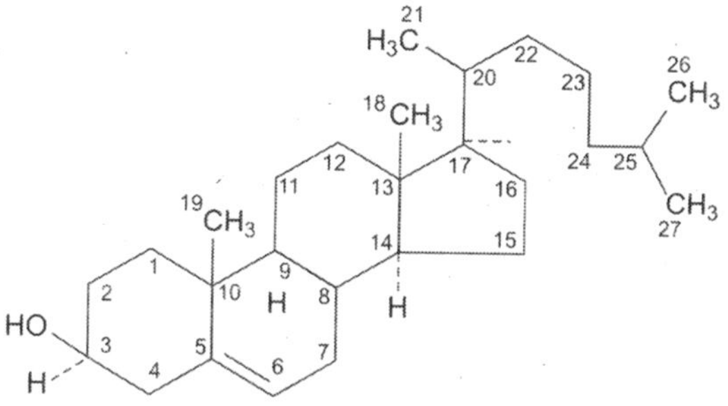

Cholesterol (animal sterol) $C_{27}H_{46}O$

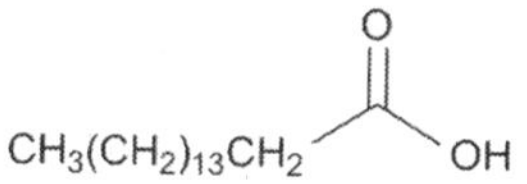

CH$_3$(CH$_2$)$_{13}$CH$_2$

Palmitic acid ($C_{16}H_{32}O_2$) or [CH$_3$(CH$_2$)$_{14}$CO$_2$H]

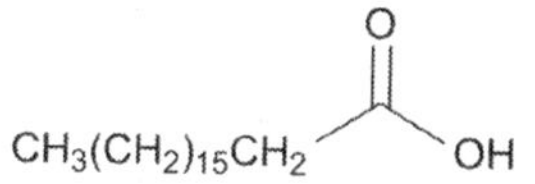

CH$_3$(CH$_2$)$_{15}$CH$_2$

Stearic acid ($C_{18}H_{36}O_2$) or [CH$_3$(CH$_2$)$_{16}$CO$_2$H]

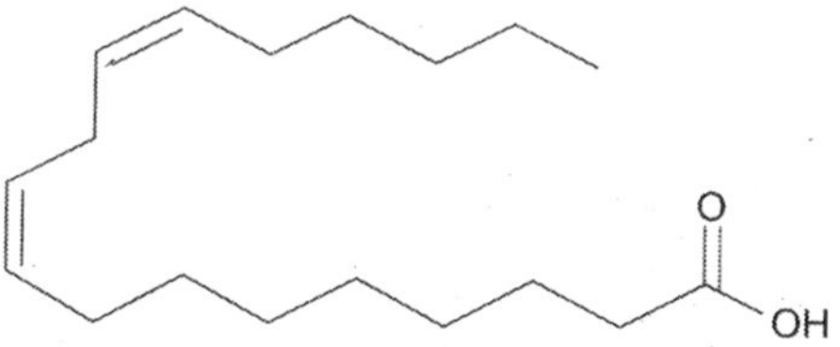

Linoleic acid ($C_{18}H_{32}O_2$) or [CH$_3$(CH$_2$)$_4$CH=CH–CH$_2$.CH=CH(CH$_2$)$_7$CO$_2$H]

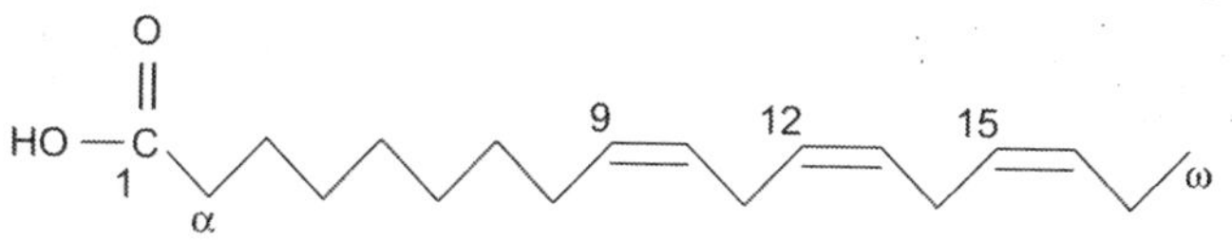

Linolenic acid ($C_{18}H_{30}O_2$) – [H$_3$C(–CH$_2$–CH=CH)$_3$–(CH$_2$)$_7$–COOH]

a. **Drying oils:** The drying oils possess glycerides of saturated acids with 2 or 3 double bonds like oleostearic acid and linolenic acid. These possess a property of slowly absorbing oxygen from air and to polymerise leading to the formation of a transparent elastic film or coating within 4–5 hours on the surface. These are useful in the manufacture of paints and oil cloth (linseed oil and hemp seed oil).

b. **Nondrying oils:** The nondrying oils possess triolein. They get rancid due to oxidation on exposure to light and storage during which process they are decomposed to glycerol and saturated and unsaturated fatty acids. The former get decomposed to ketones while the latter get oxidised to aldehydes and acids with a few carbon atoms (olive oil and almond oil).

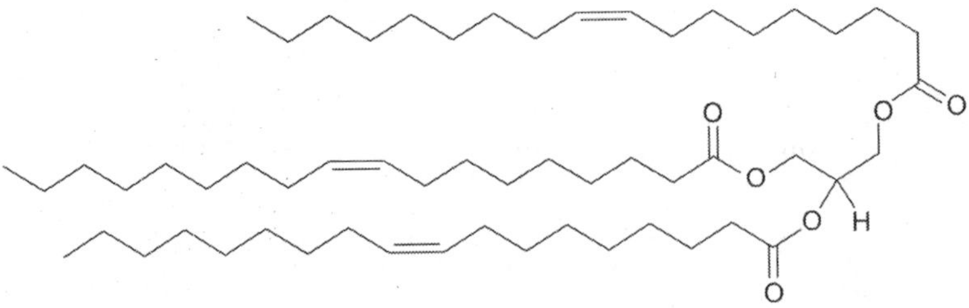

Triolein or 1, 2, 3-(9Z-octadecenoyl)-glycerol ($C_{57}H_{104}O_6$)

c. **Semidrying oils:** The semidrying oils have a lower/higher content of linolenic acid when compared to the drying/nondrying oils. Under excess hydrogen under pressure they get hydrogenated and if heated during cooking, some amount of glycerol escapes out due to hydrolysis and produces acrolein which may cause headache and eye trouble (sunflower oil and cotton seed oil).

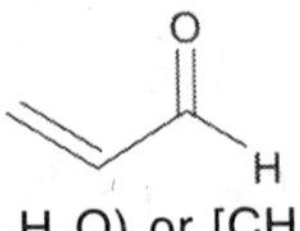

Acrolein (C_3H_4O) or [$CH_2=CHCHO$]

The fats and oils are used externally as emollients in treating wounds, burns, sunburn, eczema, dandruff, etc. as they have a protective action on the skin. Internally they can also be used as mild laxatives (castor oil). Some oils are used in the treatment of leprosy (chaulmoogra oil). These can also be used as food supplements, as vehicles and in the preparation of ointments and liniments. These also find a use in avitaminosis as some oils contain fat soluble vitamins like A, D and E.

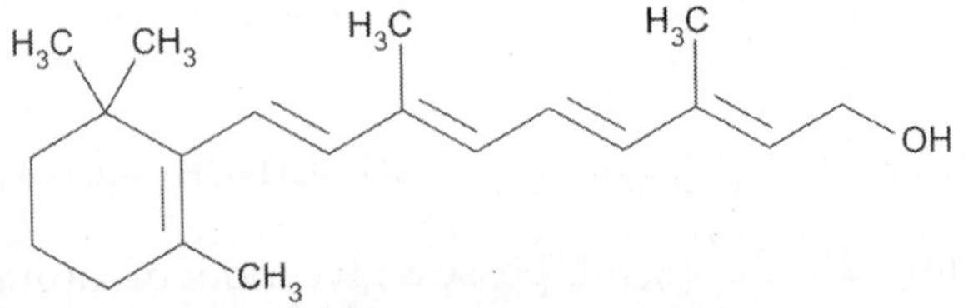

Vitamin A: Retinol ($C_{20}H_{30}O$)

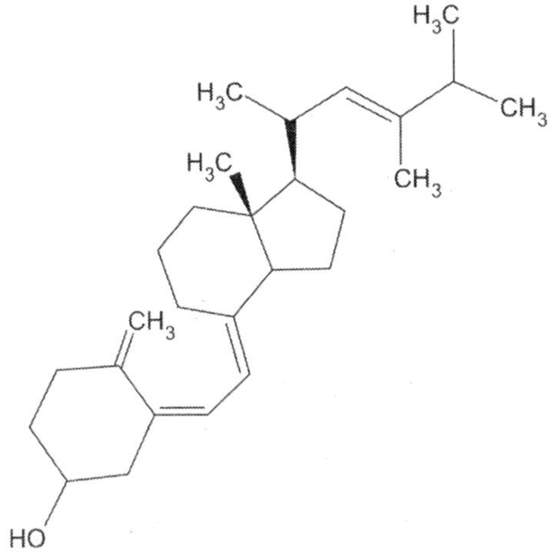

Vitamin D: Ergocalciferol or calciferol ($C_{28}H_{44}O$)

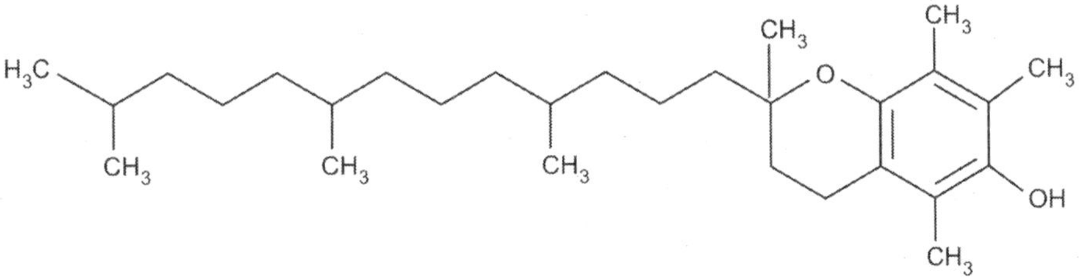

Vitamin E: Tocopherol ($C_{29}H_{50}O_2$)

Waxes

The waxes are solid esters of long-chain fatty acids (palmitic acid) with aliphatic or alicyclic higher molecular weight monohydric alcohols (other than glycerol). These are water-insoluble due to the weakly polar nature of the ester group. Waxes are similar to fats in their physical properties and are solids, semisolids or occasionally liquids. These are the esters of fatty acids and alcohols with a high molecular weight. The fatty acids that occur in waxes are similar to those in fats. The true waxes have alcohols other than glycerol while steryl esters have sterols. The component fatty acids and alcohols usually possess 24–36 carbons. The hydrocarbon chains in the waxes are completely reduced and are insoluble in water and are highly resistant to atmospheric oxidation. The waxes are chemically inert and are not digested by the enzymes, but split slowly with hot alcoholic potassium hydroxide. They are useful in the preparation of furniture polish. The waxes in insects, birds and furred animals serve as water barriers. These also help as a protective coating on the leaves and fruits, e.g. bees-wax (from bees), spermaceti (from the head of sperm whale), carnuba wax (from Brazilian palm) and lanolin (from the sheep wool). These are not suitable as food because the enzymes which can hydrolyze waxes are not present in our digestive system. These are mainly of three types, namely: true waxes—which are the esters of higher fatty acids with acetyl alcohol or higher straight chain alcohols; cholesterol esters are the esters of fatty acid with cholesterol; and vitamin A and vitamin D esters are palmitic or stearic acid esters of retinol (vitamin A) or vitamin D respectively.

Compound Lipids

These are marked by the presence of some additional groups or elements besides fatty acids and alcohol. The additional groups may have either a protein or elements like phosphorus, sulphur and nitrogen. The most important groups of compound lipids are phospholipids and glycolipids. The most important groups of compound lipids are phospholipids and glycolipids. Other compound lipids are: Lipoproteins, amino lipids, and sulpholipids (sulphatides).

Phospholipids (Phosphatides)

The phosphatides are the esters of fatty acids with glycerol containing an esterified phosphoric acid and a nitrogen base. These are present in larger amounts in the nerve tissue, brain, liver, kidney, pancreas and heart.

These contain glycerol, phosphoric acid and fatty acids and are fats in which one of the fatty acids has been replaced by phosphoric acid. The important phospholipids are lecithin, cephalin, plasmogen, phosphoinositide and phosphosphingoside. Lecithin in animals is needed for the normal transport and utilisation of other lipids in the liver. This is an important component of lipoproteins and occurs in the yolk of the egg. The enzyme lecithinase is present in bee venom and cobra venom. It dissolves in ether and alcohol but insoluble in acetone. Upon exposure to air, it becomes darker in colour. Cephalin occurs in tissues of animals in association with lecithin and also occurs in soybean oil. In cephalin, choline is replaced by ethanolamine, colamine or serine. Stearic acid, oleic acid, linoleic acid and arachidonic acid are the fatty acid components of cephalin. Plasmogen is present in the seeds of higher plants and abundant in the brain and muscles of animals. The molecular structure is similar to lecithin or cephalin except that a complex aldehyde is attached to the alpha-carbon of glycerol. This dissolves in all types of lipids. Phosphoinositide is widely distributed in plants as monophosphoinositide and is also reported to be in brain tissues as diphosphoinositide. Phosphosphingoside occurs in nervous tissues and is absent in plants and microbes. Sphingosine or phosphosphingosine replaces glycerol.

Biologically, these increase the rate of fatty acid oxidation, and act as the carriers of inorganic ions across the membranes. They help in blood clotting and also act as prosthetic group to certain enzymes. They also form the structures of the membranes, matrix of the cell wall, myelin sheath, microsomes and mitochondria.

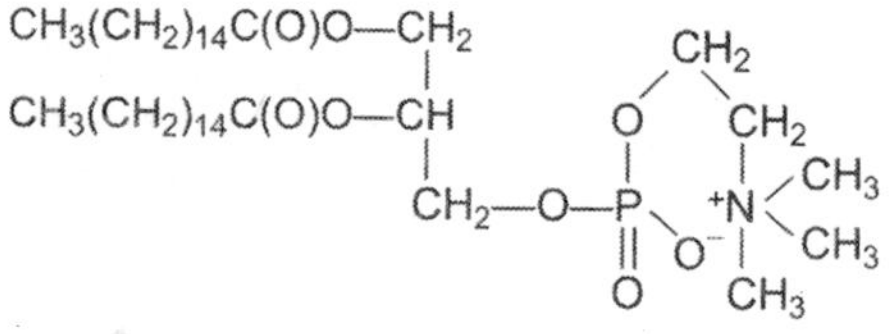
CH3(CH2)14C(O)O—CH2
CH3(CH2)14C(O)O—CH
CH2—O—P
CH2
CH2
O
O
O⁻
+N
CH3
CH3
CH3

Lecithin ($C_{40}H_{80}NO_8P$)

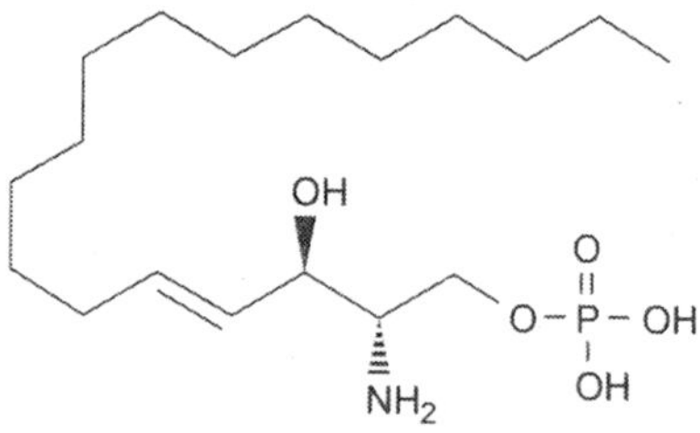
OH
NH2
O
O-P-OH
OH

Sphingosine ($C_{18}H_{37}NO_2$)

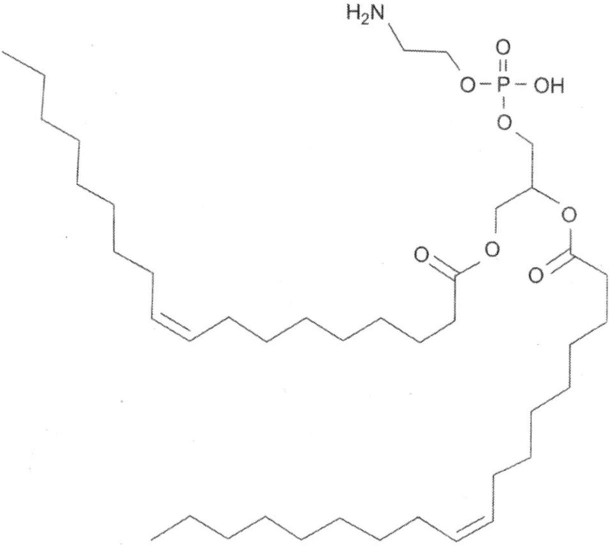
H2N
O
O-P-OH
O
O
O
O
O

Cephalin ($C_{41}H_{78}NPO_8$)

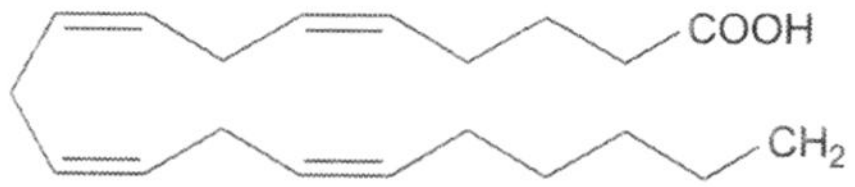
COOH
CH2

Arachidonic acid ($C_{20}H_{32}O_2$)

Phospholipids on the basis of the type of alcohol present, are classified into three types: Glycerophosphatides (glycerol is the alcohol group, e.g. cephalin [phosphatidyl ethanolamine]); lecithin [phosphatidyl choline], phosphatidyl serine, plasmalogens and phosphatidic acid); phospho-inositides (inositol is the alcohol, e.g. lipositol [phosphotidyl inositol]; and phosphosphingosides (sphingosine is an amino alcohol, e.g. sphingomyelin).

Glycolipids (Glycosphingolipids)

These lipids contain an amino alcohol [sphingosine or iso-sphingosine] attached with an amide linkage to a fatty acid and glycosidically to a carbohydrate moiety [like a sugar, amino sugar and sialic acid].

These are represented by phosphosphingosides associated with carbohydrates and occur in plant seeds. The common carbohydrate units are galactose, arabinose and fructose. These are represented by cerebrocides and ceramides. The former are mainly associated with myelin sheath of nerves and white matter of the brain while the latter serve as antigens.

These are further classified into: Cerebrosides and Gangliosides. The former contain galactose, a high molecular weight fatty acid and sphingosine. These are the chief constituents of myelin sheath. These are differentiated by the type of fatty acid, e.g. kerasin [with lignoceric acid], cerebron [with cerebronic acid (hydroxyl-lignoceric acid), nervon (with an unsaturated homologue of lignoceric acid, called nervonic acid), oxynervon (with hydroxyl-nervonic acid), etc. The latter are the glycolipids that occur in the brain. The gangliosides contain ceramide (sphingosine + fatty acids), glucose, galactose, N-acetylgalactosamine and sialic acid. Some also contain di-hydrosphingosine (or gangliosine) in place of sphingosine. Most of these contain glucose, 2 molecules of galactose, 1 molecule of N-acetylgalactosamine and up to 3 molecules of sialic acid.

Derived Lipids

These are the hydrolytic products of lipids and lipid like compounds such as sterols, carotenoids, essential oils, aldehydes, ketones, alcohols and hydrocarbons. These are the solid waxes which occur abundantly as alcohols or esters of fatty acids and are highly soluble in fat solvents. These do not get saponified. Sterol distribution is wider in plants, animals and microbes, and also occurs in cell membranes and cellular components.

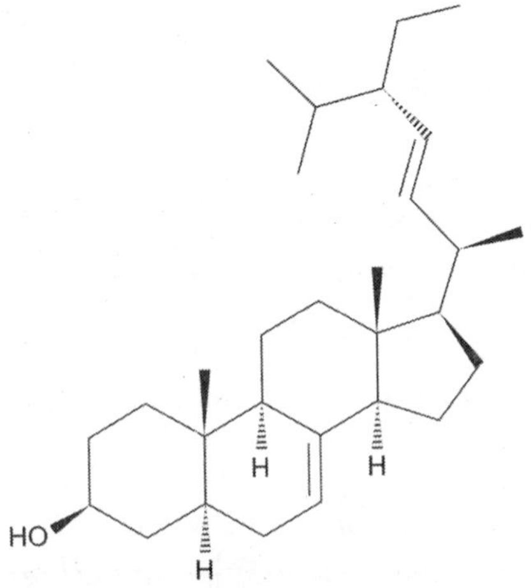

Spinasterol ($C_{29}H_{48}O$)

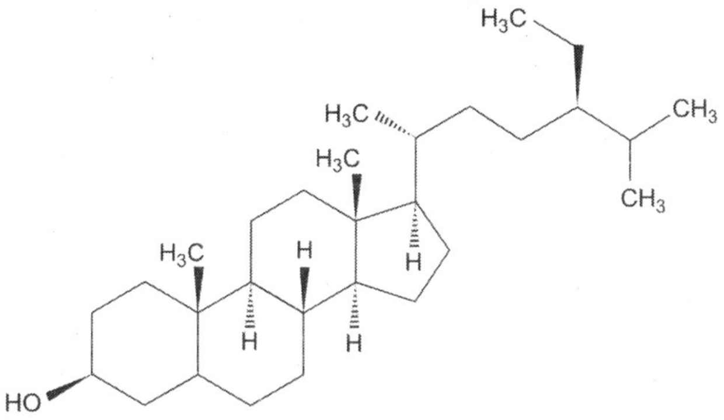

Sitosterol ($C_{29}H_{50}O$)

The best known sterols are cholesterol (in animals), spinasterol (in spinach), cabbage stigmasterol (in coconut and soybean) and sitosterol (in the seeds of cereals). Carotenoids are the important plant pigments and essential oils can be isolated from pine, peppermint, lemon, eucalyptus and rose. These include: Fatty acids, saturated fatty acids, and others. Essential fatty acids, refined and hydrogenated oils, and steroids. Castor oil, cod liver oil, shark liver oil, linseed oil, cocoa butter, kokum butter, beeswax, wool fat, hydnocarpus oil, lard oil and olive oil are described below.

CASTOR OIL

Synonyms

Ricinus oil, Oleum ricini, Aceite de Ricino (Colombia), Zejt ir-Riegnu (Maltese), Zait al kharwaa (Arabic), Erand oil (Tamil-from Sanskrit, *Eranda*), Aamudam (Telugu).

Synonyms for Castor

Castor oil plant (English), Erandam or Vatari (Sanskrit), Ricin (French), Gemeiner Wunderbaum (German), Arand (Hindi and Punjabi), Khirva (Arabic), Bedanjir (Persian), Bheranda or Sadabheranda (Bengali), Eri (Assamese), Erandi (Gujarati and Maharashtrian), Aamudamu chettu (Telugu), Chittamani (Tamil), Haralu (Kannada), Chittamanaku (Malayalm), Endaru (Sinhalese), Kesusi (Burmese), Miniak-jarah (Malayese).

Biological Source

Castor oil is a fixed vegetable oil obtained from the seeds (castor beans) of *Ricinus communis* L. (Family: Euphorbiaceae). The name *Ricinus* is a Latin word for *tick* and is so named because the seed has red markings (bloody) and a bump (caruncle) which resembles the head of certain dog-ticks and *communis* in Latin means 'common'. The common name 'castor oil' comes from its use as a replacement for 'castoreum', a perfume made from the perineal glands of the beaver (*castor* in Latin). It also has another name, palm of christ or *Palma Christi* because of its ability to heal wounds and cure ailments. The plant is the most poisonous in the world according to Guinness Book of World Records (2007 edition) due to presence of ricin, although the reports of actual poisoning are rare.

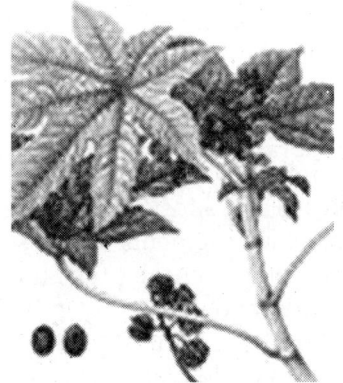

Ricinus communis

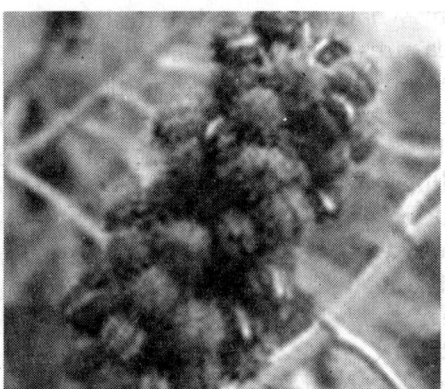

Plant in fruit

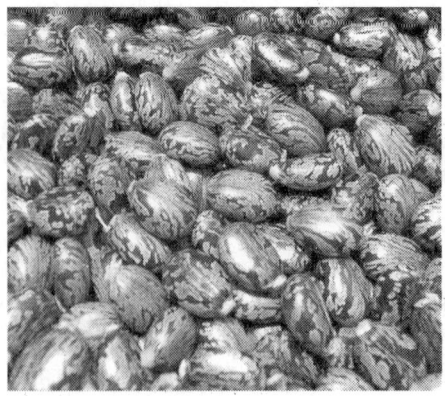

Castor seeds

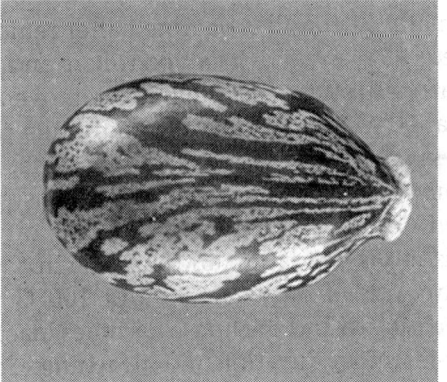

Single seed

Geographical Source

Castor is a native of India which is widely naturalised and cultivated and is common and apparently wild in the jungles. It is also cultivated throughout India, chiefly in Tamil Nadu, West Bengal and Maharashtra and grows wild in most tropical and temperate countries. Two varieties are known, a perennial bush with large red seeds yielding about 40% of oil in the tropics and a smaller annual herb with small grey seeds with brown spots and yielding about 37% of oil in the temperate regions. The plant is indigenous to South-eastern Mediterranean basin, Eastern Africa and India but is widespread in tropical regions of the world. The principal castor producing countries are Brazil, India, China, Russia, South America and Thailand.

Characters of Seeds (Beans)

The seeds show considerable differences in size and colour. They are oval, somewhat compressed ventrally, the dorsal surface being convex. The seed measures 8–18 mm in length and 4–12 mm in breadth. The testa is very smooth, thin, glossy and brittle. The colour may be a more or less uniform grey, grey-brown or black, or may be variously mottled with reddish-brown or black spots and lines. Tegmen is white, membranous adhering to large, yellowish-white oily endosperm. A small, often yellowish, caruncle is usually present at one end covering the micropyle, from which runs the line-like raphe to terminate in a slightly raised chalaza at the opposite end of the seed. The testa is easily removed to disclose the papery remains of the nucellus surrounding the endosperm. Within the latter lies the embryo, with two thin, flat, papery cotyledons, a conical hypocotyl and a radicle directed towards the caruncle. The taste is oily and acrid.

Collection and Preparation

Usually castor oil is obtained after removing the seed coat. Sometimes, the seeds are placed in grooved rollers and crushed when the testa (outer seed coat) becomes loosened and is removed by blowing in the air current. The cleaned seeds are decorticated, hulls removed and the kernels are cold-pressed at room temperature by suitable hydraulic presses (oil-expellers) maintaining the pressure of 1–2 tons per square inch. About 30% of the seed oil is thus extracted out. The oil is filtered but it contains ricin (a poisonous principle) and enzyme lipase. Steam is passed into the oil at a temperature between 80 and 100°C when ricin gets coagulated and precipitated and the lipase becomes inactive. The oil is filtered and is refined by steaming, filtration and bleaching. Cold expression yields medicinal oil

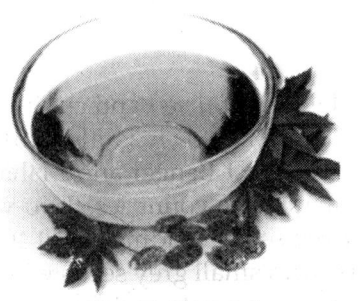
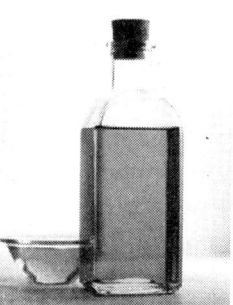

Pure castor oil

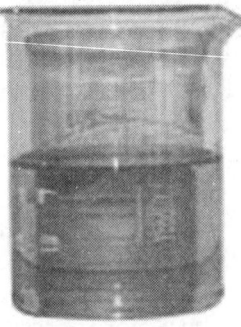

Bleached castor oil

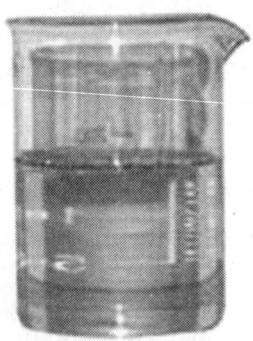

Sulphated castor oil

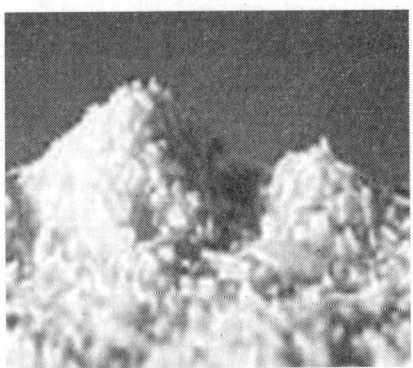

Hydrogenated oil

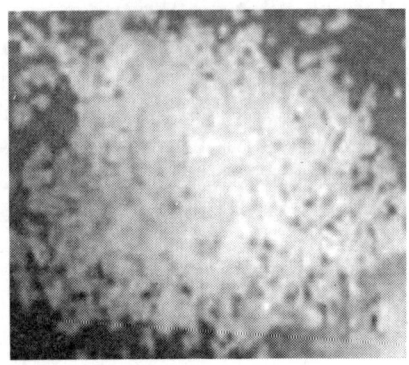

Castor oil crystals

and known in commerce as 'cold drawn oil' (used for medicinal purposes). Remaining oil of the seeds is extracted by hot expression or solvent extraction methods. This oil is not suitable for medicinal purposes and is only of industrial significance. The oil cake or the pomace is a by-product.

Chemical Constituents

The pure oil is clear or viscid fluid almost colourless to very pale yellow and with mild or slight odour and highly nauseable and disagrreable taste (cold-drawn oil). The fixed oil is 45% and is soluble in alcohol. It has a boiling point of 313°C and specific gravity of 0.96. It dissolves freely in alcohol, ether and glacial acetic acid. Castor oil consists of ricinolein which is a mixture of the triglycerides of ricinoleic, isoricinoleic acids along with oleic, stearic, palmitic and dihydroxystearic acids. The fixed oil also contains a toxalbumose ricin, lipase and protein. The oil is viscid and the purgative action is said to be due to ricinolein and tristearin, the glyceride of dihydroxystearic acid. The cake left after expression contains an extremely poisonous toxin known as ricin (a deadly water-soluble protein, lectin), which make it unfit for use (violently purgative, causes agglutination and haemolysis of RBCs, haemorrhage in the digestive tract and damage to liver and kidneys) as cattle feed but it can be used as a fertiliser.

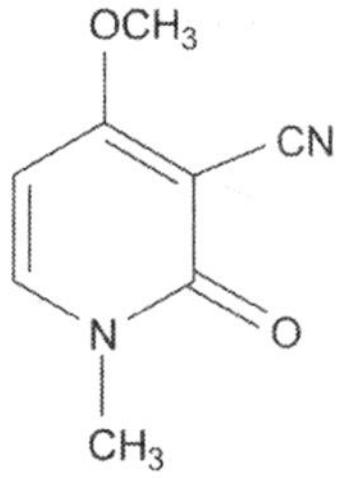

Ricinine or ricinin ($C_8H_8N_2O_2$)

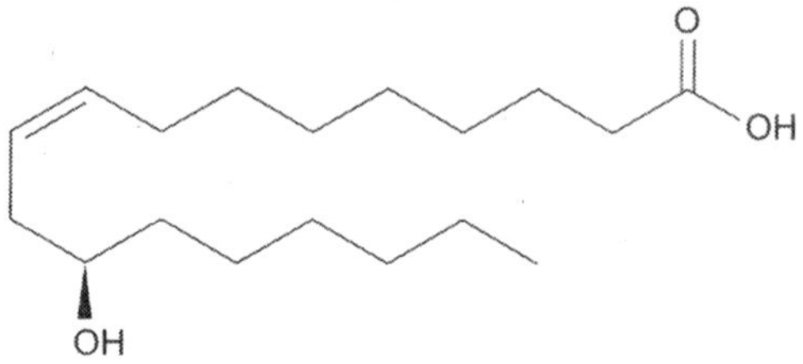

Ricinoleic acid ($C_{18}H_{34}O_3$)

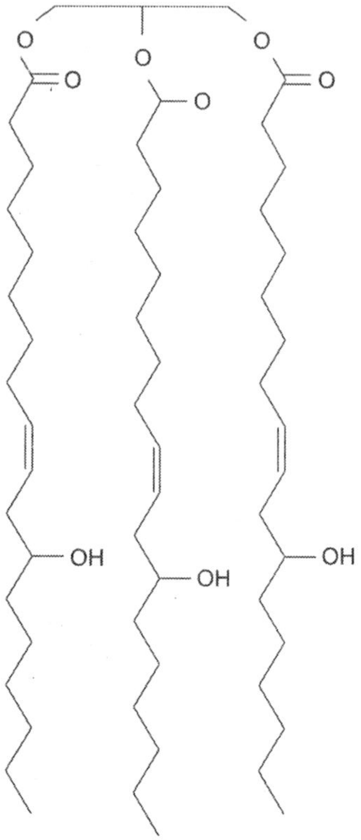

Ricolenic acid

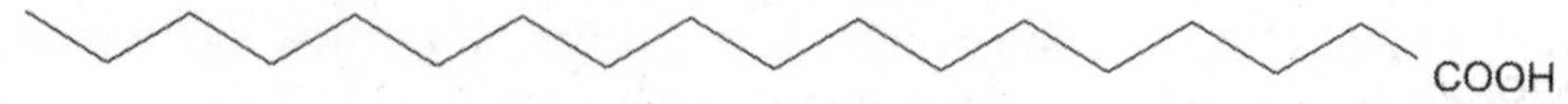

Stearic acid ($C_{18}H_{36}O_2$)

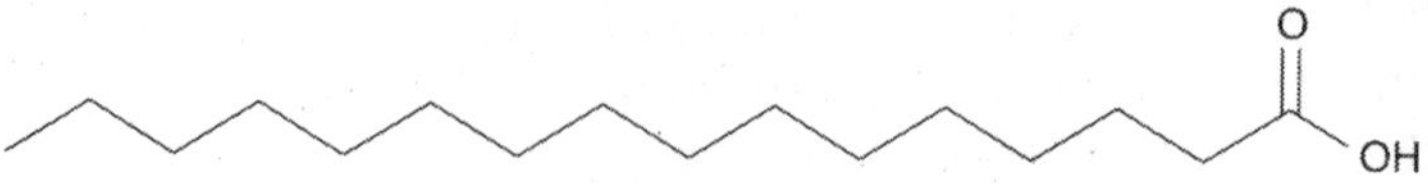

Palmitic acid ($C_{16}H_{32}O_2$)

$$CH_3(CH_2)_7-CH=CH(CH_2)_7C(O)O-CH_2$$
$$CH_3(CH_2)_7-CH=CH(CH_2)_7C(O)O-CH$$
$$CH_3(CH_2)_{14}C(O)O-CH_2$$

Tristearin ($C_{57}H_{110}O_6$)

History of Castor Oil

The seeds of castor have been found in Egyptian tombs which date back to 4000 BC and the oil was used mostly to fuel lamps. The Greek travellers and Herodotus (called it as *kiki* – 4th centruy BC) also noted the use of the oil for lighting, body ointments and improving the growth and texture of hair. Theophrastus and Dioscorides (1st century) not only described the plant but also gave an account of extraction and said that it is not fit for food, but used in medicine externally and that the seeds are extremely purgative. Pliny also described it to be a drastic purgative. It is understood that Cleopatra used the oil to brighten the whites of her eyes. The Ebers Papyrus, the ancient Egyptian medical treatise (1552 BC) describes the oil as a laxative. Egyptian doctors used the oil to protect the eyes from irritation. In United States, the oil has been used medicinally since the days of the pioneers. In India, since 2000 BC the use of the oil in wick lamps, as a facial oil and local medicine as a laxative, purgative and cathrtic in Unani, Ayurvedic and other systems of medicine has been well-documented. The Ayurvedic medicine considers the oil as the *'king of medicinals'* for curing arthritis. Gerard (1597) called *Oleum ricinum* (Ricinus or Kik) and said that it can be used externally in skin diseases. In China, the seed and the oil have been used in local medicine for dressings and internal use. In the early civilisations, the oil was used in the rituals of sacrifice to please the gods. Under the regime of Benito Mussolini, the Italian dictator, the oil was known to have been used as an instrument of coercion by the paramilitary to cause the death of the opponents by forced ingestion of the large amounts of the oil to trigger severe diarrhoea and dehydration. In Canary Islands, the fresh leaves are used as an external application by nursing mothers to increase the flow of milk.

Medicinal Uses

Castor oil, once widely used as a domestic purgative is now more restricted to hospital use for administration after food poisoning and as a preliminary to intestinal examination. The oil is a non-irritant purgative and after reaching the duodenum it is decomposed by the pancreatic juice into ricinoleic acid which irritates the bowels and stimulates the intestinal glands and the muscular coat thus causing purgation. It acts in 4 to 5 hours causing liquid stools without pain or griping and has a sedative effect too on the intestines. The Food and Drug Administration (FDA) of USA has categorised castor oil as 'generally recognised as safe and effective' (GRASE) as a laxative with its major site of action, the small intestine. Ricinoleic acid is absorbed into the blood and tissues and excreted along with the human milk which when sucked by the babies imparts its purgative action. This also exerts anti-inflammatory effects. Ricinin is a violent irritant of the intestines, kidneys and bladder and gives rise to inflammation of the bile duct and very often causes jaundice and dysuria. The pure oil is administered either plain or in emulsion with mucilage in inflammatory conditions of the bowels, in diarrhoea of children. In simple diarrhoea of adults it is mixed with opium. It is also useful in irritable conditions of the system among the debilitated persons and for young children. It is also used for lying-in women after childbirth and before the childbirth to facilitate delivery, in operations for lithotomy, in peritonitis, in dysentery, and inflammatory diseases of the urinary organs. The oil is best given floating in milk, strong coffee, dry ginger water or omum water. In small doses, the oil is great service to soften the faeces and lubricate the passages in painful affections of the rectum and haemorrhoids (piles). In sore nipples, the oil is smeared over freely each time the child is removed from the breast. It is used as an enema in constipation. The oil is also used to expel worms, in complaints of ringworm and itch. It is used to remove the foreign bodies in the eyes and ears. The oil is much praised for its efficacy in chronic articular rheumatism, colic, sciatica and lumbago. A poultice of the crushed seeds promotes suppuration, helps in the maturation of the boils and reduces the gout as well as rheumatic swelling. As the oil is an excellent solvent of pure alkaloids like atropine, cocaine, etc. it is used in ophthalmic surgey. The oil can also be used in many disorders like breast pain and gallstones.

In folk medicine, it is used in skin problems, burns, sunburns, skin cuts and abrasions, etc. It has also been used to remove the styes in the eye and as a rub for abdominal complaints, headaches, muscle complaints, inflammation, skin eruptions, lesions and sinusitis. It has also been noted for its ability in acne healing. The oil has been used to induce childbirth in pregnant women, but the use requires consultation of a medical practitioner. In South Egypt, women use a full large spoon of castor oil to prevent the pregnancy for one year.

Non-medical Uses

Castor oil is put to many other uses industrially in transportation, cosmetics, illumination, lubrication of machinery, hydraulic and brake fluids, adhesives, making of soaps, candles, paints, dyes, coatings, pomatum, inks, lacquer, refrigetation lubricants, paper making, leather dressing, cold resistant plastics, waxes, polishes, greases, rubbers, washing powders, waxes, machine oils, pigments, nylon and perfumes, etc. It is also a useful lubricant in jet, diesel and race-car engines and high voltage capacitors. Earlier, it was used by the Egyptians as an ointment thousands of years ago and in India for lighting the rail road lanterns as recently as 1895. It is also employed as an emollient in preparation of lipsticks and as sulphorecinolate in tooth formulation being a strong bactericide. Turkey red oil (sulfated castor oil) was the first synthetic detergent after ordinary soap and is used in the formulation of lubricants and dyes. The oil is used as a food additive, flavouring, and candies, as a mold inhibitor and in packaging. The important minor use of the oil is in the manufacture of fly-papers.

The side effects that require medical attention include confusion, irregular heart beat, muscle cramps, skin rash and weakness. The other less serious side effects are belching, diarrhoea and nausea. If used moderately, the oil is normally safe. However, pregnant women, lactating women and people suffering from intestinal blockages, acute inflammatory intestinal disease, appendicitis or abdominal pain should not take castor oil without the approval of the medical practitioner.

COD LIVER OIL

Synonyms

Oleum morrhuae, Oleum Jecoris Aselli, Cod oil, Lebertran (German), Huile de Foie de Morue (French), De higado de bacalao (Spanish), Oleo de figado de bacalhai (Portuguese), Olio de fegato di merhizzo (Italian), Huodao fukuan (Chinese).

Synonyms for Cod

Torsk, Kabliau (Danish), Bakalar, Bakalarom (Czech), Voor de mal houden (Dutch), Cabillaud (French), Kabeljau (German), Vakalaos, Bakaliaros, Bakalaos (Greek), Bacalhau (Portuguese), Treska (Russian), Abadejo, Bacalao (Spanish), Kabeljou (Swedish), Triski, Triska (Ukrainian).

Biological Source

Medicinal cod liver oil is a fixed oil prepared from the fresh liver of the codfish, *Gadus callarias* (=*Gadus morhua morhua*, *G. arenosus*, *G. callarias*, Baltic cod, Variable cod), *G. morrhua* L. (=*Gadus morhua callarias* is the accepted name, Atlantic cod) and other species of *Gadus* (Family: Gadidae) under conditions which give a palatable oil containing due proportion of vitamins.

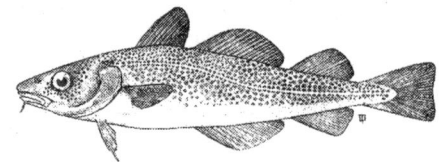

G. morhua—Baltic cod

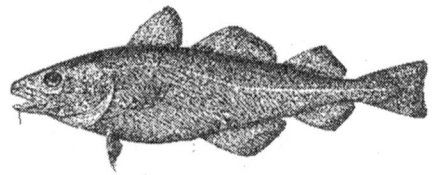

G. callarias—Atlantic cod

Geographical Source

Cod fish inhabits the cooler and deeper waters of Northern Atlantic Ocean, and cod liver oil is a by-product of the fishing industry. Large quantity of oil is prepared in coastal regions of USA, Norway, Japan, Poland, Scotland, Iceland, Germany, Denmark and Great Britain.

Collection and Preparation

The livers of the cod fish are removed while the fish are still fresh during the fish processing by hand gutting or mechanical splitters, taking care to exclude the gallbladder. They are then washed and the oil is extracted either by direct steam process or by subjecting them to a gentle heat in iron pots or by cold expression or electrolysis. The steaming takes place in closed containers in carbon dioxide atmosphere to prevent oxidation. The first fraction called the 'ordinary refined oil' is marketed for medicinal purposes. The second fraction called 'common cod oil' is not used medicinally. The oil is refined by chilling in tin vessels at a low temperature of minus 5°C; and the precipitated stearin or solid fat is separated from the lighter vitamin-containing oil by decantation and filtration. Finally, the oil is adjusted to definite vitamin-content (50 units per gram) by admixture, if necessary, of different lots with higher or lower vitamin levels.

Characters

Cod liver oil is a thin, pale-yellow liquid that has a distinctive, mild sardine-like flavour to an intense odour of a fish but not rancid odour and a fishy taste. It is slightly soluble in alcohol and completely soluble in chloroform, ether, carbon disulphide and ethyl acetate. It has a specific gravity of 0.918

to 0.927 at 25°C. The medicinal value of oil is due to vitamin A and vitamin D group. 1 gm of oil contains not less than 255 mcg of vitamin A and 2.125 mcg of vitamin D. The oil contains glyceryl esters of oleic, linoleic, gadoleic, myristic, palmitic and other acids. Cod liver oil also contains 7% eicosapentanoic acid and 7% docosahexanoic acid. Both of them are omega-3 fatty acids.

Chemical Constituents

Cod liver oil has high levels of omega-3 fatty acids, EPA and DHA. It also contains fat soluble vitamin A, vitamin D, traces of iodine and bromine, organic compounds, jecolein, therapin, palmatin, biliary acids, cholesterin, the alkaloids aselline and morrhuine, etc. The oil is a mixture of glycerides of fatty acids, predominantly oleic acid, gadoleic acid and palmitoleic acid. Vitamin A represents the growth promoting and anti-xerophthalmic element while vitamin D represents the anti-rachitic element of the oil.

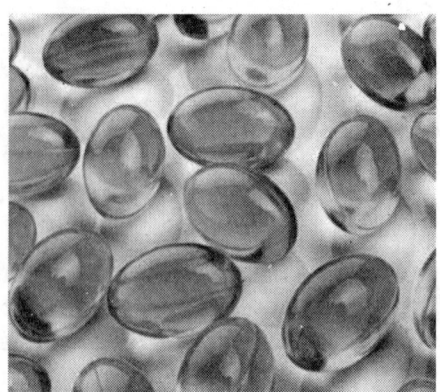

Gelatin capsules of oil

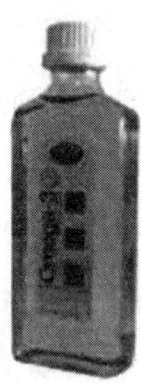

Pure cod liver oil

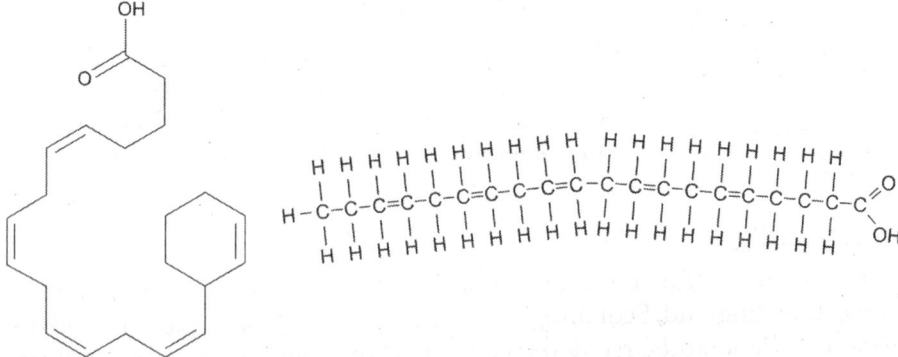

EPA (eicosapentaenoic acid)—omega 3 fatty acid ($C_{20}H_{30}O_2$)

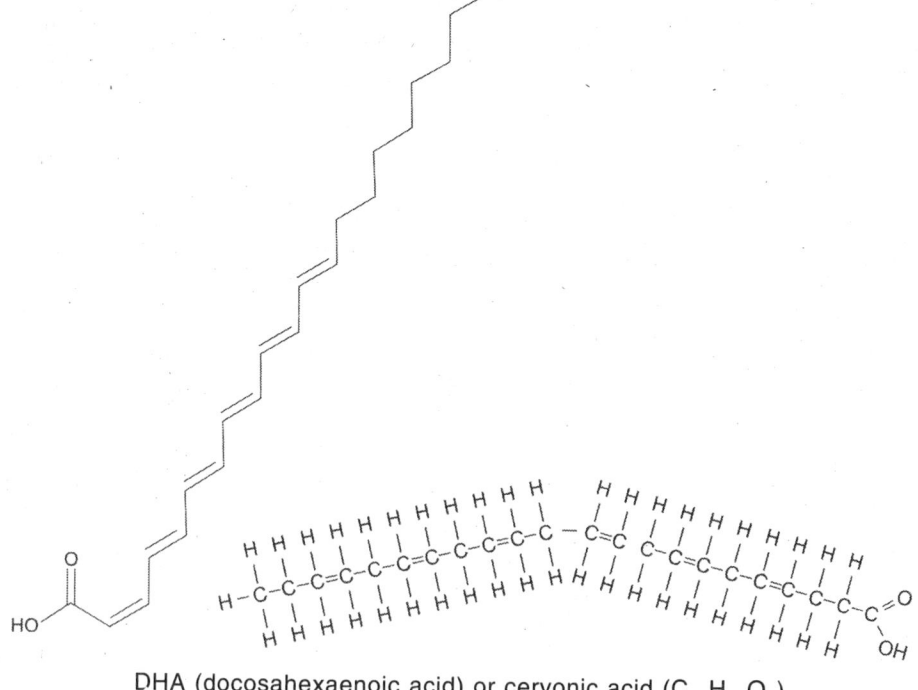

DHA (docosahexaenoic acid) or cervonic acid ($C_{22}H_{32}O_2$)

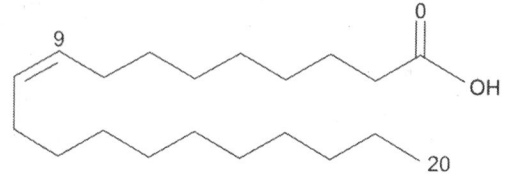

Gadoleic acid ($C_{20}H_{38}O_2$)—eicosenoic acid

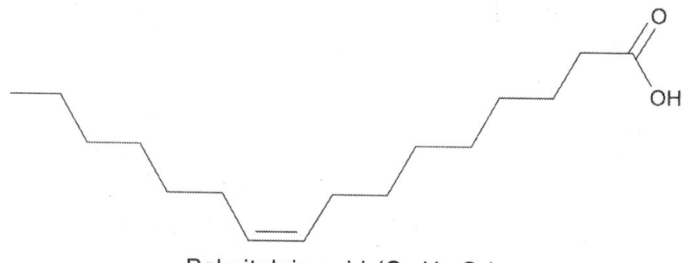

Palmitoleic acid ($C_{16}H_{30}O_2$)

History of Cod Liver Oil

The cod liver oil first became established in the poor fishing communities of North of England, Scotland, Ireland, Northern Europe, Iceland, Norway, Newfoundland and Greenland several centuries ago where they used it to protect themselves against the rigour in the intense cold that they were exposed to, in addition to fuel their lamps, soften the leather and also to make the textiles. It was also used in the animal feed which resulted in the glossy coats and the healthy constitution of the animals. This observation encouraged them to consume cod liver oil themselves. The island nation of Iceland far north in the icy Atlantic is truly remarkable in that the people who live there have withstood the challenges of the harsh weather and long seasons of darkness because of cod liver oil which has always been an important part of their diet. They recognised early the importance of vitamin A, vitamin D and the essential omega-3-fatty acids found in the cod liver oil and it was used as a panacea for everything that affected their health and daily activities. The people in the Iceland as on today live longer than any other people on earth and they have less heart disease and high blood pressure than any other culture in the world. They also have the lowest mortality rate and their women give birth to healthy babies with a well-developed immune system and optimal brain and eye functions. The regular use of cod liver oil has supported the overall health of these people for thousands of years. In the fishing communities, the fishermen used it to rub it on their aching joints and troublesome condition of the skin. Some fishermen when they were out at sea to fight colds, are reputed to have eaten raw fish liver soaked between the two slices of bread. In Nigeria, the oil is used as a rub for a healthy glow of the skin of the babies. Cod liver oil was a traditional medicinal drink for Newfoundlanders, and a song was made by Johnny Burke (1851–1930), a balladder from St. John's, Newfoundland. Cod liver oil is known since at least 1615, it has been recommended medicinally since 1783. The earliest recorded medical use of cod liver oil dates back to 1789 and is credited to Dr. Darbey, Machester Infirmary, where he used it for treating rheumatism. The oil was recognised as a specific remedy against rickets as early as 1824 in the German medical literature. The oil was also a folk remedy used for centuries for arthritis and gout and also as a spring tonic among the fishermen families in Norway, Iceland, Scotland and Newfoundland. We have the stories told by our grandparents that by taking their daily dose of cod liver oil they were releived of their rheumatism, aching muscles and stiff joints. It was commonly used to treat rickets during 1890s. During Second World War, the oil was imported from Iceland and distributed to pregnant and breast-feeding mothers and children under the age of five and people over forty to protect against malnutrition. The research carried out on the EPA and DHA in cod liver oil and other fishes has led to the view that this is beneficial to the heart and circulatory system.

Medicinal Uses

Cod liver oil is the source of vitamin A and vitamin D. The oil is used in formulating oleovitamin A and vitamin D products and topical emollients containing these vitamins. The sterol solution of the sodium salts of the fatty acid from cod liver oil known as sodium morrhuate is administered as a sclerosing agent. The oil is used as a nutritive and growth stimulating agent in rickets, malnutrition and tuberculosis especially in children. The oil is widely employed to ease the pain and stiffness of the joints in arthritis. It has a positive effect on heart, bone and brain and also helps nourish the skin, hair and nails. The oil is effective in the treatment of household burns and leaves no blisters. It is used as a complementary measure for long-term treatment of multiple sclerosis. When used during the pregnancy it lowers the risk of type I diabetes in the offspring. In nursing mothers, it improves the breast milk, promotes the development of the brain and increased the amount of vitamin A helping prevent the infections. The oil is one of the most reliable food source of DHA, EPA, vitamin A and D needed for a healthy skin, strong bones and teeth, healthy joints, cardiovascular system, nervous system and prevention of depression and mood disorders. Vitamin A of the oil is essential for the immune system, growth of the bones, night vision, and cellular growth, resistance to bacterial and viral infections and testicular and ovarian function. Vitamin D in the oil is useful for the absorption and utilisation of calcium and potassium required for the skeletal growth while Eicosa Pentaenoic Acid (EPA) and Docosa Hexaenoic Acid (DHA) affect a variety of physiological processes and reduce the risk of coronary heart disease, reduce the inflammation throughout the body, helps good eyesight, healthy nervous system and skin, and essential for the development of the normal brain in unborn babies. Research has shown that consumption of 1–2 tablespoons of oil helps to prevent diseases like cancer, diabetes, arthritis, musculoskeletal pains, problems of the kidneys and high cholesterol.

Adverse Effects

A tablespoon of cod liver oil contains 136% of the preformed vitamin A (or retinol). This accumulates in the liver and can reach harmful levels which are sufficient to cause hypervitaminosis A (which harms the bones: bone mineral density becomes low). Pregnant women should necessarily consult a doctor when they want to take the oil because of high amount of retinol in it. Too much intake of the oil can also make asthma worse. Other side effects include: Large doses of omega-3 fatty acids (in the form of cod liver oil) can stimulate the production of glucose which contributes to high levels of long-term blood sugar levels. The excess consumption of the fish oil leads to bleeding gums and nose bleeds. The oil has a capacity to lower the blood pressure which has been well-documented. One of the most common side effects is diarrhoea. A high intake of omega-3 fatty acids also decreases the ability of the blood to clot and increases the risk of haemorrhagic stroke. Taking too much of fish oil also interferes with sleep and thus contributes to insomnia. Other effects are acid reflux, belching and constant vomiting.

Other Uses

Cod liver oil was sometimes used as the liquid base for the traditional red ochre paint in Newfoundland, the coating of choice for use on out-buildings and work buildings associated with cod fishery industry. Vikings used the oil as a lubricant in ships.

Adulteration

The common adulterants are seal oil and other fish oils the detection of which is highly difficult.

SHARK LIVER OIL

Synonyms

Oleum selachoidi, Oleum squalae, Machhi-ka-tel (Hindi), Meenaenne (Tamil), Langue d'oil (French), Olio de fegato squalo (Spanish).

Synonyms for Shark

Tagana (Hindi), Samudrada dodda menu (Kannada), Sora menu (Telugu), Sor (Hindi), Haj (Danish), Haaien (Dutch), Squale, Requin (French), Der Hai, Der Haifisch, Hai, Haifisch (German), Ayogdh no (Greek), Squalo, Lo squalo (Italian), Tubarao, Esqualo (Portuguese), Akula (Russian), Hajar, Hajfisk (Swedish), Akuli, Likhvar (Ukrainian), Jalkirat (Sanskrit).

Biological Source

Shark liver oil is the fixed oil obtained from the fresh or carefully preserved livers of various species of the shark, mainly *Hypoprion brevirostris* Poey (*Negaprion brevirostris* is the valid name, Requiem shark) and *Galeorhinus zygopterus*. Other species include *Squalus carcharius* (White shark) found on the sea shores of Indian coastal towns. These are caught for food and live in cold, deep oceans. It is also obtained from several other species of sharks namely *Centrophorus squamosus* Bon. (=*Squalus squamosus*, *Lepidorhinus squamosus*, *Centrophorus foliaceus*, Leaf scale gulper shark, Deep sea shark), *Squalus acanthius* L.(=*Squalus acanthius*, *Acanthius americanus*, Piked dogfish, Cape shark, Spurdog, Dogfish shark) and *Cetorhinus maximus* (Basking shark).

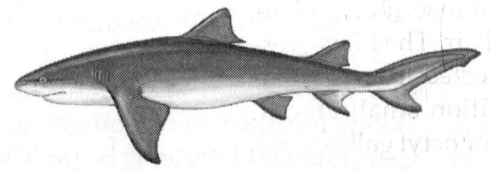

Negaprion brevirostris—Requiem shark

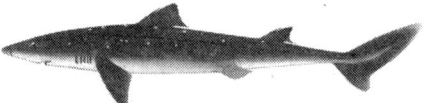

Squalus acanthius—Piked dogfish

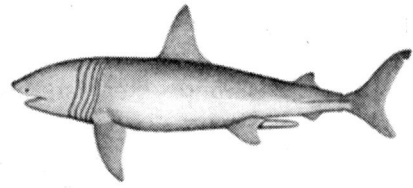

Cetorhinus maximus—Basking shark

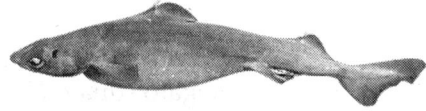

Centrophorus squamosus—Leafscale gulper shark

Geographical Source

Many Northern European countries and Greenland, Norway are producing shark liver oil on a large scale. In India shark liver oil is obtained on commercial scale in Tamil Nadu, Maharashtra and Kerala.

Collection and Preparation

Livers removed from the shark are thoroughly cleaned, freed from fatty material and adhering tissues (such as gallbladders). The cleaned livers are minced and heated in a boiling pot at a temperature not exceeding 80°C. The oil thus extracted which floats on the top is separated, washed and is treated with dehydrating agent to remove traces of water. Then the oil is taken to the vacuum still for dehydration and chilled to separate stearin. It is then centrifuged to get the clear oil after removing the suspended materials in it. Deodourisation is achieved by steaming under vacuum which removes about 0.02% of the aldehydic and ketonic impurities to protect the oil from oxidation. The clear oil is manipulated further to adjust the desired strength of vitamin A as per requirement (normally 600 units of vitamin A in 1.0 gm) and sometimes fortified with vitamin D (not less than 85 units) if desired. All through the process, special care is taken to minimise its exposure to sunlight and air as the oil is sensitive to light and air. The oil is preserved and stored in well-filled, air-tight containers protected from light and in a cool place, to avoid the loss of vitamins. In addition small amounts of different antioxidants (like dodecyl gallate and/or octyl gallate) can also be used. With a little variation, the principle involved in oil extraction is uniform in almost all the cases.

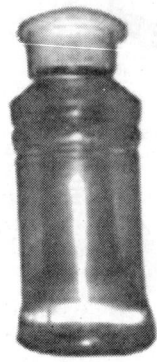

Deep sea shark liver oil

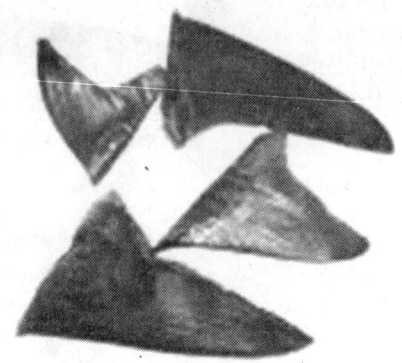

Liver of shark

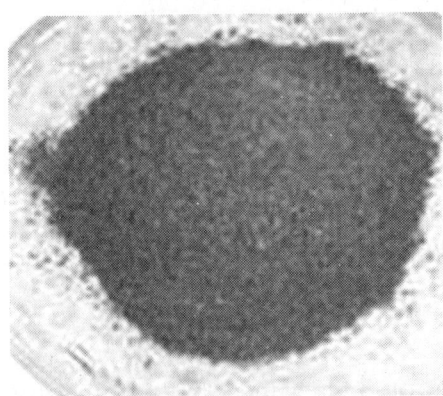

Steamed shark liver oil

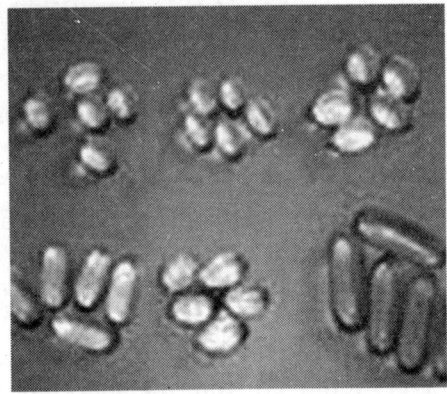

Gelatin capsules of oil

Characters

The oil is a fine amber coloured oily liquid (pale yellow to brownish-yellow in colour) having characteristic fishy odour, but not rancid. Taste is bland or fishy like cod liver oil but more strong and disagreable. If the oil is left for a more time, it deposits a white granular substance, stearin to which the name squalin is applied. It is insoluble in water, slightly soluble in alcohol and miscible with other solvents like petroleum ether, solvent ether and chloroform. The oil is richer in iodine and phosphorus than cod liver oil but contains less bromine and sulphur. The oil has an acid value not more than 2, a saponification value ranging between 15 and 200 and an iodine value ranging from 160 to 350.

Chemical Constituents

Shark liver oil contains vitamin A, concentration of which varies from 15000 to 30000 units per gram of the oil. The oil also contains glycerides of saturated and unsaturated fatty acids. The oil also contains alkylglycerol, pristane, squalamine, squalene, vitamins A, D and E, omega-3 fatty acids, triglycerides, glycerol ethers, cholesterol and fatty alcohols and some natural trace elements like copper, zinc and iron.

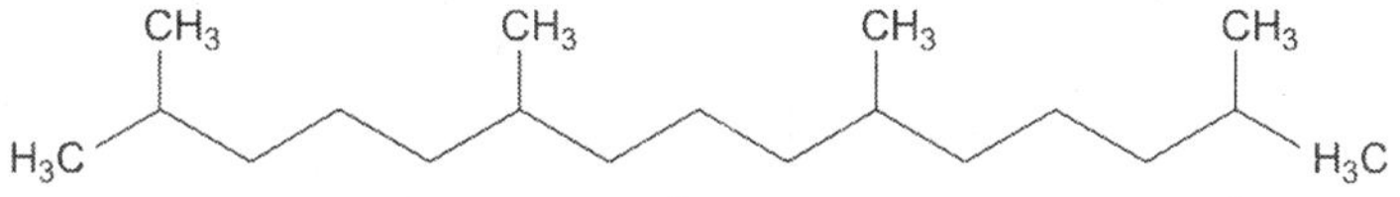

Pristane ($C_{19}H_{40}$)

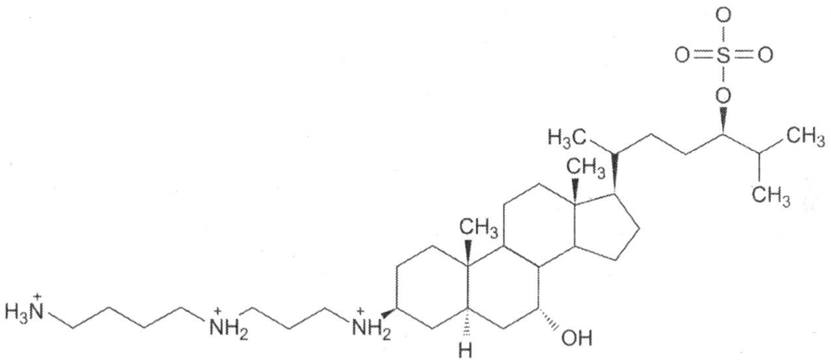

Squalamine ($C_{34}H_{65}O_5N_3S$)

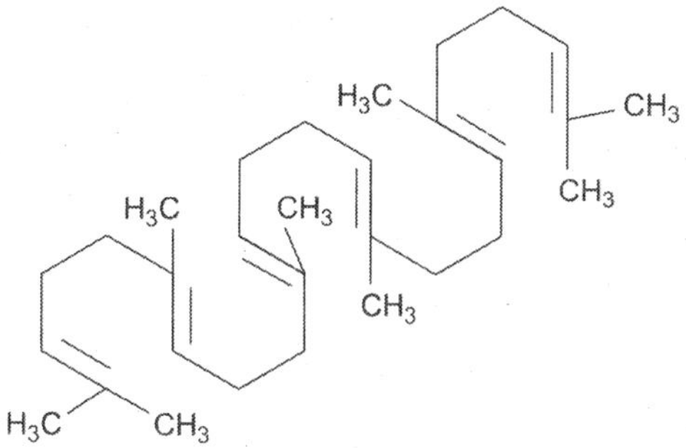

Squalene ($C_{30}H_{50}$)

History of Shark Liver Oil

Shark liver oil has been used for centuries as a folk remedy for general health by the fishermen. Initially, it was employed by the Scandinavian fishermen to treat certain diseased conditions of skin. Hundreds of years ago, Japanese fishermen called the liver oil from the deep sea sharks as *samedawa* meaning 'cure all'. In China, the use of oil was recorded in their ancient pharmaceutical book, *'Honzukomuko'*. In Norway and Sweden, the oil was traditionally used externally to heal wounds and to protect the skin from sun. Internally it was used to give stamina and also heal the irritation of the respiratory and alimentary system. In Micronesia, it was long used for many sicknesses and diseases and also used as a tonic. The Spanish seamen regularly took the 'oil of the great fish' to resist cold and illness.

Medicinal Uses

The oil is a rich source of vitamin A and it is used in the treatment of xerophthalmia (abnormal dryness of the surface of the conjunctiva) which occurs as a result of vitamin A deficiency. The oil is also used daily as a nutrient, demulcent and alterative in cachexia, pulmonary consumption, atrophy of the body, scrophulous affections of the joints and bones especially in rickets, ophthalmia, abscesses, suppurating glands, ulcerations, discharges from the nose or ears and skin diseases. It is also used in the mesenteric affections of children, in obstinate constipation, in stricture of the rectum, in chronic hydrocephalus, in the advanced stages of spasmodic coughs such as whooping cough, lung affections, in chorea, epilepsy and neuralgia. It is used in chronic rheumatism causing atrophy, in some types of paralysis and in leprosy. It is used for healing wounds, sores, irritations of the respiratory tract and alimentary canal and the swollen lymph nodes. As preparation H, it is an active ingredient of haemorrhoid creams. The oil is rich in alkylglycerols with anticancer properties which are found in breast milk and bone marrow. The oil strengthens the immune system, hay fever, sinusitis and other allergies. It also eases joint pains from arthritis, maintains healthy skin, has anti-angiogenesis properties and works against bad effects of radiation. It helps reduce cholesterol, prevents deep vein thrombosis, prevents scarring in wound healing, and supplies to the cells oxygen. The oil has an antioxidant property and protects the body from toxic substances and helps in leaching mercury from the bodies. It helps in controlling the blood sugar levels in diabetes, helps to achieve a complete recovery in asthma patients. The oil has also been shown to be of a great benefit in conditions of chronic fatigue syndrome, fibromyalgia and postviral syndrome. Some believe that the oil from deep water sharks may prove useful in fighting cancer and boosting the immune system. The oil is used as a moisturiser in lip balms to prevent chapping. The oil is always taken along with a vehicle and not on an empty stomach as it causes nausea. The diet during the course should be plain and nutritious such as bread, fresh roasted meat along with vegetables, fruits and liquids in a moderate quantity. The rich food like pastries, fat, meat cream should be avoided.

Side Effects

The contraindications have not yet been identified. But, when used for a short-term, the oil is safe in adults. Sometimes, minor side effects related to the stomach and intestines have been reported. Liver injury also has been reported rarely. If taken in higher doses the oil may increase the levels of cholesterol. The oil can also cause pneumonia in people who accidentally breathe it into the lungs. Especially when one first starts taking the oil mild digestive upset such as nausea, diarrhoea and indigestion may occur. There are no known serious side effects from taking the oil at recommended doses.

LINSEED OIL

Synonyms

Flax seed oil, Oleum lini, L'huile de lin (French), Olio di lino (Italian), Leinol (German), Oleo de linhaca (Portuguese), Binale ka thel (Hindi), Linolei (Danish), Lijnolie (Dutch), Linfroolija (Swedish), Winterlein, Chih-ma.

Synonyms for Linseed

Linseed, Flax plant (English), Atasi (Sanskrit, Telugu and Kannada), Lincultive (French), Gemeiner Lein or Flachs (German), Alsi or Tisi (Hindi), Masina (Bengali), Javas (Gujarati), Alashi (Konkan), Alashi-virai (Tamil), Zaghu or Tukhmizaghira or Roghani zaghira (Persian), Bazarul-kattana (Persian).

Biological Source

Linseed (flax seed) is the dried ripe seed of *Linum usitatissimum* L. (Family: Linaceae). Seeds contain not less than 25% of fixed (drying) oil. The Latin name, *linum* is derived from the Greek, *limon* while its common name, *flax* is Middle English, originally from Old English, *fleax* and is related to the German, *flachs* which means '*to plait*' or '*interweave*', in connection with the fibres being spun into thread.

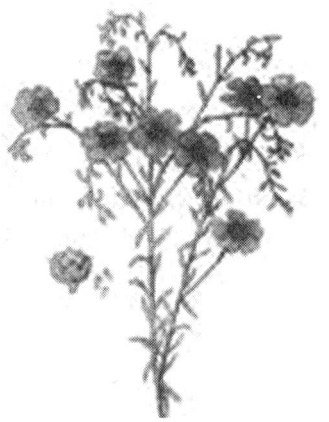

Linum usitatissimum

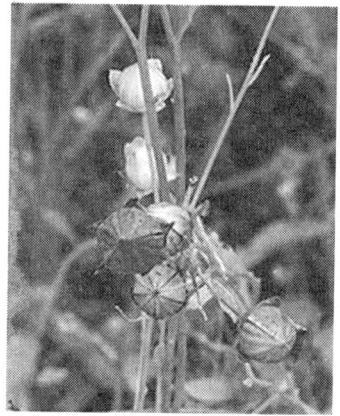

Plant with capsules

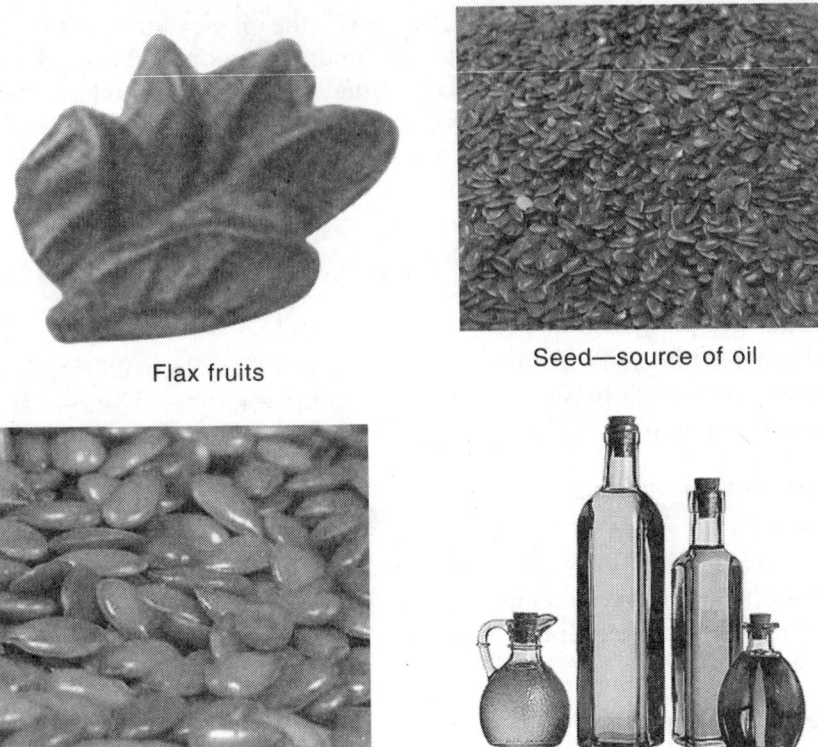

Flax fruits

Seed—source of oil

Seeds of flax

Oil

Geographical Source

The plant is a native of Egypt extensively cultivated in India chiefly in West Bengal, Bihar and Uttar Pradesh. It is cultivated in South America, India, USA, Russia, Argentina, Holland and Canada. It is cultivated chiefly in the temperate regions of the eastern and western hemispheres. At present, the major flax producing countries for fibre are the Soviet Union, Poland and France.

Characters of the Seed

The seeds are ovate or ovate-lanceolate, compressed (flat). The seed is obliquely pointed at one end and round at the other, 4–6 mm long and 2–2.5 mm broad. The testa is chestnut-brown, glossy and finely pitted with a pale-yellow linear raphe along one edge. Internally, the seed coat is brown and the endosperm is yellowish-green. The odour is slight and the taste is mucilaginous and oily.

Collection and Preparation

The seeds are separated by thrashing, cleaned, crushed through oil seed rolls, moistened and the crushed moist seeds are heated to 85–90°C in steam jacketed troughs. When the seed's tissues are sufficiently softened, the material is pressed through heated hydraulic press at a pressure of 3300 to 5000 pounds per square inch (cold pressing). The oil thus expressed is filtered and treated with alkali to remove free fatty acids. The oil is bleached by using either Fuller's earth or charcoal. The refined oil thus obtained is chilled to separate any waxy material.

The manufacture of the linseed oil comprises the following steps: Heating the crude linseed oil to an increased temperature lower than the boiling point of water—adding a heated inorganic acid to the oil and mixing—separation of the precipitated materials—adding a heated aqueous solution of the alkali to the oil and mixing the oil—discharge of the soap formed— and rinsing the oil with hot water until a clear rinsing water is obtained.

Characters

Linseed oil is a clear to yellowish to dark-grey or yellowish-brown drying oil with a characteristic odour and bland taste; much commercial oil has marked odour and acrid taste. Pure fresh oil is colourless while the commercial oil is dark yellow. On exposure to air, the oil dries up to a transparent varnish chiefly of linoxyn.

Chemical Constituents

The fixed oil is a mixture of many triglycerides derived from fatty acids and contains about 30–40% of linolein, 25% protein and 15% of mucilage (6% in the testa) along with proteins, amygdalin, resin, wax, sugar and ash (3 to 5%). The ash contains sulphates and chlorides of potassium, calcium and magnesium. Linseed oil has a high iodine value as it contains considerable quantities of the glycerides of unsaturated acids. The fatty acids present include linolenic acid (51.9–55.2%), linoleic acid (14.2–17%), oleic acid (18.5–22.6%) along with some saturated acids like myristic acid, stearic acid (3.4–4.6%) and palmitic acid (about 7%).

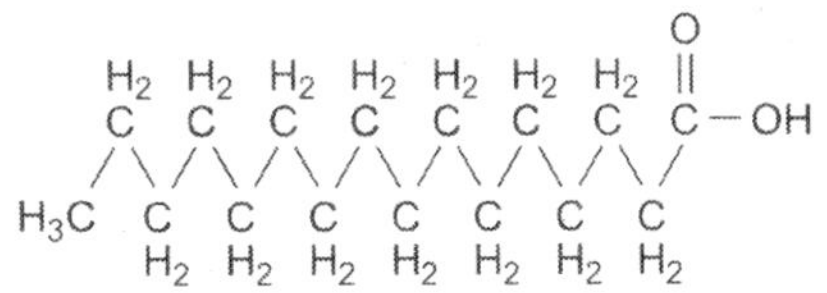

Palmitic acid or hexadecanoic acid $CH_3(CH_2)_{14}COOH$ or $(C_{16}H_{32}O_2)$

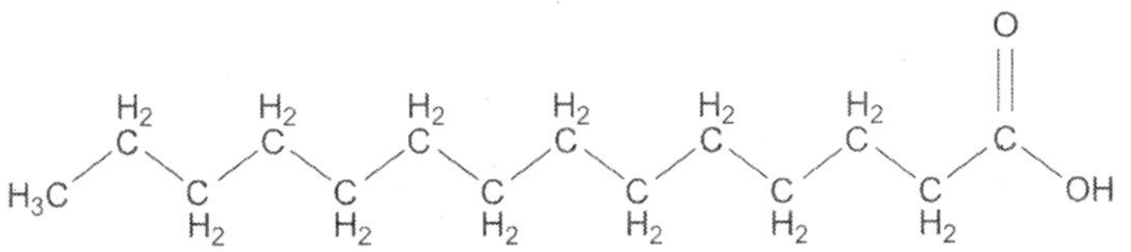

Myristic acid or tetradecanoic acid $CH_3(CH_2)_{12}COOH$ or $(C_{14}H_{28}O_2)$

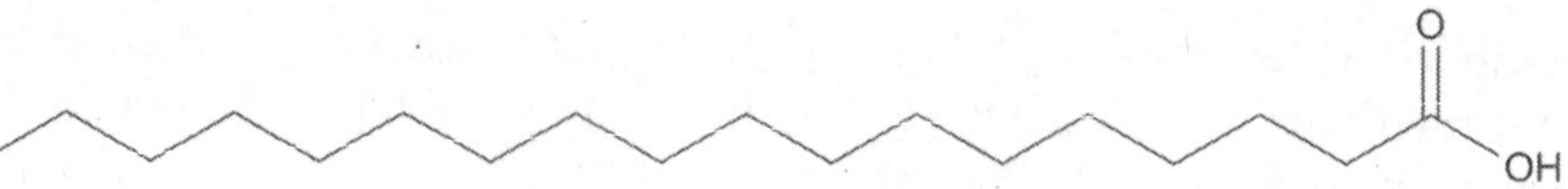

Stearic acid or octadecanoic acid $CH_3(CH_2)_{16}COOH$ or $(C_{18}H_{36}O_2)$

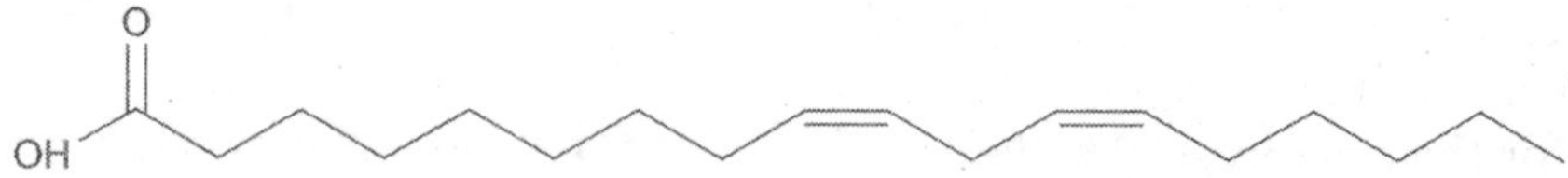

Linoleic acid or octadecadienoic acid $(C_{18}H_{32}O_2)$

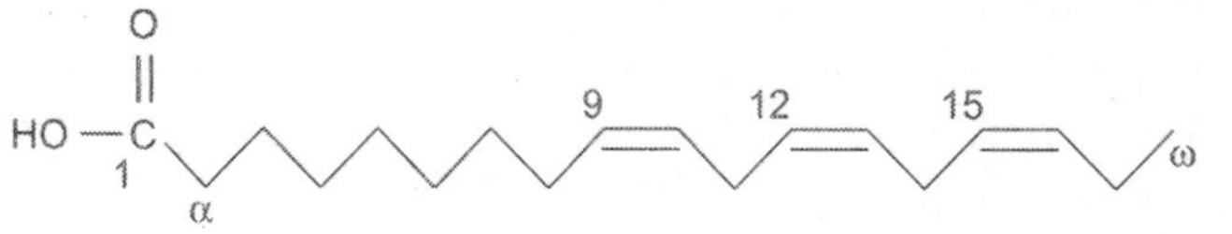

Linolenic acid or octadecatrienoic acid
$CH_3(CH_2CH=CH)_3(CH_2)_7COOH$ or $(C_{18}H_{30}O_2)$

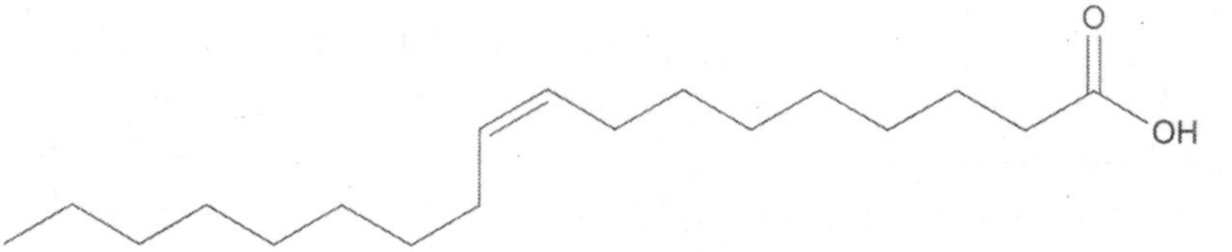

Oleic acid or octadecenoic acid $CH_3(CH_2)_7CH=CH(CH_2)_7COOH$ or $(C_{18}H_{34}O_2)$

History of Linseed Oil

Common flax was one of the first crops domesticated by man, and is thought to have originated in the Mediterranean region of Europe. Archeological remains indicate that several plants were first cultivated almost about the same time in Mesopotamia which included flax, emmer wheat, barley, einkorn wheat, peas, lentils, chickpeas and bitter vetch. The people of the Stone Age living near the Swiss Lake produced flax and utilised the fibre and the seed. The linen cloth made from flax was used to wrap the mummies in the early Egyptian tombs (5000 BC). The Babylonians were the earliest people to cultivate flax as a source of food and irrigation ditches were formed along the Tigris and Euphrates rivers of the Fertile Crescent (2000 BC) to ensure a good water supply for the flax fields. Homer (8th century BC) in his epic poem, *the Iliad,* wrote that linen was used for cord and sail-cloth and this was an indication that the Greeks cultivated flax plants and also consumed the seeds. The 'Father of Medicine', Hippocrates (460–377 BC), also recognised the medicinal value of flax in relieving many intestinal disorders upon prescription to patients. The early colonists in the United States grew flax for their home use. The plant has been known to be cultivated for its seed since very ancient times and it is one of the oldest cultivated plants known to man. The 8th century King of France, Charlemagne regarded flax very highly for its health benefits and also made a detailed entry pertaining to the cultivation and use of flax for food and medicine in his medical law books and also ordered his subjects to consume it to maintain good health and also to prevent disease. The excavations of the most ancient Egyptian tombs have come up with flax seeds as well as the flax fibre cloth woven from the plant. The commercial production of flax began in 1753. Even today, few still grow flax to make linen for their own use. The first linen mentioned in the Bible was spun from flax according to historians and archaeologists. The linseed oil has been used medicinally by human societies since pre-history. It is believed that the first ancestors of the human race as long ago as 8500 years ago, ate the flax and some wild grasses as a part of their diet. In ancient times, the diet of early humans contained every part of the flax plant.

The plant has been cultivated for its fibre, for at least five millennia. The wall paintings of ancient Egypt depicted the spinning and weaving of linen. The flax fibre was processed into a fine white fabric as early as 3000 BC and this was used to wrap the mummies of the ancient Egyptian Pharaohs. It has been also used as a cool and comfortable fiber in the middle east for centuries, as mentioned several times in the Bible. It was also greatly valued as a commodity by Ancient Greeks and Romans. The flax has been introduced to Northern Europe by Finnish traders. It was known that the *'Father of the Nation'*, Mahatma Gandhi once said, *'whenever flax seeds become a regular food item among the people, there will be better health'*. Flax is the emblem of Northern Ireland used by its Assembly. It also appeared on the reverse of the British one pound coin to represent Northern Ireland in 1986 and 1991. Flax is also seen on the badge of the Supreme Court of the United Kingdom representing the Northern Ireland. Common flax is also the national flower of Belarus.

Medicinal Uses

The oil is used in liniments and also as a demulcent, emollient and laxative. The oil is also an expectorant, diuretic. The seeds are aphrodisiac and the roasted seeds are astringent. The mucilage from the seed extracted by cold water is used for the irritable conditions of conjunctiva of the eye. Along with honey it is used for cough and colds. The powdered seed cake is called *Linum contusum* is popular as linseed meal. The poultice of the meal is used as a soothing application to ulcerated and inflamed surfaces, boils, carbuncles, abscesses, etc. It is also used as a mild counter-irritant for the deep seated inflammations like pneumonia, bronchitis, broncho-pneumonia, pleuritis, pericarditis, peritonitis, arthritis, pelvic cellulitis, etc. Linseed oil is prescribed internally in 'painter's colic', piles and a good laxative. With lime water in equal proportions, it is a popular remedy for burns and scalds as 'carron oil'. The infusion of the seed called linseed tea with licorice and sugar is internally used as a demulcent in cold, cough, bronchitis, irritations of urinary organs, cystitis, gonorrhoea, stranguary, as injection to the vagina, bladder and the rectum.

Other Uses

In addition, the stem fibres find a use in the manufacture of linen cloth. The best quality lint is made from the retted and finely carded fibre. Linseed oil is used as an impregnator in varnish and wood furnishing, as a pigment binder in oil paints, as a plasticiser and hardener in putty and in the production of linoleum. It is edible but is a minor constituent of nutrition because of its strong odour. It is also used as a traditional protective coating for the raw willow of cricket bats, for cue shafts (billiards) and surf boards.

Adulteration

The common adulterants are corn meal, wheat middlings, cake meal and foreign weed seeds. It is also adulterated with cotton seed oil, sunflower oil, resin, mineral oils, mustard oil and fish oils.

COCOA BUTTER

Synonyms

Theobroma oil, Cacao butter, Butter of cacao, Oleum Theobromatis, Butyrum Cacao, Oleum concretum e Semine Theobromae Cacao, Beurre de Cacao (French), Kakao butter (German).

Synonyms for Cocoa

Cocoa plant, chocolate tree, Chocolate, cocoa, Nicaraguan cocoa shade (English), Cacaoboom (Dutch), Kakao (Finnish and Swedish), Cacaoyer, Cacaotier, Cacao (French), Kakaobaum, Kakaopflanze (German), Cacao amarillo, cacao criollo, Cacao forastero (Spanish), Keke shu (Chinese), Cacau (Portuguese), Coklat (Indonesian), Maikona gaha (Sinhalese), Kona maram, Kakkavo (Tamil), Kokkoo (Malayalam), Kho kho (Thai), Kokoe (Burmese), Pokok coklat (Malaysian), Planta del cacao (Italian).

Biological Source

Cocoa butter is a fixed oil (fat) extracted from the roasted seeds (cacao beans—about 40–50%) of *Theobroma cacao* L. (Family: Sterculiaceae). *Theobroma* in Latin means the *'food of the Gods'*.

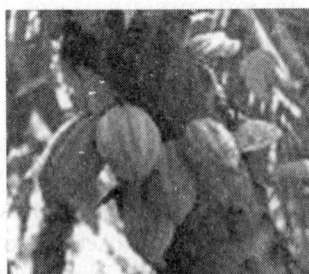

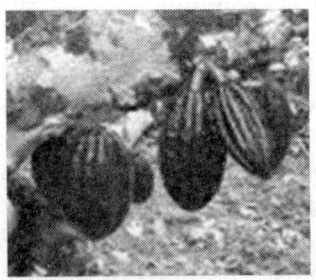

Theobroma cacao—fruits   Mature fruits of cacao

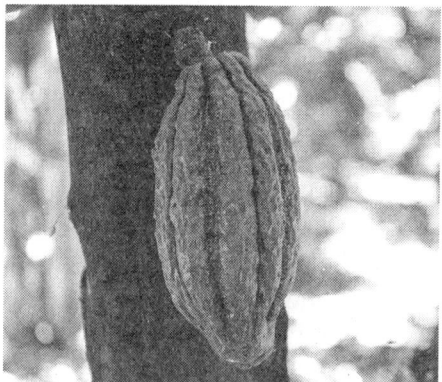

Single fruit-unripe

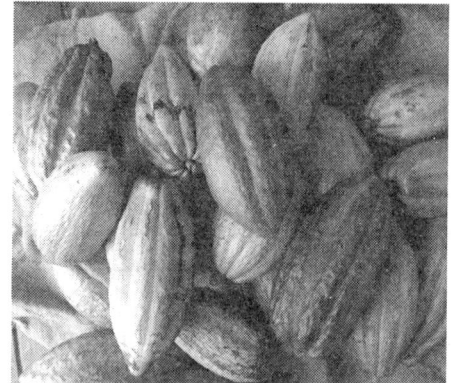

Ripe fruits—different stages

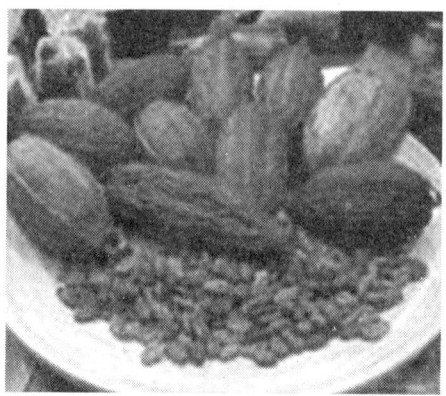

Dry fruits and beans

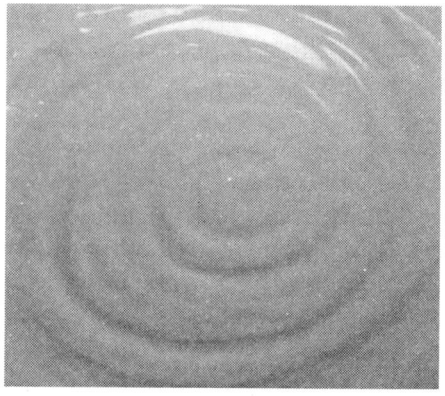

Cocoa chocolate

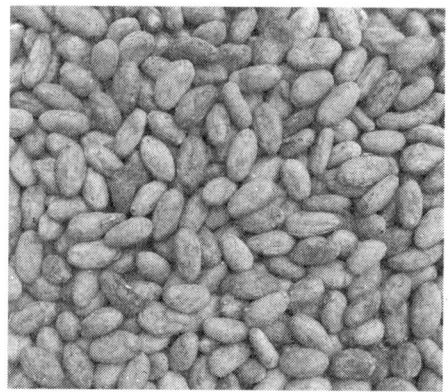

Cocoa beans

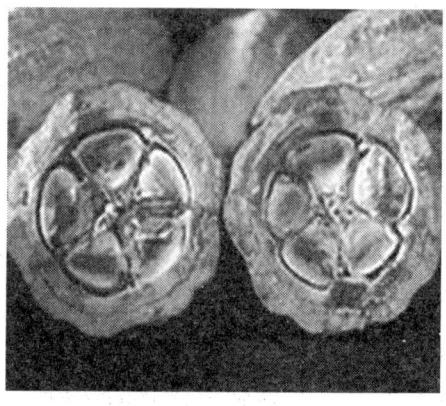

Split opened fruit

Geographical Source

Cocoa is produced in Ecuador, Colombia, Brazil, Venezula, Guiana, West Indies, Indonesia, Malaysia, Dominican Republic (outside Africa) and Cameroon, Nigeria, Ivory Coast and Ghana (West Africa).

Collection and Preparation

The cocoa seeds are separated from the pods and are allowed to ferment wherein the seeds change their colour from white to dark reddish-brown due to enzymatic reaction (chocolate liquor). Fermentation occurs in tubs, boxes or cavities in the earth, the process lasts 3–9 days, and the temperature is not allowed to rise above 60°C. The seeds are then roasted at 100–140°C, when they lose water and acetic acid and acquire their characteristic odour and taste. Roasting facilitates removal of seed coat. The seeds are cooled as rapidly as possible and testa removed by a 'nibbling' machine. The nibs or kernels are separated from the husk by winnowing. The kernels are then fed to hot rollers which yield a pasty mass containing cocoa butter. This is further purified to give cocoa butter. Butter can also be extracted by the broma process. Finally, it is deodourised to remove its undesirable taste.

Characters

Cocoa butter is a yellowish white or a pale-yellow pure, edible vegetable fat that has a mild chocolate flavour and aroma and bland chocolate-like taste. It is brittle at temperatures below 25°C. It melts between 35 and 37°C. The refractive index of the butter is 1.44556–1.44573. It has an iodine value of 34.8, an acid value of 1.68 and saponification value of 197.7. The oil is freely soluble in ether, chloroform and benzene and boiling dehydrated alcohol and slightly soluble in 95% alcohol. Its saponification value is not less than 188 and not more than 195. Its iodine value is not less than 33 and not more than 38. The butter displays polymorphism with crystals possessing different melting points.

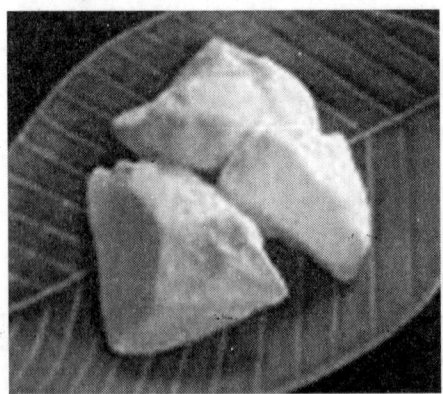

Cocoa butter

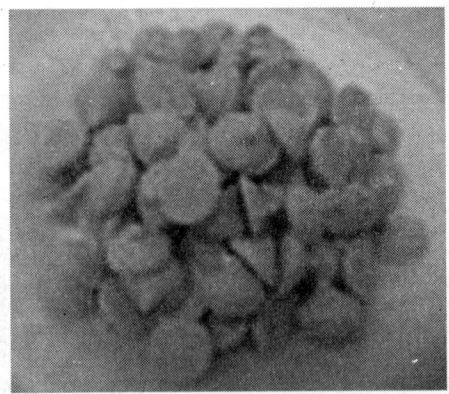

Cocoa powder—as flakes

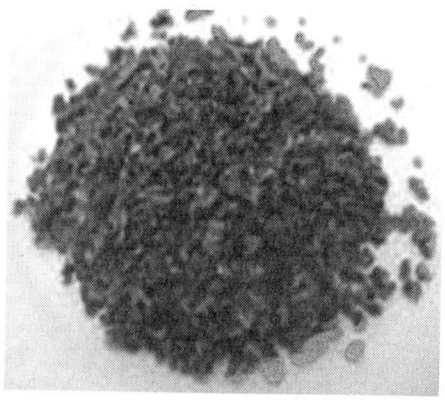
Raw cocoa nibs

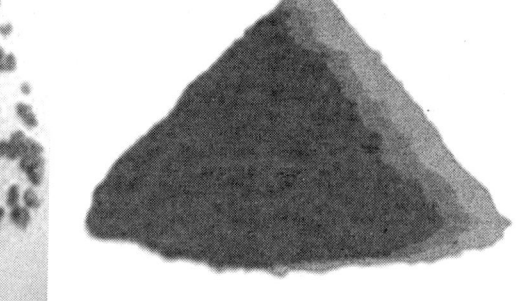
Cocoa powder

Chemical Constituents

The solid fixed oil consists chiefly of the glycerides of oleic, stearic and palmitic acids. Because of its high content of oleostearin, it is also used as a source of stearic acid. It is one of the stable fats known which contains natural antioxidants that prevent rancidity. The percentage of the constituents—non-saponifiables is 0.2–0.4%, total saturated fats is 57–64%, free fatty acids is 1.08%, total monosaturated fats is 29–43% and total polysaturated fats is 1–5%. The main fatty acids of the butter are represented by oleic acid (29–38%), palmitic acid (22–29%), linoleic acid (1–4%), stearic acid (24–37%), capric acid (0–10%), myristic acid (0–4%), arachidic acid (1%), palmitoleic acid (0–2%), and linolenic acid (0–1%).

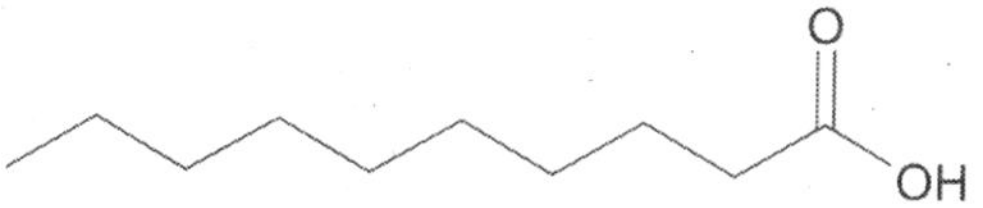

Capric acid or decanoic acid $CH_3(CH_2)_8COOH$ or $(C_{10}H_{20}O_2)$

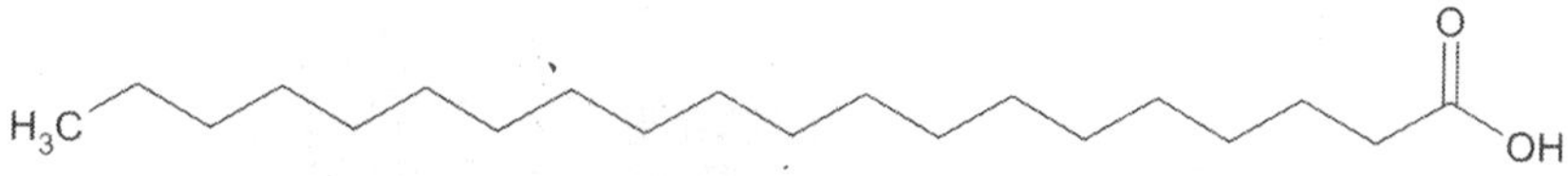

Arachidic acid or eicosanoic acid $CH_3(CH_2)_{18}COOH$ or $(C_{20}H_{40}O_2)$

History of Cocoa

Cocoa butter has been used for centuries in Africa for its moisturising properties and healing properties, where it has been used to protect and also condition the skin which has been damaged by the sun and the wind. Cocoa tree was originally named *kakawa* and according to historical records; the people of Mesoamerican civilisation along the Mexican Gulf coast cultivated the tree in 1000 BC. They used the beans for making drinks for consumption by the elite class. Later, the tree came to be known as *cacao* from proto-Mixe-Zoqueqn family of languages, during Olmec civilisation (1150–300 BC). Later, this culture moved to Mayan civilisation by the Izapan civilisation of the lowlands of Chialas of Mexico, Peten of Guatemala and Belize. Historians believe that the word, *chocolate* or *chocolatl* originate from the Nahuatl word, *xocoatl* or *cacahuatl* meaning *'bitter water'*. Some believe that it is a combination of the Mayan words, *choco* and *haa* and the Nauhatl term, *atl* which resulted in the term *'chocolate'*. There is also another theory according to linguists that the word *chicolatl* originated from the word, *chico-li* meaning *'to beat'* or *'to stir'* and not *chocoatl*. It was a Swedish who gave the cocoa plant its binomial, *Theobroma cacao* which literally meant the *'food of the Gods'*. During 450–500 AD, clay vessels were made for drinking the chocolate, as a status symbol by Mayans. At the end of Mayan civilisation (200 BC to 1550 AD) cocoa beans had become a major Mesoamerican commodity. We know that chocolates are made from cocoa beans that have been cultivated for millions of years in the South American rainforests. The archaeological surveys account for the physical residues of chocolate in some Mayan pots which suggest that Mayans drank chocolate some 2600 years ago. It is also believed that the cocoa plant was cultivated in the Amazon for more than 4000 years. Archaeological evidence comes from the recovery of cocoa beans at Uaxactun, Guatemala (1947) and also from the preserved wood fragments of the cocoa tree at Belize sites (1981) and Pulltrouser area (1984). Similarly, the residue analysis from the ceramic vessels from an early classic period (460–480 AD) tomb at Rio Azul in North-Eastern Guatemala has revealed the presence of theobromine and caffeine. History also accounts for the worshipping of the cocoa tree by the Mayans and Aztecs who offered chocolate to the God as an offering. The cocoa beans were brewed along with maize and capsicum which resulted in a spicy bitter-sweet drink which after fermentation was used for the ceremonies by Aztecs (1500 AD). Aztecs also treated cocoa beans as currency and paid their taxes too, and the beans were used as a currency throughout Mesoamerica by the time the Aztec empire fell (1376–1520 AD). Mythically, the cocoa tree has been linked to Quetzacoatl, the God of agriculture of Mexicans. Chocolate came to Europe in the 16th century by a Spanish explorer, Don Hernan Cortes (1519). The tradition of drinking hot chocolate began in Spain where the drink was served to travelers and was a common drink with the nobility. Christopher Columbus introduced the chocolate into Spain (1502). The cocoa tree was introduced to the Asia in 1560 and to the Africa in 1590. The chocolate was served in the Spanish court during 1600 to 1650 and it arrived in London in 1657. Later, the drink entered France, and was introduced to England in the 17th century by Sir Hans Sloane. Initially, the brew was sold as medicine by apothecaries in England. C. J. Van Houton, a Dutch chocolate master invented the 'cocoa press' (1828) which helped to squeeze out cocoa butter from the beans through an alkalising process called 'dutching'. The first large scale production of chocolate bar was by J. S. Fry and Sons who introduced the use of cocoa powder (1847). Later, in 1853, it was Cadburys who manufactured the chocolate and became the supplier to Queen Victoria, and emerged as one of the leading chocolate manufacturers in the world as we know it today. The milk chocolate was introduced into the market by Henri Nestle and Daniel Peter (1879) in Switzerland by blending cocoa powder and condensed milk along with cocoa butter and cocoa solids.

Medicinal Uses

Cocoa butter has nutritive, stimulant, antiseptic and diuretic properties. The oil is used pharmaceutically in the making of suppositories and also as excipient for pills (oral medicine in capsule form) and as an emollient it is an ingredient of many products in cosmetics, soaps and lotions. It is also recommended as a moisturiser for the prevention of stretch marks in pregnant women, in the treatment of chopped skin and lips. It is a natural preservative. Theobromine in the butter is a diuretic. It is used to prepare biscuits, chocolate, bakery products, pharmaceuticals, ointments and toiletries. It is an additive in cosmetics, shampoos and soaps. It is used to add flavour, scent and smoothness to chocolate, tanning oil, topical lotions, creams and soap. It is used in conditions of eczema and dermatitis as it helps as a barrier between the skin and the environment and also helps in retaining the moisture (body care lotions and moisturisers). The butter also contains cocoa mass polyphenol (CMP) which inhibits the production of immunoglobulin IgE known to aggravate the symptoms of dermatitis and asthma. Butter when used in massaging the skin helps relieve stress, boost the immune system and inhibits the growth of cells of cancer and tumours in addition to preventing the heart disease and eases the arthritis and helps treating conditions such as psoriasis, fibromyalgia and chronic fatigue syndrome according to recent research. The butter is rich in vitamin E which helps to soothe, hydrate and balance the skin and provides collagen assisting with wrinkles (stretch marks in pregnant women) and signs of ageing. The butter is a folk remedy for burns, cough, dry lips, fever, malaria, rheumatism, snake bite and wounds.

Adulteration

Wax, stearin and tallow are the common adulterants in cocoa butter. Mano kernel oil is used as a substitute.

Alternative to Cocoa Butter

The global production of cocoa is in decline due to the failure of the crop, diseases and aging plantations which lead to fluctuations in the price and the necessity for the cocoa industry to find high quality cocoa butter alternatives. The studies in this direction explore the potential of a wild mango, *Mangifera sylvatica*, an under-utilised fruit in South-East Asia, as a new cocoa butter alternative (CBA). The analysis showed that the wild mango butter has a light coloured fat with a similar fatty acid profile (palmitic acid, stearic acid and oleic acid) and triglyceride profile (POP [1,3-dipalmitoyl-2-oleoyl-glycerol], SOS [1,3-distearoyl-2-oleoyl-glycerol] and POS [1-palmitoyl-2-oleoyl-3-stearoyl-glycerol]) to cocoa butter. The thermal and physical properties of CBA are also similar to cocoa butter. In addition, wild mango butter comprises 65% SOS (1,3-distearoyl-2-oleoyl-glycerol) which indicates its potential to become a Cocoa Butter Improver (an enhancement of CBA).

KOKUM BUTTER

Synonyms

Goa butter, Kokum oil, Mangosteen oil, Black kokum, Cocum (French, Spanish and Italian), Kokam (German), Kokum butter (Indian).

Synonyms for *Garcinia*

Red mango, Mate mangosteen, Indian berry, Indian tallow tree (English), Kokam, Bhirand kokum (Hindi), Birandel ratamba, Kokambel, Kokan (Gujarati and Maharashtrian), Murgal mara (Tamil), Murgina-huli-mara, Dhupadamara, Murgala, Murginahalli, Punarpuli, Ratambi (Kannada), Punampuli (Malayalam), Beerunda (Konkani), Brindao (pulp of the fruit) or Amsel (bark of the tree) or Ratambasal (Goanese), Vrikshamla, Vrichhamala (Sanskrit), Bhirand, Kokam, Kokambi (Marathi), Kokkam (Malayalam), Garushinia indika (Japanese), Brindonnier (French).

Biological Source

Kokum butter is the fat expressed from the seeds of *Garcinia indica* (=*Garcinia purpurea*), (Family: Clusiaceae=Guttiferae). The genus *Garcinia* is named after Laurentiers (Jacques) Garcin (1673–1751), a French explorer, physician

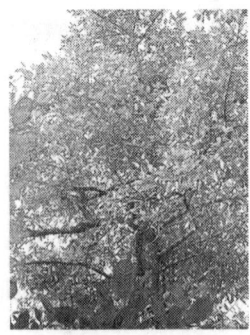

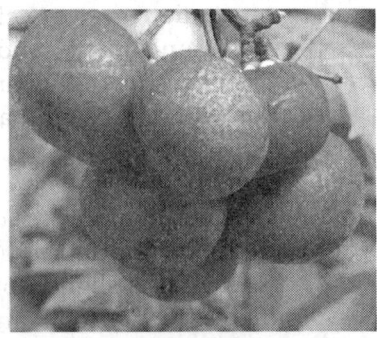

Garcinia indica   Fruits

and a priest who lived in India and collected it as well as first described it. He wrote the first article on the medicinal properties of the fruit in 1697.

Geographical Source

The plant is indigenous to Thailand, Cambodia and China. The plant is a native to the western coastal region of Southern India. In India it grows in the evergreen forests of Konkan (Mangalore), Malabar (Kerala) and Canara (Karnataka) districts of Western India and Assam, Khasi, Jantia hills, West Bengal and Gujarat.

Collection and Preparation

Raw kokum butter is a white coloured fat with a creamish-yellow or even slight-grey tint which is extracted by traditional rural/cottage industry sized oil mills. The fruits are collected manually by hand picking. The branches are shaken with long sticks and the fallen fruits are collected. These are broken by sticks to separate the seeds, picked up by hand. The seeds are gathered from the natural forest habitats. The seeds are cleaned to remove the dust, dirt and foreign matter. The seeds are dried to reduce the moisture content. These are decorticated by wooden mallets. The final product is obtained by crushing the kernels and boiling the pulp in water (in a steam boiler) and skimming off the fat from the top or churning the crushed pulp with water. Pure oil is obtained after double filtration and is cooled to create kokum butter slabs and cubes of different sizes and weight. This is a time consuming process and the yield is about 25% of raw butter.

The kernels from the seeds are churned and boiled in water with caustic soda. This yields hard soap which is decomposed by sulphuric acid leaving tristearin as stearic acid, myristic acid and oleic acid. The melted fat is separated by skimming with hot water twice and decolourised with animal charcoal or Fuller's earth. The seeds contain 30% of fat. After refining, the fat is equivalent to vanaspati ghee.

Characters

This is a white to light grey or yellowish solid fat with a neutral odour and taste. It is hard and brittle and exceptionally stable. It has an earthy scent. It solidifies below 39°C and its melting point is 39–42°C. It has a saponification value of 191 and an iodine value of 36.9.

Chemical Constituents

Kokum butter contains glycerides of stearic acid (40–45%), oleic acid (40–50%), hydroxyl capric acid (10%), palmitic acid (5–8%) and linoleic acid (2–4%). The fat is slightly bitter. It contains free fatty acids (0.08%), non-saponifiables (0.9%), total saturated fats (52–68%), total monosaturated fats (30–42%) and total polysaturated fats (0–2%). It also contains antioxidant vitamin E. The butter is often substituted for cocoa butter because of its more uniform triglyceride composition. Its high fatty acid content improves the stability of the emulsion and offers thickness without stiffness.

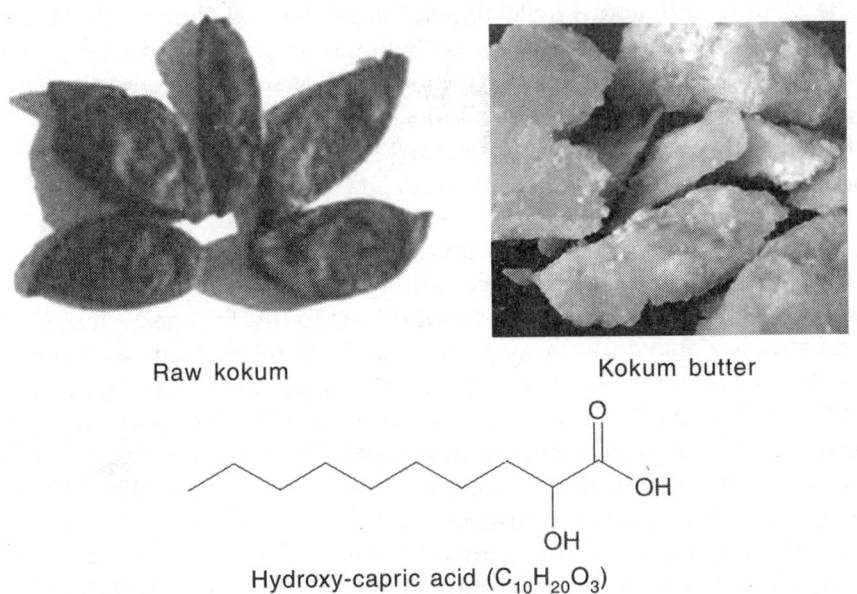

Raw kokum   Kokum butter

Hydroxy-capric acid ($C_{10}H_{20}O_3$)

History of *Garcinia*

The place of origin is unknown but is believed to be the Sunda Islands and the Moluccas Islands, and it can be found throughout South East Asia. According to Corner, the tree was first domesticated in Thailand or Burma (Myanmar). According to Alphonse De Candolle, the mangosteen species is certainly wild in the forests of the Sunda Islands and of the Malay peninsula. The plant is cultivated in Thailand, Kampuchea, Southern Vietnam and Burma, and throughout Malaya and Singapore. It was introduced into Ceylon (Sri Lanka) in 1800 and into India in 1881. In India, it is confined to four areas namely, the Nilgiri hills, the Tinnevelly district of Southern Madras (Tamil Nadu), the Kanya Kumari district at the southernmost tip of the Madras Peninsula (Tamil Nadu) and in Kerala state in South Western India. The fruit has been mentioned in traditional Chinese medicine dating back to 1368–1644 AD during the reign of the Ming dynasty. The rind has been used to cure infections by the South East Asian populations for centuries and the poultice was used to treat the skin problems and the extract of the white pulp was used to bring down the fever. The best bibliography of the historical references to *Garcinia* was assembled by Cora L. Feldkamp (1946) and the compilation includes 'references on all aspects of the mangosteen—botany, culture, diseases and pests, varieties, composition, nutritional value, cookery, toxic effects, uses and economics'. The records indicate that the first introduction of the mangosteen in the UK during the 18th and 19th century goes back to Anton Pantaleon Hove (Hoveau). He procured the plants along with some better strains of cotton seeds from Gujarat, India, and sent it to Plymouth, England (1789) which was moved to Kew. This was the introduction of mangosteen into Western Hemisphere. The other reference was an 18th century publication, 'a description of the mangostan (Molucca Islands) and the bread fruit' by John Ellis (1775) which contains a sketch of the bread fruit and the mangosteen. Ellis made a reference to Laurent Garcin, a French naturalist who travelled in India and collected and described mangosteen in particular and Linnaeus honoured his work and named mangosteen after him as *Garcinia*. David G. Fairchild (1903) referred mangosteen fruit, *Garcinia mangostana*, as the '*queen of tropical fruits*' and also 'the finest fruit in the world'. Mangosteen is the national fruit of Thailand.

Medicinal Uses

The seeds yield a concrete oil known as kokum oil or kokum butter. The butter is a specific remedy in dysentery and mucous diarrhoea. It is also used in phthisis and scorbutic diseases. It is often recommended as a substitute for cod liver oil and is a good substitute for cocoa butter. It is also eaten by poor people as a ghee substitute. Kokum butter is nutritive, demulcent, astringent and emollient. It contains compounds that help in the regeneration and repair of skin cells and as such it is used in skin lotions, creams, body butters, soaps, cosmetics and toiletry. It is used as a local external application to ulceration, fissures of lips, hands and also wounds and sores accompanied with inflammation. It is used in the preparation of ointments and suppositories. It is also a good moisturiser for skin in summer. The butter is well known to counteract the heat in summer particularly Gujarat and Maharashtra where it is used as a sherbat. It has the same quality of tamarind and enhances the dishes made of potatoes, okra (Lady's finger) and lentils. It is used as edible oil in fish curries, in pickles and chutneys. The fruit extract is traditionally used to relieve gastric problems like acidity, flatulence, constipation and indigestion. Its juice acts as a stimulant for appetite and has also anthelmintic properties. The infusion is used in ayurvedic medicine to treat piles, dysentery and infections. The fruit contains rich amounts of antioxidants which promote cell repair. The butter is known to strengthen the cardiovascular system and stabilise the liver function. The hydroxy citric acid in the fruit fights cholesterol and curbs lipogenesis. The butter can also be used as edible oil. Xanthone found in the pericarp of the fruit has about 28 health benefits therapeutically; it is also anti-neuralgic, helpful for the diseases of the gums and also in glaucoma. One of the most popular preparations of Malabar Tamarind is a Goan speciality, called *solkadi*, in which coconut milk and kokum are used. It can be had as a drink after meals to aid digestion or along with rice and vegetables.

Other Uses

The seed contains 23–26% oil, which is solid at room temperature. It is used in the preparation of chocolate and sugar confectionery. The tree is ornamental with a dense canopy of green leaves and red-tinged, tender, young leaves.

BEE'S WAX

Synonyms

Yellow bee's wax, Yellow wax (English), Gelbes Wachs (German), Cire jaune, Cire d'abeilles (French), Cera flava, Encerar (Spanish), Shamah al nahl, Shama (Arabic), Siktha or Madhujama (Sanskrit), Mom (Persian and Hindi), Mina (Gujarati), Mum or Myana (Maharashtrian), Maena (Kannada and Konkani), Taenmazhaeu or Mellugu (Tamil and Malayalam), Mynum (Telugu), Miettie (Sinhalese), H'pa-noung (Burmese), Lilin (Malaysian), Bazi (Chinese), Bijenwas (Dutch), Cera d'api (Italian), Wosk (Polish), Cera de abelha (Portuguese), Vosk bock (Russian), Bal mumu, Bulmumu (Turkish).

Synonyms for Honeybee

Hive bee (English), Madhumakkhi (Hindi), Teneteega (Telugu), Bhramaramu (Sanskrit), Abelha de mel, Abelha comum (Portuguese), Honungsbi (Swedish), Miel de abejas, Abeja melífera (Spanish), Honningbie (Norwegian), Azhilchin z°giy (Mongolian), Miele d'api (Italian), Melissa i imeri, Melissa i koini, Melissa i meliforos (Greek), Honigbiene, Die Honigbiene (German), Abeille domestique, Abeille commune (French), Honigbij, Honingbij (Dutch).

Biological Source

Bees wax is a natural wax produced in the beehive of honeybees and is obtained by melting and purifying the honeycomb of the genus *Apis, Apis mellifera* L. and other bees. The female worker bees have 8 wax-producing mirror glands on the inner sides of the sternites (the ventral shields of the body segments) on 4 to 7 abdominal segments. The size of these glands depends on the age of the worker bee. The bees use the wax to build the honeycomb in which the young are raised and honey and the pollen are stored.

Geographical Source

West Indies, California, Chile, Africa, Madagascar and India produce bee's wax.

Collection and Preparation

Wax is secreted by worker bees in cells on the ventral surface of the last four segments of their abdomen. The wax passes out through pores in the chitinous plates of the sternum and is used, particularly by young workers, to form the comb.

Yellow beeswax is prepared, after removal of the honey, by melting the comb under water (residual honey dissolving in the water and solid impurities sinking), straining, and allowing the wax to solidify in suitable moulds.

White beeswax is prepared from the above by treatment with charcoal, potassium permanganate, chromic acid, chlorine, etc. or by the slow bleaching action of light, air and moisture. In the latter method, the melted wax is allowed to fall on a revolving cylinder which is kept moist. Ribbon-like strips of wax are thus formed which are exposed on cloth to the action of light and air, being moistened and turned at intervals until the outer surface is bleached. The whole process is repeated at least once, and the wax is finally cast into circular cakes.

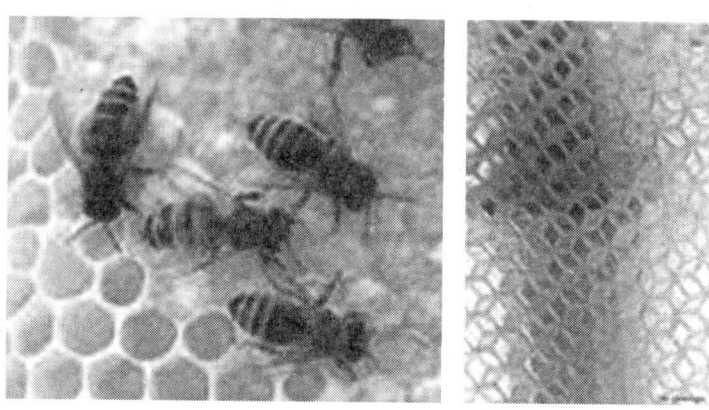

Yellow beeswax from honeycomb

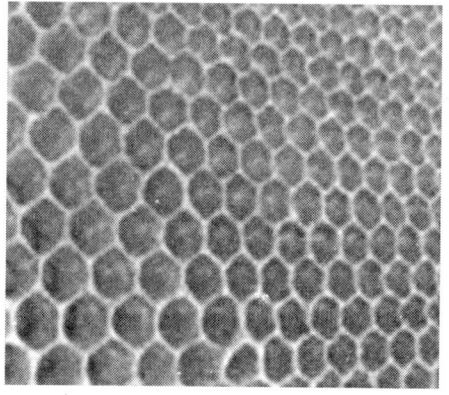

Honeycomb—the source

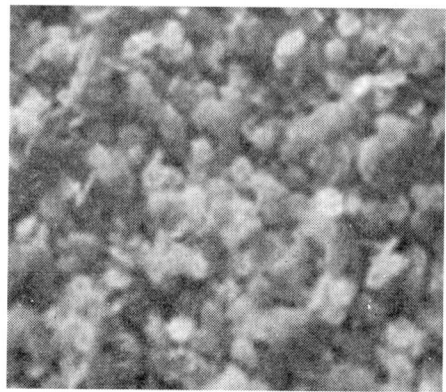

Natural beeswax

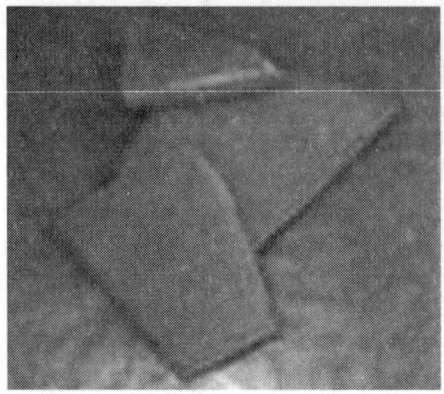
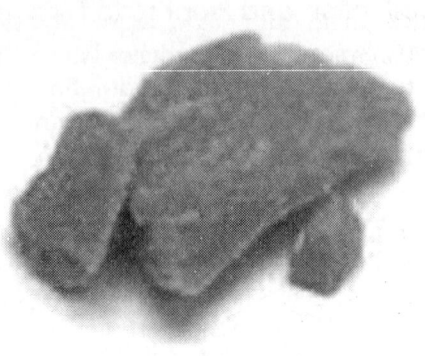

Pure raw wax   Commercial wax

Characters

Beeswax $[CH_3(CH_2)_{24}CO_2 - (CH_2)_{29}CH_3]$ is a tough, solid, non-crystalline material varying in colour from yellow to brownish-yellow or greyish-brown. It occurs as molded cakes, flakes or scales, brittle when cold and exhibits a dull granular form when broken. It melts between 62 and 66°C and is lighter than water having specific gravity between 0.958 and 0.970 g/cm^3 at 25°C. The flash point is 254–274°C and the saponification value is lower (3–5) for European type and higher (8–9) for Oriental type. It has a honey-like odour and tastes faint. Beeswax is insoluble in water but is soluble in hot alcohol, ether, chloroform, carbon tetrachloride, warm fixed oils and volatile oils. The wax is nearly white but becomes yellowish or brown by incorporation of pollen oils and propolis. The scales are about 3 mm across and 0.1 mm thick and about 1100 make a gram of wax. The aroma of beeswax is due to 48 hydrocarbon compounds and out of 100 volatile constitutens in it only 41 have been identified. This is generally classified into two types namely, the European type and Oriental type. The best substitutes are hydroxy-octa-cosanyl-hydroxy stearate and Japanese wax.

Chemical Constituents

The empirical formula is $[C_{15}H_{31}COOC_{30}H_{61}]$. The main components of beeswax are palmitate, palmitoleate, hydroxypalmitate and oleate esters of long chain (30–32 carbons) aliphatic alcohols and two principal components triacontanylpalmitate $(CH_3(CH_2)_{29}O-CO-(CH_2)_{14}CH_3)$ and cerotic acid $(CH_3(CH_2)_{24}COOH)$ in the ratio of 6 : 1. The beeswax mainly contains an ester myricin (Miricyl palmitate) up to an extent of 78%, free wax acids (14%) especially cerotic acid and its homologus along with cerin, two alcohols, aromatic substances and colouring matter. The percentage of the contents of beeswax is hydrocarbons (14%), monoesters (35%), diesters (14%), triesters (3%), hydroxy monoesters (4%), hydroxy polyesters

(8%), acid esters (1%), acid polyesters (2%), free acids (12%), free alcohols (1%) and unidentified substances (6%).

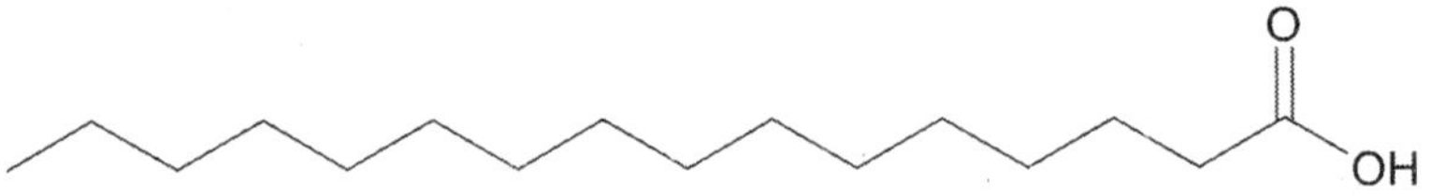

Palmitic acid or hexadecanoic acid $CH_3(CH_2)_{14}COOH$ or $(C_{16}H_{32}O_2)$

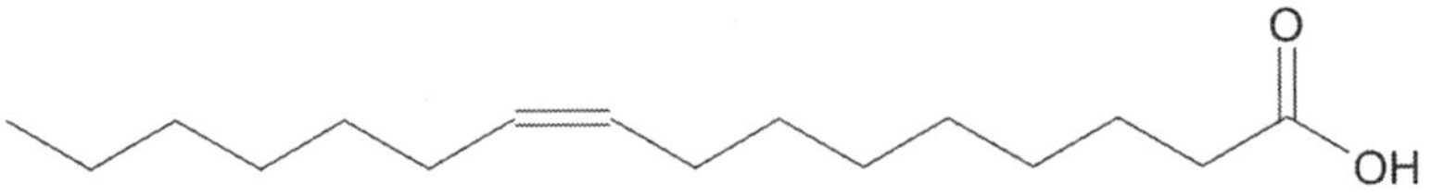

Palmitoleic acid or hexadec-9-enoic acid $[CH_3(CH_2)_5CH=CH(CH_2)_7COOH]$ or $(C_{16}H_{30}O_2)$

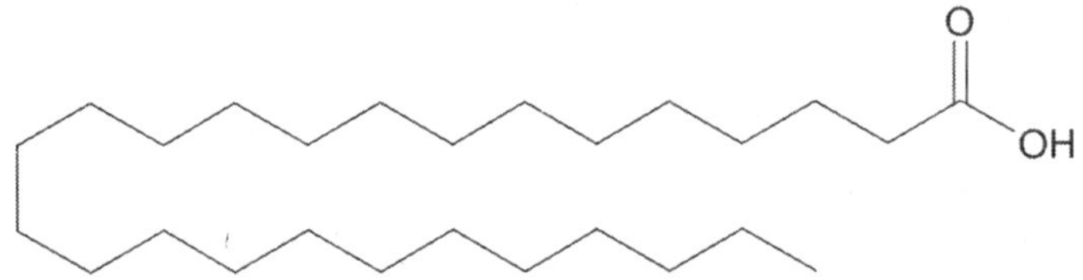

Cerotic acid (hexacosanoic acid) $(C_{26}H_{52}O_2)$ or $[CH_3(CH_2)_{24}COOH]$

History of Beeswax

This was ancient man's plastic and for thousands of years was used as a modelling material to create sculpture and jewelry molds in the lost-wax casting or *Cire perdue*. This casting of metals by Greeks and Romans involved a coating of wax model with plaster, melting of the wax and filling the space with the molten metal. This method is still used by the jewellers, goldsmiths and sculptors and also in dentistry. Romans sent their messages on writing tablets coated with beeswax, written on the smooth surface with a stylus and after it had been read, it was erased and reused for sending a reply. Egyptians used it in ship building. Romans used it as a waterproofing material for painted walls. In the middle ages it was used as a form of currency. It was also used in making English longbow. It was used as a sealing material and/or a stabiliser and a lubricant for bullets and fire arms.

Medicinal Uses

Beeswax has nonallergenic properties that can make it a useful skin protection from airborne allergies. It is a good electric insulator. It provides slight anti-inflammatory and antioxidant qualities which can benefit the body. It contains natural moisturisers that make it useful as a skin and lip balm. Sometimes, it may be applied to minor burns or other skin damage to help the skin heal. This barrier also helps to protect the skin from environmental toxins and irritants, which will not suffocate the skin but allows it to breathe. It can also be mixed with honey and olive oil that can serve as a natural treatment against eczema and psoriasis. Because it has vitamin A, it improves hydration to the skin and also promotes cell regeneration.

Yellow beeswax is used as a hardening agent for the preparations of ointments cerates and plaster. It is an ingredient of paraffin ointment and yellow ointment. In cosmetics, beeswax is used for the preparation of lipsticks and face creams. It is a skin enhancer, skin moisturiser, liver protector, cholesterol stabiliser, pain reliever, antiseptic (clears acne), lip healer, eliminator of stretch marks, and relaxer. There is insufficient evidence for its effectiveness against anal fissures, diaper rash, haemorrhoids (piles), ring worm, jock itch, fungal skin infection, ulcers, diarrhoea, hiccups, and other conditions.

Non-medical Uses

The food uses of beeswax include glazing of the fruits, candies and baked goods. It is a natural ingredient of chewing gum. It is used as a coating for cheese to protect it as it ages. The wax is used for making the candles and used as a lubricant or as a wood polish and shoe polish. Beeswax candles are preferred in Eastern Orthodox Churches, for the Easter Candles and candles used in Roman Catholic Churches. It is an ingredient of moustache wax and hair pomades. Earlier, it was used in the manufacture of cylinders in the phonographs. Solid beeswax has many uses. It is used to fill the worm-holes in the furniture, in Batik making and egg decoration, in lace making, as a waxing thread in sewing, in waxing fishing lines for free floating, etc. It is a thickening agent in herbal oils, in pine needle baskets, to finish iron work, to flux molten lead, in candy creations, in pulling metals into thin wires, in metal fabrication, etc.

Adulteration

The common adulterants are tallow, resin, colophony, hard paraffin, ceresin, stearic acid, Japan wax (from the fruits of *Rhus*), spermaceti, caranuba wax and other fats and waxes.

WOOL FAT

Synonyms

Anhydrous Lanolin, Adeps lanae anhydrous, Aloholes lanae, Wool wax, Wool grease, Lanoline, Wool alcohol, Soof al kharoof (Arabic), Tukovy (Czech), Das Lanolin (German), Grasa de lana (Spanish), Ullfett (Swedish).

Synonyms for Sheep

Sheep, Domestic sheep, Wild sheep, Urial, Feral sheep (English), Muflon (Czech), Far (Danish), Moeflon (Dutch), Mouton (French), Muflao (Portuguese), Tamfar, Fawr (Swedish), Mesha (Sanskrit), Gorre (Telugu),

La oveja (Spanish), Ovtsy (Russian), La pecora (Italian), Schafe (German), Bhed (Hindi).

Biological Source

Lanolin is derived from Latin, *lana* meaning 'wool' and *oleum* meaning 'oil', coined in 1885 by German physician, Mathias Eugenius Oscar Liebreich (1838–1908). Anhydrous wool fat (anhydrous lanolin) is a purified cholesterin; a fat prepared from the wool (fleece) of the sheep, *Ovis aries* L. (Class: Mammalia, Order: Ungulata, Family: Bovidae), secreted by the sebaceous glands of wool bearing animals. This is also found in the skin hair of the humans, feathers of the fowls, wool of domestic sheep and different parts of other animals.

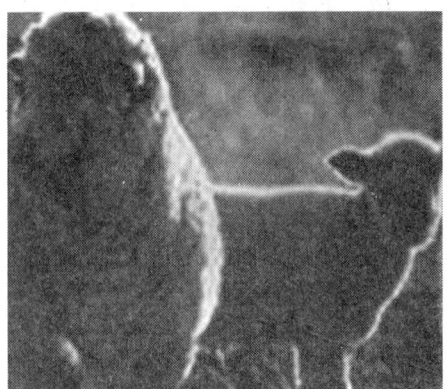
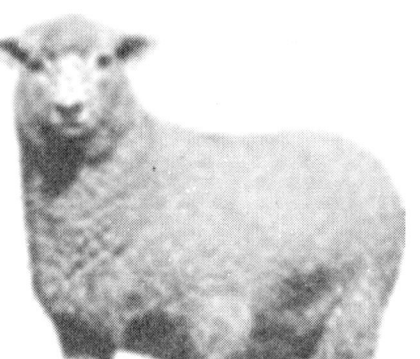

Source of wool fat—sheep   Sheep—source of lanolin

Collection and Preparation

Raw wool contains considerable quantities of 'wool grease' or crude lanolin, the potassium salts of fatty acids and earthy matter. During extraction, a large pot is taken with water until full. The raw wool is pushed into water gently. One to three tablespoons of salt is added to water. Keep it over an open fire outdoors. Keep the wool boiling over a period of several hours. Add more water to avoid the burning of the wool. Remove the wool from boiling water and keep it in a clean and waterproof area. Continue the boiling of water until all the water gets evaporated. The substance that remains is lanolin. Pour the lanolin through cheesecloth to remove any impurities. Pour it into a bowl and leave it to cool. Upon cooling, scrape off the lanolin and place it into sterilised jars, and it is ready to use. Raw lanolin is separated by 'cracking' with sulphuric acid from the washings of the scouring process and purified to fit it for the medicinal use. Purification may be done by centrifuging with water and by bleaching.

Characters

Purified wool fat is a uniform, greasy, light-yellowish, homogeneous, tenacious, unctuous solid not readily becoming rancid with a slight characteristic odour. This is a mixture of esters of fatty acids with high molecular weight alcohols. It melts at about 36–42°C. It is insoluble in water but forms very stable emulsions. It is sparingly soluble in alcohol more so when it is boiling. It is readily soluble in chloroform, ether, carbon disulphide, acetone, and benzene or petroleum ether. The saponification value ranges from 90 to 102 and the specific gravity is 0.932 to 0.945 at 15°C.

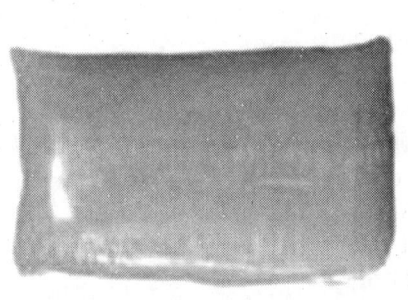

Anhydrous lanolin

Solid lanolin

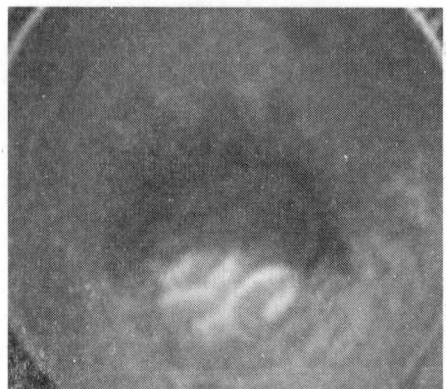

Lanolin grease

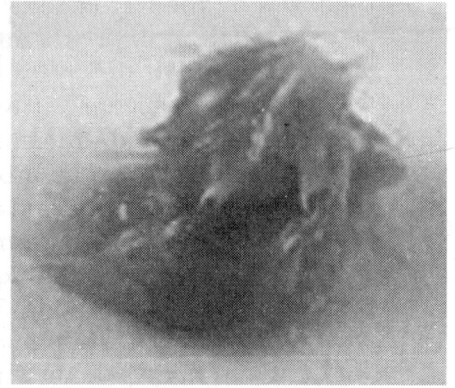

Pure lanolin

Chemical Constituents

This is not a true fat and lacks glycerides (glycerol esters). It primarily consists of sterol esters instead. Its waterproofing property helps sheep in shedding water from their coats. Lanolin contains cholesteryl and isocholesteryl alcohols together with many esters of lanoceric acid, lanopalmitic acid, carnaubic acid, myristic acid, oleic acid and cerotic and palmitic acids.

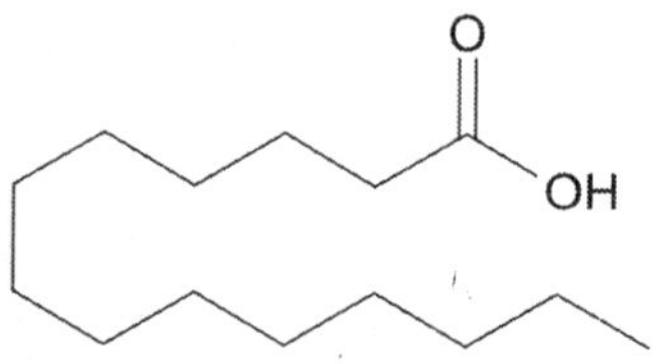

Myristic acid ($C_{14}H_{28}O_2$) or [$CH_3(CH_2)_{12}COOH$]

History of Wool Fat

Lanolin is used since very ancient times in cosmetics and dermatology as well as in industry like fabrics, lubricants and preparation of ink. The ancient Greeks were the first to extract crude wool fat from the sheep's wool. Documentation from 700 BC describes a process of boiling wool in water followed by the extraction of the top layer of grease. A more refined method was discovered in 60 AD by the Greek physician, Dioscorides, which consisted of pouring wool washings into a receptacle several times until froth developed and a layer of wool wax was collected after the froth disappeared. This product was called 'oesypus' by Dioscorides and it became widely cited in several ancient medical texts and pharmacopeias. Otto Braun, a German, patented a method for centrifuging the liquid derived from wool washings and the term lanolin was coined. This discovery was followed by the large scale production of lanolin in Germany and was spread to UK in the 19th century. The use of sheep's wool fat is ancient and was handed down by Pliny in his Natural History and it was reintroduced by Liebreich (1885) as a therapeutic agent. It is employed as a non-irritating and efficient ointment base and has its own marked advantage that it can be mixed with aqueous mixtures and glycerin. Stellwagon and Liebreich and others believe it to be absorbed more rapidly than any other fat. Modern methods of extraction from wool washings involve sophisticated techniques like modified centrifugation, solvent extraction and acid cracking. The crude wool grease is then purified and modified in different ways to produce different products and derivatives. In China, Wujiang Jinyu Lanolin Co. Ltd, has been a professional manufacturer in anhydrous lanolin, industrial lanolin, refined lanolin, pharmaceutical lanolin and its derivatives since 1991.

Medicinal Uses

Chemically, lanolin is similar to wax and can be used as a skin ointment, waterproof wax, as a raw material in shoe polish and textiles like yarn or felt. Medical grade lanolin is used as a cream to soothe the skin as it is hypoallergenic and bacteriostatic. It is an emollient used on sore and cracked nipples of breastfeeding mothers. It can be used to treat chapped lips, diaper rash, dry skin, itchy skin, minor incisions, minor burns and abrasions. It can also be used in shaving creams, as an ointment base, etc. In folk medicine, it is used in the nose to treat head colds. It is used as a raw material for the production of vitamin D_3. Lanolin is generally found in the baby oils, eye care products, diaper rash products, haemorrhoid (piles) ointments, lotions and creams, medicated shampoos, make-up products (lipsticks and foundations), make-up removers and shaving creams, etc. It is used in different types of colour cosmetics, hair care, skin care, soaps, topical applications and baby products.

Non-medical Uses

Anhydrous lanolin is used as a lubricant for brass instrument tuning slides and for making the woolen garments, waterproof and diaper covers. Commercially, it is used in rust preventing coatings, to create slippery coating on the propellers and stern gear and to prevent corrosion on stainless steel. In shipping equipment, it is used to create slippery surfaces on the propellers and stern gear to which barnacles cannot adhere. Commercial products like lanocote (with about 85% lanolin) are used to prevent corrosion in marine fasteners (when two different materials are in contact with each other and salt water). It is also valuable as a lubricant grease where corrosion would be a problem. The base ball players often use it to soften the base ball gloves. Lanoloin is also a popular additive to moustache wax. When mixed with neatsfoot oil, beeswax, and glycerol, lanolin is used in various leather treatments (as in saddle soaps and leather care products). Lanolin poisoning may occur when the products are swallowed accidentally, but it is not a health hazard.

Side Effects

Normally, side effects are possible (but do not always occur) that may occur in medicines that contain wool fat. In case of glaucoma and chest infection, one must consult a doctor immediately.

Adulteration

The common adulterants are mineral fats like soft paraffin, animal or vegetable fats and oils.

HYDNOCARPUS OIL

Synonyms

Chaulmoogra oil, Gynocardia oil, Oleum chaulmoograe, Kalaw tree oil, Gynocardia oil.

Synonyms for *Hydnocarpus*

Tuvaraka, Turveraka, Tuvrak, Kushtavairi (Sanskrit), Jangli Almond (English), Chaulmoogra, Jangli badam, Calmogara, Chalmogra (Persian and Hindi), Kadu Kawath (Marathi), Kadu kawata or Kowtee (Maharashtrian), Niradimutt, Maravetti, Maravattai, Marotti (Tamil), Kodi, Maravatty, Marotti, Nirvatta and Nivetti (Malayalam), Mirolhakai, Suranti, Toratti, Garudaphala (Kannada), Niradi-vittulu (Telugu), Makulu, Ratakakunta (Sinhalese).

Biological Source

Chaulmoogra is botanically known to the world as *Taraktogenos kurzii*, *Hydnocarpus kurzii*, *Hydnocarpus wightiana*, and *Hydnocarpus laurifolia* (Family: Achariaceae). This is the fixed oil obtained by cold expression from the fresh ripe seeds of *Hydnocarpus wightiana* Blume. (=*H. laurifolia*), *H. anthelmintica* Pier., *H. heterophylla* and other species of *Hydnocarpus* and also of *Taraktogenos kurzii* King. (Family: Achariaceae). There are about 40 species found in the rain forests from India to Philippines and Celebes.

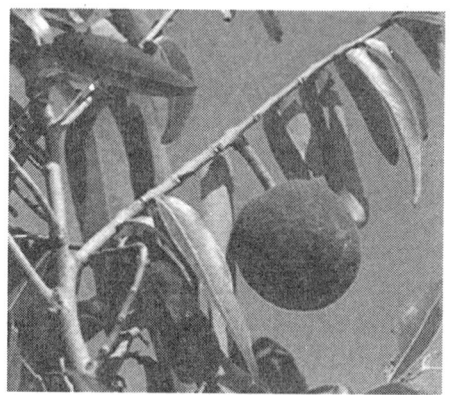

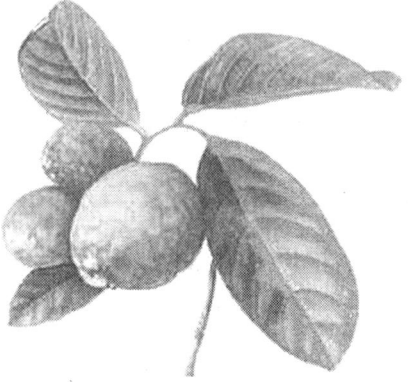

Hydnocarpus wightiana   *Taraktogenos kurzii (=H. kurzii)*

Geographical Source

Chulmugra seeds are the seeds of *Taraktogenos kurzii* King, a tree that grows in Myanmar (the then Burma). *Hydnocarpus* seeds are derived from *Hydnocarpus wightiana* Blume, a tree growing in South-East and South-West India, belonging to family Achariaceae. The plant is indigenous to India, Myanmar (Burma), Indonesia, Malaysia and Philippines. In India, it grows in the tropical forests along Western Ghats, along the coast from Maharashtra to Kerala, Assam, Tripura, and often planted on the sides of the road in hilly areas. The tree is also found in South-East Asia, chiefly in Indo-Malayan region. It is also cultivated in Sri Lanka, Nigeria and Uganda.

Characters of the Seed

The seeds of *T. kurzii* are irregularly ovoid, about 2–3 cm long and 1–1.5 cm wide, with a smooth and brittle testa. The seeds contain an abundant oily, dark brownish endosperm. Embedded within the endosperm is an embryo with 2 large, foliaceous, 3-nerved cotyledons and a terete radicle. The seeds of *H. wightiana* are similar to those of *T. kurzii*, but are smaller in their size about 2 cm long.

Collection and Preparation

During the extraction of chaulmoogra oil, the seeds are collected by the natives of Myanmar from the ripe fruits, cleaned, washed and dried in the sun. The seed contains 40–45% fixed oil, chaulmoogra oil. The seeds are mechanically decorticated (shelled) during which process; the outer seed coat (testa) is cracked and removed. The collected kernels are beaten to a paste. The paste is then put into square jute bags (about 30 cm square and 5 cm thick). The bags are piled up and the fixed oil is expressed by a hydraulic process (this method is followed in Chittagong even today). The cold-drawn oil is filtered and stored in well-closed containers protected from light. Hydnocarpus oil is also collected by a similar process from the seeds of *H. wightiana* and *H. anthelmintica* to be legitimately substituted for chaulmoogra oil, if it agrees in physical and chemical properties designating its source.

Characters of both the Oils

The two oils, chaulmoogra oil and hydnocarpus oil are very similar in their physical characters and chemical constituents. The latter is yellow to brownish yellow oil or a soft fat with a slight characteristic odour and somewhat acrid taste. The specific gravity is between 0.950 and 0.960, melting point ranges between 20 and 25°C and the refractive index between 1.472 and 1.476 (at 40°C). The oil has an acid value not more than 25, saponification value ranges between 198 and 204 and iodine value is 93–103.

Chemical Constituents

Chaulmoogra oil contains primarily unsaturated acids like hydnocarpic acid (45%) and Chaulmoogric acid (25%). Small quantity of glycerides of palmitic acid is also found in the oil.

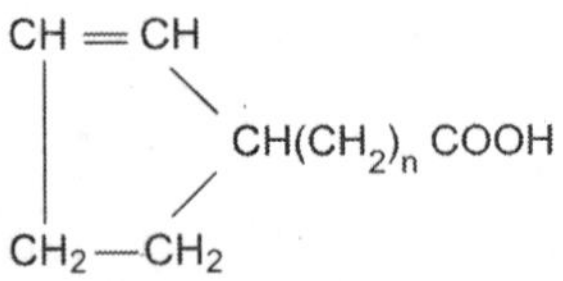

$$CH = CH$$
$$CH(CH_2)_n \, COOH$$
$$CH_2 - CH_2$$

Hydnocarpic acid (n = 10)
Chaulmoogric acid (n = 12)

Hydnocarpic acid ($C_{16}H_{28}O_2$) and chaulmoogric acid ($C_{18}H_{32}O_2$)

History of Hydnocarpus Oil

Chaulmoogra oil was used by the Chinese for leprosy from at least 14th century and about a century ago it began to be used for the same purpose by the Western physicians. The oil had been used in India and China to treat leprosy and other diseased skin conditions. Frederic John Mouat (1854), an English doctor working in Calcutta, reported the possible use of chaulmoogra oil in treating leprosy, and the oil or its derivatives were the chief medication by the 1920s. Roger Adams, a chemist and a teacher, was known for determining the chemical constitution of many natural substances including chaulmoogra oil.

Medicinal Uses

The cyclic unsaturated fatty acids (hydnocarpic acid and chaulmoogric acid) present in the oil possess strong antibacterial effect on micrococci of leprosy and destroy *Myobacterium leprae* and thus have a positive cure for leprosy. This was described in the ancient Hindu and Chinese documents. Esterification of these acids enhances the bactericidal action and thus, the ethyl esters and salts of hydnocarpic and chaulmoogric acids have been used in the treatment of leprosy. The esterified oil and the esters of the derived acids are all employed only for external application in rheumatism, psoriasis and tuberculosis. This is also the source of Ethyl Chaulmoograte. The oil has antimicrobial properties and has been used the formulations to help treat eczema, psoriasis, arthritis, sprains, bruises and skin inflammations. The oil can be included in creams, lotions, balms, ointments, lip balms, massage oils and wound care balms. The oil is used locally in rheumatism, phthisis, tuberculosis and an effective dressing for scaly eruptions, chronic skin diseases and even syphilis. A seed paste is a home remedy for ringworm and scabies. The infusion of the seed is used as a disinfectant for vaginal infections in gonorrhoea and foetid discharge after child birth. The bark of the plant contains tannins beneficial in fevers.

Side Effects

Chaulmoogra oil is unsafe when it is taken by mouth because it contains cyanide (cyanogenic glucosides) and might cause poisoning. It can cause cough, difficult breathing, spasm in the throat, and damage to the kidneys, visual disorders, pain in the head and muscles and also paralysis. It can also cause irritation of the skin.

SPERMACETI

Synonyms

Spermawax, Oleum ceti (Latin), Tuk z vorvanì (Czech) Spermaceti, Hvalrav (Danish) Walrat, Das Walrat, Cetaceum (Dutch and German) Blanc de baleine, Spermaceti, Blanc de cachalot, Adipocere (French) Spermatokiros, Leiko tis falainas, Leiko toi fisitira, Lipos kitois (Greek) Spermaceti, Bianco di balena (Italian) Eespermacete, Branco de cachalote, Branco de baleia (Portuguese), Spermatet (Rumanian) spermatset (Russian) Esperma de ballena, Spermaceti, Blanco de ballena (Spanish) Ispermeçet (Turkish).

Synonyms for Sperm Whale

Ýspermeçet balinasý (Turkish), Pottfisk (Swedish), Ballena esperma (Spanish), Bolshoi plavun (Russian), Cachalote (Portuguese and Spanish), Paus sperma (Malay), Kigutilissuaq (Korean), Makko-kujira (Japanese), Capidoglio (Italian), Ikan paus sperma (Indonesian), Pottfisch (German), Cachalot (French), Kaizilot, Potvis (Dutch), Pot whale, Sperm whale, Spermacet whale (English).

Biological Source

Spermaceti (from Greek, *sperma* means the 'seed' and from Latin, *cetus* means 'whale') is a concrete solid or semiliquid waxy substance contained in the large cavity in front of the cranium near the upper jaw of sperm whale, *Physeter macrocephalus* L. (=*Physeter catadon*, a largest living toothed whale (an odontocete), a largest living predator, the deepest diving animal, with loudest sound produced by any animal and with the largest brain of any animal) and other species of *Physeter* (Class: Mammalia; Order Cetacea; Family: Physeteridae) found in the Indian, Atlantic and Pacific oceans. It is obtained mixed with sperm oil or oleum ceti. Part of the spermaceti of commerce is obtained from the bottle-nosed whale, *Hyperoodon rostratus* and *H. restrains*. The crude sperm oil is secreted in a special large cylindrical organ in the upper region of the huge jaw and above the right nostril. The spermaceti organ help adjust the whale's buoyancy, aids in echolocation and sexual selection. Spermaceti is found in various parts of its body in small proportions dissolved in its blubber.

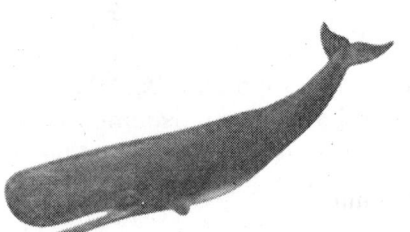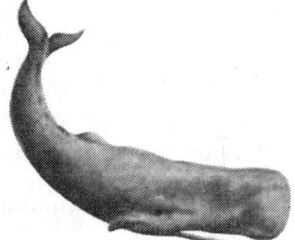

Physeter macrocephalus   Sperm whale

Geographical Source

Sperm whales are found in the Pacific, Atlantic and Indian oceans. These gregarious animals inhabit Pacific ocean, the Indian archipelago and the Chinese and Australian seas.

Collection and Preparation

This large whale which attains a length of about 20 to 30 m is killed. In the head there is a special cavity filled with a semifluid substance which is dried and exposed to strong pressure to remove the sperm oil just sufficient to fill as many as 10 large barrels. The oil from the head of the killed animal is removed by buckets or by pumping. The oil, on cooling deposits about 10 to 11% of spermaceti wax which is melted in warm water, strained to remove the impurities and boiled with weak caustic soda solution, washed with warm water and finally allowed to solidify into spermaceti wax. For pharmaceutical use, spermaceti is further refined by boiling with alcohol. This gives white scaly mass of crystalline material.

Characters

Spermaceti occurs in concrete, translucent, pearly white crystalline masses, with a mild bland taste and a faint fatty odour which can be easily indented or scraped by the nail, slightly greasy, pulverisable, fusible and combustible. It is hard and shining which becomes yellow and rancid by exposure to air. It has a neutral reaction. It is insoluble in water and cold alcohol but dissolves in fixed and volatile oils, sulphuric acid, ether, chloroform and boiling rectified spirit (alcohol) and forms crystalline masses as it cools. It melts near 42–50°C and congeals near 45°C having acid value not more than 1, saponification value 125.8–134.6 and iodine value 3–44. It has a specific gravity of 0.905 to 0.945 at 25°C and refractive index of about 1.4333 at 80°C. A botanical alternative is a derivative of jojoba oil, jojoba ester, a solid wax very similar to spermaceti chemically and physically.

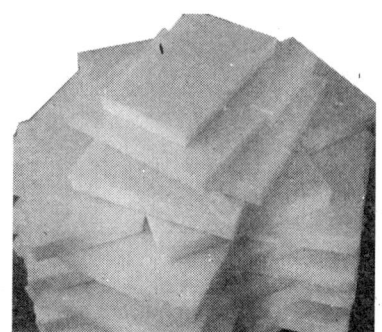

Spermaceti wax

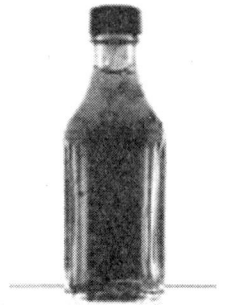

Pure oil

Chemical Constituents

Spermaceti [$CH_3(CH_2)_{14}CO_2\text{-}(CH_2)_{15}CH_3$] contains 85% of the total esters comprising chiefly of mixture of cetyl esters with cetin or cetyl palmitate ($C_{15}H_{31}.COO\text{–}C_{16}H_{33}$), lauro-stearic acid, cetyl myristate and cetyl stearate.

It contains acetylic alcohol (ethal or cetyl hydrate or cetyl alcohol $C_{15}H_{33}OH$) along with palmitic acid. The former can be obtained from spermaceti by saponification with alcoholic solution of potassium hydroxide, diluting with hot water and filtering and crystallising which forms brilliant colourless crystals melting at 49.5°C. It is commonly adulterated with stearic acid, stearin, tallow and paraffin wax.

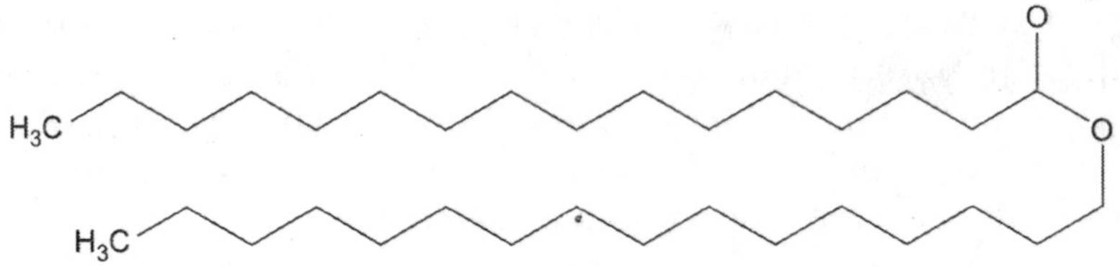

Cetyl palmitate or hexadecyl hexadecanoate
$CH_3(CH_2)_{14}CO_2(CH_2)_{15}CH_3$ or $(C_{32}H_{64}O_2)$

History of Spermaceti

In the late 18th century, the growth of the whaling industry brought a first major change in the making of the candles since the Middle Ages, when spermaceti, a wax obtained by crystallising the sperm whale oil became available. Like beeswax, which was earlier utilised in candle making, spermaceti did not emit a repugnant odour when burnt, and also did not soften or bend in the summer heat. Earlier historians noted that the first standard candles were made from spermaceti. Joseph Morgan (1834), an inventor, introduced a machine which allowed continuous production of molded candles by the use of a cylinder with a movable piston which ejected the solidified candles. Further development occurred in 1850 with the production of paraffin wax from oil and coal shales. The art of producing candles from the oil of sperm whales began in America around 1748 and the process was introduced by Jacob Rodriques Rivera, a Sephardic Jew, in Newport, Rhode Island.

Medicinal Uses

Spermaceti is used as an emollient and in the preparation of cerates and ointments, especially cold creams. It is a demulcent and protective and is used in domestic practice for cough, colds, catarrhal affections and irritation of intestinal mucous membranes and urinary affections. It is also used in blisters and ulcers. It is an ingredient in cosmetics, leather working and industrial lubricants (machine oils). It is also used in making fine wax candles, pomades, in soaps, in dressing of the fabrics and as a pharmaceutical excipient.

Non-medical Uses

The sperm oil is a popular lubricant and works well for the fine, light machinery like sewing machines, watches, etc. as it is thin, does not dry out and corrode metals. It is also used in heavy machinery like locomotives and steam-powered looms as it can withstand high temperatures. The oil has a widespread use in aerospace industry because of its very low freezing point. A coat of the oil is used to protect the metals from rust and provides temporary protection for metal components in fire arms as it does not dry out.

Adulteration

Often a mixture of esters of saturated fatty alcohols and fatty acids is used as a substitute.

LARD OIL

Synonyms

Lard (purified fat of the hog), Adeps, Charbee (vernacular), Oleum adipis, Ades preseparatus, Axungia porci (Porcina), Prepared (hogs) lard (Brazilian), Adeps suillis, Schweine-schmalz (German), Axonge, Graisse de porc, Huile de saindoux, Huile de lard (French), Ladhi toi sialoi (Greek), Aceite de manteca de cerdo (Spanish).

Synonyms for Pig

Pig, Feral pig, Domestic pig, Old world swine, Razorback, Wild hog, Swine (English), Kuhukuhu (Maori), Kune-kune (Maori – New Zealand), Wildschwein (German), Suvar (Hindi), Varah (Sanskrit), Pandi (Telugu), Chancho (Spanish), Le cochon (French), Suino (Italian), Sor (Kashmiri).

Biological Source

Lard is the purified internal fat of the abdomen of pig/hog (wild boar), *Sus scrofa* var. *domesticus* Gray. (= *Sus scrofa, Sus domesticus*: Order: Ungulata, Family: Suidae), a member of the pig family. It is the fresh fat, especially that fat over the mesentery, omentum, kidneys and its external membranes of winter-killed hogs.

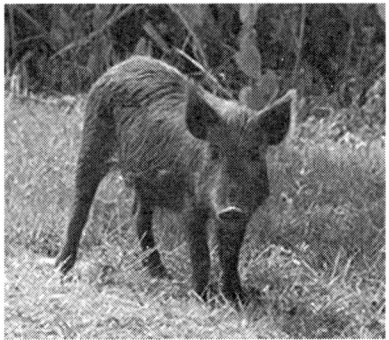
Source of lard-wild animal

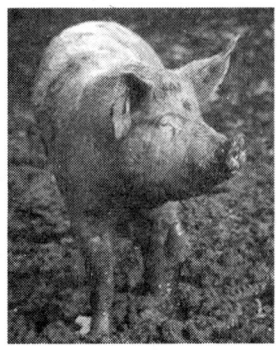
Domesticated animal

Geographical Source

Its original distribution ranges from France to European Russia. It has been introduced into Sweden, Norway, USA, Canada, N. Asia, Japan, Indonesia, S. America, New Guinea, New Zealand, Australia and other Islands.

Collection and Preparation

Lard is a soft, creamy, white solid or semisolid fat with butter-like consistency, obtained by rendering (or melting) the fatty tissue of hogs. Lard varies with the type of the method of production and the fat-bearing animal parts used during production. Steam-rendered or wet-rendered lard is made by injecting the steam under pressure into a closed vessel containing the fats of hog. The open-kettle-rendered or dry-rendered (enclosed system) lards, darker in their colour, are made by melting the fat in steam-jacketed vessels (the residue is called cracklings). Neutral lard is prepared by melting the leaf (from around the kidneys) and back fat at about 49°C (120°F). Continuous rendering involves grinding, rapid heating, and the separation of the fat from the cells by centrifugation.

It is first exposed to the air, cut into thin slices, beaten in a mortor and converted into a uniform mass. Then it is put into a vessel with water and heated till the fat melts and separates from the membranous matter and strained. To remove the odour, alum and common salt is added to the lard. For medicinal purposes lard is prepared from the abdominal fat known as 'flare', from which it is obtained by treatment with hot water at a temperature not exceeding 57°C. The lard has a tendency to become rancid and thus benzoinated lard is prepared by adding 1% Siam benzoin to the purified lard. The addition of benzoin tends to retard the development of rancidity. After preparation, it is soft, creamy-white, solid or semisolid with butter-like consistency.

Characters

Lard is a soft yellowish to colourless oil with a characteristic aroma, bland taste, non-rancid and neutral reaction. It dissolves entirely in ether, benzene, chloroform, petroleum benzin, and carbon disulfide, slightly in alcohol and insoluble in water. It has an acid value of not more than 1.2, a lower melting point (40°C) to form a clear liquid and a higher iodine value (52–66). It should be kept cool in well-closed containers impervious to fat.

Chemical Constituents

Lard is a fat from pig in both its rendered and un-rendered forms, which is a semisoft, white fat derived from the fatty parts of the pig, with a high saturated fatty acid content and no trans fat. Rendering is by steaming, boiling, or dry heat. It contains 50 to 60% of olein (oleum adipis—$(C_{17}H_{33}COO)_3C_3H_5$ or $(C_{57}H_{104}O_8)$) and 38% of palmitin $(CH_3(CH_2)_{14}CO_2H$ or $C_3H_5(OOC_{16}H_{31})_3)$, margarin and stearin (Tristearin $(C_{17}H_{35}COO)_3C_3H_5$ or $C_3H_5(C_{18}H_{35}O_2)_3$ or $(C_{57}H_{110}O_6)$). Of the fatty acids present, oleic acid (44–47%) and palmitic acid (25–28%) are predominant but appreciable amounts of stearic acid (12–14%) and linoleic acid (6–10%) are also present. Thus, lard contains about 40% of solid glycerides such as stearin and palmitin and about 60% of mixed liquid glycerides such as olein. These fractions are sometimes separated by pressure at 0°C and sold as 'stearin' and lard oil, respectively. Lard has a specific gravity of 0.917–0.938 at 20°C, an iodine value of 45–75, an acid value of 3.4, a saponification value of 190–205 and a smoke point of 121–218°C.

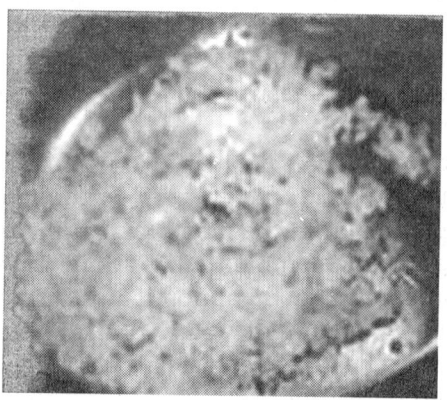

Lard   Purified lard oil

History of Lard Oil

Lard has always been an important cooking and baking staple in cultures where pork is an important dietary item. During the 19th century, lard was used as butter in North America and other European nations. Lard was used widely as a substitute for butter during World War II. It was common in many people's diet until the industrial revolution because it was cheaper than most of the vegetable oils. By late 20th century, lard had been considered less healthy than vegetable oils, but has been regarded as a food for the poor people. But, in the 1990s and early 2000s, the special culinary properties of lard became widely recognised by chefs and bakers which led to rehabilitation of this fat. Lard was once widely used in the cuisines of Europe, China and the New World and is still has a significant role in the British, Central European, Mexican and Chinese cuisines. It is a traditional ingredient in mince peas and Christmas puddings, lardy cake and for frying fish and chips in the British cuisine. Traditionally, it is one of the main ingredients in the Scandinavian pate leverpostei and in Catalan cuisine; it is still used to make cocoa bases and typical cakes as ensaimades.

It was once very common in Europe and North America in the areas where dairy fats and vegetable oils were rare as a spread on bread. Lard was often consumed mixed into cooked rice along with soy sauce to make lard rice in Taiwan and Hong Kong as well as mainland China.

Medicinal Uses

Benzoinated lard is used as an emollient and protective. A more common use however, is as a vehicle in the preparation of ointments as an ointment base. It is used in the preparation of benzoated lard employed for preparing the ointments. Lard oil is obtained by expressing the fixed oil from lard at a low temperature when stearin gets separated from olein. Sometimes, it is used to prepare the nitrate of mercury ointment.

Non-medical Uses

It is used as a lubricant, cutting oil, wool oil, an illuminant (in light houses), in perfumery and also in the manufacture of soap. Rendered lard can be used to produce biofuel. Lard is used in many cuisines as a cooking fat or as a spread similar to butter. It is an ingredient in sausages and fillings, and the preparation of pastry. Lard is one of the few edible oils with a high smoke point. Pure lard is useful for cooking since it produces little smoke when it is heated, and has a distinct flavour when combined with other foods. Often, lard is treated with bleaching and deodourising agents, emulsifiers and antioxidising agents to make it more consistent and prevent the spoilage. Formerly, lard and other animal fats were used as an anti-foaming agent in industrial fermentation processes like brewing.

Adulteration

This is often adulterated with cotton oil and paraffin oil.

OLIVE OIL

Synonym

Oleum olivae.

Synonyms for Olive

Olive, Europen olive, Wild olive, Iron tree, Common olive, Olienhout (Africanus), Oleastro (Italian), Olivier.

Biological Source

Olive oil is a fixed oil which is expressed from the ripe fruits of *Olea europaea* L. (Family: Oleaceae). The richness of the oil in the tree is reflected in its botanical name, *Olea europea* as the word 'oleum' in Latin means 'oil'.

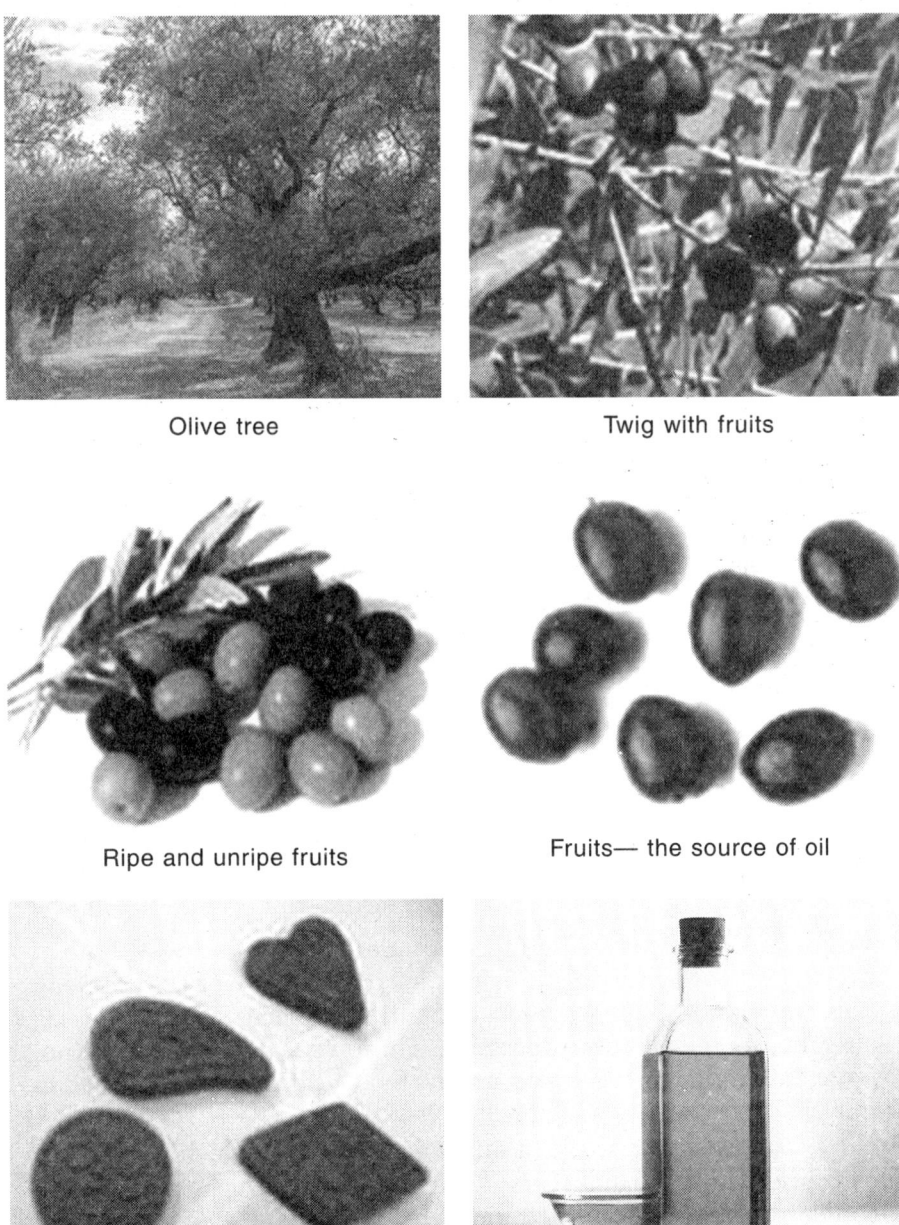

Olive tree

Twig with fruits

Ripe and unripe fruits

Fruits— the source of oil

Natural oil as cakes

Olive oil

Geographical Source

The plant appears to be a native of Palestine. It is now grown in Southern Europe and Mediterranean region. It is also cultivated in USA and Australia.

Italy, Spain, France, Greece and Tunisia produce 90% of the world production. The leading producers of extra virgin oil are Liguria, Tuscany, Umbria and Apulia in Italy. The wild tree has its origin in Turkey (older Asia Minor) and spread to Africa, Australia, Japan and China.

Collection and Preparation

It is prepared by crushing and pressing ripe fruits called 'Olives'. The entire olive consists of 20–30% oil and the fruit pulp has 60–80% oil. In the modern factories hydraulic presses are widely used to squeeze oil out of the fruit under low pressure. This type of technique is called cold pressing (physical method) and it generates a very little amount of heat, because of which it gives the best quality oil called 'Virgin olive oil'. The further pressing gives low quality oil. The oil that comes from the last pressing is called olive residue (pomace) and is generally used for cosmetics, medicines, etc.

Characters

Olive oil is a pale yellow liquid, which sometimes has a greenish tint. The oil has a slight odour and a bland taste. Olive oil is practically insoluble in alcohol. It is miscible with organic solvents such as chloroform and ether. It is stored at a temperature not exceeding 40°C. The extra virgin oil is derived from the first pressing and possesses the most delicate flavour and antioxidant properties.

Types of Olive Oil

The International Olive Oil Council (IOOC) has released the Trade Standard Applying to Olive Oils and olive-Pomace Oils, and the council has provided the descriptions for different types of oils. The descriptions are as follows:

- *Virgin olive oil:* This is the most popular variety and well known cooking oil used for cooking with a surprisingly lower acid content. This is prepared by mechanical and physical means, and there is no alteration to the oil after processing. This oil has a free acidity of not more than 2 gm per 100 grains, and no food additives are permitted in this oil.
- *Extra virgin olive oil:* This is a much better variety which is made by cold pressing the fruits. This is edible oil which has a free acidity content of no more than 0.5 gm per 100 gm, and no additives are permitted in this oil. This is considered to be the best for our body.
- *Pure (ordinary) olive oil:* This is a combination of both refined and virgin oils which contains a higher acidic content. This has a free acidity content of no more than 3.3 gm per 100 gm, and this oil is unsuitable for use, does not contain any additives. This is sometimes sold as 'refined clove oil'.
- *Lampante virgin oil:* This is extracted by mechanical (virgin) methods but not suitable for human consumption without further refining. This

oil is not recommended for cooking purposes, and is used as a fuel, for industrial purposes, for technical use and can be refined to make it edible.

The USDA (United States Department of Agriculture) released the US standards for Grades of it in 1948. These are still followed in the US. The USDA grades olive oil in the following four categories, namely: US Grade A (US-Fancy), US Grade B (US-Choice), US Grade C (US-Standard), and US Grade D (US-Substandard). This has caused the problems for consumers in purchasing the right kind of olive oil. This grading is done on the basis of the free fatty acid content (calculated as oleic acid according to the Official and Tentative Methods of Analysis of the Association of Official Agricultural Chemists), the absence of defects (degree of freedom from cloudiness at 60°F), odour (typical olive oil odour and its variation to off-odours), and flavour (typical olive oil flavour and its variation to off-flavours). It has given a 100 point score sheet for the olive oil in which free fatty acid content, the absence of defects; odour and flavour have weights of 30, 30, 20 and 20 respectively.

Chemical Constituents

Olive oil contains about 75% oleic acid, a mono-unsaturated fatty acid. It also contains palmitic acid (8–20%) and linoleic acid (4–20%). The untreated extra virgin olive oil is of the highest quality and has an organoleptic rating of 6.5, low acidity (1% or less) than the untreated oil with a rating of 5.5 and 2% acidity. The oil consists of saturated fats like palmitic acid (7.5 to 20%), stearic acid (0.5 to 5%), arachidic acid (less than 0.8%), behenic acid (less than 0.3%), myristic acid (less than 0.1%), monosaturated fats like oleic acid (55 to 83%), palmitoleic acid (0.3 to 3.5%), polyunsaturated fatty acids like linoleic acid (3.5 to 21%), linolenic acid (less than 1.5%) and unsaturated fats. In addition, it has omega-3 fat (less than 1.5 g), omega-6 fat (3.5 to 21 g), vitamin E (93%) and vitamin K (59%). It has a melting point of minus 6°C, a boiling point of 300°C and a smoke point of 190°C (virgin) to 210°C (refined). The specific gravity is 0.9150 to 0.9180 at 20°C (virgin and refined), viscosity of 84 at 20°C (virgin and refined), an iodine value of 75 to 94 (virgin and refined), an acid value of 6.6 and the saponification value of 184 to 196 (virgin and refined). It has food energy of 880 kcal per 100 g.

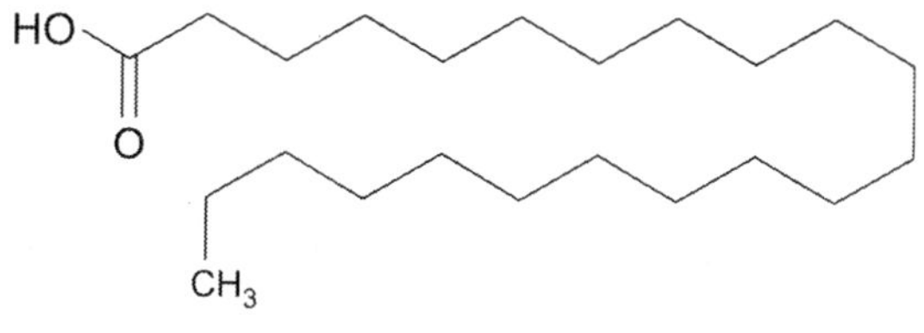

Behenic acid or docosanoic acid $C_{21}H_{43}COOH$ or $C_{22}H_{44}O_2$

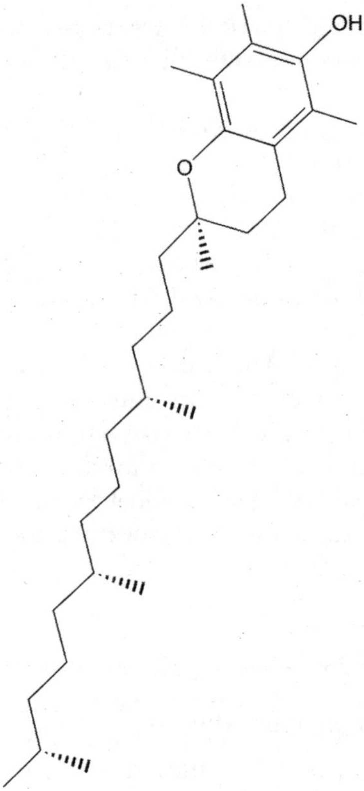

Vitamin E or alpha-tocopherol ($C_{29}H_{50}O_2$)

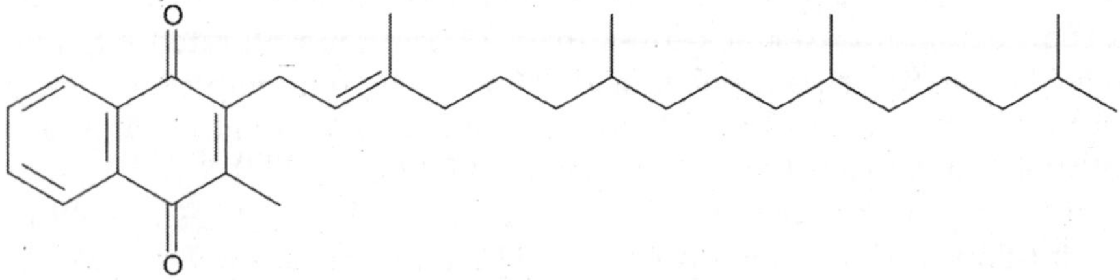

Vitamin K/K$_1$ or phylloquinone or menaquinone ($C_{31}H_{50}O_3$)

History of Olive

Olive has been used in Mediterranean countries for thousands of years and it was referred to as *'liquid gold'* by Homer. The athletes in ancient Greece rubbed it all over their bodies in rituals. It has been injected into the bones of dead saints through holes in their tombs. The olive tree has been used as a symbol of abundance, glory and peace. Its green branches were used to crown the victorious in games and war. The crown and branches were offered to deities as emblems of benediction and purification and some were found in Tutankhamen's tomb. Fossil remains of its ancestor were found near Livorno, Italy which date back to 20 million years. The cultivation of olives can be traced to 5th century BC and was first cultivated in the Eastern part of the Mediterranean in a region called the 'fertile crescent' and later moved westwards. The first cultivation began in 5000 BC and slowly spread from island of Crete to Syria, Palestina and Israel came to Southern Turkey, Cyprus and Egypt until 1400 BC. With the expansion of the Greek colonies, the culture reached Southern Italy and North Africa in 8th century BC and later spread into Southern France. Under Roman rule the trees were planted in the entire Mediterranean basin in 1st century AC. King Solomon and King David of the Hebrews gave much importance for the cultivation of olives and it is understood that King David even placed the guards to watch over the groves to ensure the safety of the trees and the precious oil. The trees were sacred in the Hellenic society of Greece that the people were condemned to death or exile when they cut down the trees. In ancient Egypt, Greece and Rome, the oil was infused with flowers and grasses to be used as medicine and cosmetics. During the excavations in Mycenae, a list was unearthed which contained fennel, sesame, celery, watercress, mint, sage, rose, juniper, etc. being added to the olive oil for the preparation of the ointments. The first recorded extraction of the olive oil is known from Hebrew Bible which took place during the Exodus from Egypt during the 13th century BC. According to a legend, the city of Athens obtained its name because Athenians considered olive oil essential, preferring the offering of the goddess Athena (an olive tree) over the offering of Poseidon (a spring of salt water gushing out of a cliff). In the permanent temple in Jerusalem, according to Jewish observance, olive oil is the only fuel allowed to be used in the Mishkan service and for anointing King of Israel (originated from King David and the last was Tzidkiyahu). In Christianity, olive oil is used for the oil of Catechumens (used to bless and to strengthen before preparing for Baptism), oil of the sick (used to confer the sacrament of anointing the sick), to confer the sacrament of confirmation (as a symbol of Holy Spirit), in the rites of Baptism, the ordination of priests and bishops and at the coronation of the monarchs. In Islam, the Quran mentions olive as a sacred plant and oil is reported to have been recommended by the Prophet Muhammad for curing over 70 diseases.

Medicinal Uses

It is more popular in North America and other parts of the world. It is actually a pure fruit juice and does not require any heat or chemicals to extract. It can be consumed immediately after pressing. Because of its high monounsaturated fat (oleic acid), vitamin E and antioxidants it is good for humans. It is known for lowering the bad cholesterol (LDL) and raising good cholesterol (HDL) and blood pressure, protection against colon, breast cancer and skin cancer and reducing the stones of the gallbladder. Olive oil is used externally as an emollient and to sooth inflamed surfaces. It is used for psoriasis, eczema, sunburn, mild burns and rheumatism. It is used as a lubricant for massage. Olive oil is used in the preparation of liniments, ointments, plasters and soaps. Given internally, olive oil acts as a demulcent and a mild laxative. The oil is useful in preventing blood clot formation, platelet aggregation and in avoiding excessive blood coagulation thereby reducing the incidence of cardiovascular diseases. It is known to decrease systolic and diastolic blood pressure. It is a good alternative in diabetes and prevents the onset and delaying of the disease. The diet rich olive oil helps in weight loss and reduces the abdominal fat and obesity. It has a key role in the development of the foetus during pregnancy. It helps in the development of the brain and bones in children, a source of vitamin E for older people, a natural oxidant which slows down the process of ageing, helps bile, liver and intestinal function and diminishes ulcers and gastro-intestinal problems like gastritis. It is a demulcent and a mild laxative and helps in softening the stools. It also acts as an ear wax softener at room temperature. It is a potent blocker of contractions of the intestine and is used to treat borborygmus. The oil contains oleocanthol which is a non-selective inhibitor of cyclo-oxygenase similar to ibuprofen. Extravirgin oil is used as a mosituriser for the skin and effective shaving oil. The most important negative health effect is the likelihood of development of breast cancer in postmenopausal women and prostrate cancer.

Side Effects

In spite of a lot of benefits, olive oil does have some side effects. The oil can cause allergic reactions in some individuals when applied on the skin, like eczema and skin rashes that prove to be itchy. Since the oil is rich in calories, overconsumption of it can cause the risk of heart diseases (not more than 2 tsp on a daily basis). The oil may react with diabetes medications and cause further drop in sugar levels which can be fatal at times. The consumption of more than the advised quantity the oil can also cause a fall in the levels of blood pressure and gallbladder blockage and other diseases. Too much of oil may have completely opposite effect on weight due to the high fat content in it. The oil should not be heated too long (more than 20–30 seconds) as it has a tendency to burn quickly to lose its beneficial properties. The oil should not be applied to wounds or cuts without consultation. When cooking the food for pregnant or lactating women, the dosage of the oil should be decreased.

Non-medical Uses

The oil offers more nutrition and flavour than other vegetable oil, remains stable when heated. The virgin oil is higher in its antioxidants and is used in dips and dressings. The refined oil is reommended for baking and frying.

The oil is valued for flavour, bouquet and colour in culinary preparations as well as a fuel for traditional lamps. It can also be used as an excellent lubricant in place of machine oil.

Religious Uses

In the Roman Catholic, Orthodox and Anglican Churches, the oil is used for the oil of catechumens (to bless and strengthen those preparing for baptism), and oil of the sick (to confer the sacrament of anointing of the sick or unction). Mixed with balsam, the oil is consecrated by bishops as sacred chrism (to confer the sacrament of confirmation—as a symbol of the strengthening of the Holy Spirit), in the ordination of priests and bishops, in the consecration of altars and the churches and also traditionally in the anointing of monarchs at their coronation. The Eastern Orthodox Christians still use the oil lamps in the churches, home prayer corners and in cemeteries with olive oil. The Church of Jesus Christ of Latter-day Saints uses virgin olive oil that has been blessed by the priesthood and this oil is used for anointing the sick.

In Jewish observance, olive oil was the only fuel that is allowed to be used in the seven-branched menorah in the Mishkan service during the Exodus of the tribes of Israel from Egypt, and later in the Temple of Jerusalem. Another use of the oil in Jewish religion was for anointing the kings of the Kingdom of Israel, originating from King David.

REVIEW QUESTIONS

1. **Essay and Short Answer Questions**
    1. What are lipids? How are they classified? Describe the different categories of lipids with examples.
    2. Write short notes on:
        a. Medicinal and non-medicinal uses of castor oil
        b. Uses of fish liver oils
        c. Cocoa butter
        d. Kokum butter
        e. Uses of beeswax
        f. Lanoline
        g. Chaulmoogra oil
        h. Spermaceti oil
        i. Lard oil
    3. Describe in detail the biological source, chemical constituents and pharmaceutical uses of linseed oil.
    4. Describe the biological source, collection and preparation, constituents and medicinal uses of clove oil.

2. **Choose the Correct Alternative**

    1. Beeswax is obtained from: [ ]
        a. *Sus scrofa*   b. *Apis mellifera*
        c. *Garcinia indica*   d. *Olea europea*

    2. Taste of kokum butter is: [ ]
        a. Acrid   b. Sour
        c. Bitter   d. Salty

    3. Volatile oil gets decomposed by: [ ]
        a. Higher temperature   b. Oxidation
        c. Light   d. All the above

    4. The following can cause allergy: [ ]
        a. Wool fat   b. Lard
        c. Spermaceti   d. Olive oil

    5. The toxic substance present in the castor oil is: [ ]
        a. Phosphorous   b. Lipase
        c. Ricin   d. Invertase

3. **Fill in the Blanks**

    1. Enzymes present in castor seeds are ....

    2. Castor oil contains phosphorous in the form of ....

    3. Cold pressing gives the best quality olive oil called ....

    4. .... is the purified internal fat of the abdomen of hog.

    5. Spermaceti is obtained from ....

4. **True or False Statements**

    1. Halibut liver oil is shark liver oil.   [True/False]
    2. Mango kernel oil is used as a substitute for castor oil. [True/False]
    3. Hydnocarpus oil is also called chaulmoogra oil.   [True/False]
    4. Linseed oil is internally prescribed for painter's colic. [True/False]
    5. Lard contains 40% of solid glycerides and 60% of mixed liquid glycerides.   [True/False]

5. **A. Match the following**

    1. Ispagol   [ ]   a. Arabic acid
    2. Tragacanth   [ ]   b. Anethole
    3. Cod liver oil [ ]   c. Aldobionic acid
    4. Fennel   [ ]   d. Bassorin
    5. Acacia   [ ]   e. Vitamin A

B. Match the following

1. Beeswax	[ ]	a.	Eczema and psoriasis
2. Lard	[ ]	b.	Ointments for sunburn
3. Olive oil	[ ]	c.	For tuberculosis and rickets
4. Shark liver oil	[ ]	d.	Cold creams
5. Cod liver oil	[ ]	e.	Paraffin ointment

C. Match the following

1. Linseed oil	[ ]	a.	Caruncle
2. Triolein	[ ]	b.	Fish liver oil
3. Solid oil	[ ]	c.	High iodine value
4. Castor seed	[ ]	d.	Cocoa butter
5. Liquid fat	[ ]	e.	Non-drying oil

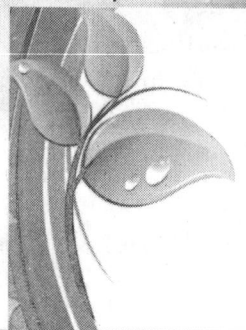

Chapter 8

Systematic Pharmacognostic Study of Volatile Oils

VOLATILE OILS (ESSENTIAL OILS OR ETHEREAL OILS)

Volatile oils are lipophile liquids which are insoluble in water and cause a characteristic smell to plants in which they occur. On being exposed to atmosphere, these evaporate quickly at an ordinary temperature. They dissolve in 1 : 200 parts of water and impart a characteristic taste and smell to water as such they are used in the production of aromatic water like rose water. These oils are readily soluble in alcohol, ether and other lipid solvents. They possess a specific gravity less than one and are lighter than water. They have a high refractive index and show optical rotation.

Volatile oils may occur in any part of the plant like leaves, flowers, bark, seeds, fruits, wood and underground parts. The characteristic plant families which contain volatile oils are Lamiaceae, Rutaceae, Myrtaceae, Lauraceae, Piperaceae, Zingiberaceae and Apiaceae. The oils occur in larger parenchyma cells in the form of special secretory structures like glandular trichomes, endogenous schizogenous oil cavities and oil canals. The oils are the products of metabolism formed directly by the protoplasm or by decomposition of the cell walls or as the products of glycosides. In some cases, they also occur in combination with resins and gums, and are referred to as oleo-resins and oleogum-resins.

These oils belong to the group terpenoids or isoprenoids and in plants occur as monoterpenes and sesquiterpenes in a high frequency. Volatile oil chemically is a mixture of many constituents in which some predominate than others as hydrocarbons, alcohols, acids, ethers, esters, aldehydes and ketones. The constituents are complex and are represented by the mixture of terpenes (mono, di or sesquiterpenes) and their derivatives and derivatives of phenyl propane. The odour and the use of a drug are determined by the predominant constituents of the oil. The oils are variable in their quality and quantity as the habitat determines their nature. The oils are isolated by steam distillation or by mechanical methods. They are extracted with either volatile or nonvolatile solvents.

On the basis of their volatile oil content many crude drugs are used both medicinally and commercially. The crude drugs in the form of a powder are used as spices, condiments and flavouring agents. Externally, the oils are used as counter-irritants in inflammation, swelling and rheumatism. The oils are also used as carminatives, digestive and spasmolytic stimulants, bactericidal and antiseptic agents, disinfectants, diuretics and anthelmintics. They are also used in the manufacture of soaps, deodourisers, and perfumery and in polishes and household cleaners. Mentha, coriander, cinnamon, lemon oil, nutmeg, eucalyptus, ginger, cardamom, tulsi, lemon grass, caraway, cumin, dill, clove, fennel and black pepper are described bellow.

MENTHA

Synonyms

Lamb mint, American mint, Lammint, Brandy mint, Paparaminta (Sanskrit), Mint, Menta, Balm mint, Curled mint, Menthe, Bohe, Peppermint, Pepparmynta, Pepermynte, Na'na, Pepermunt, Hortela, Myata, Seiyo-hakka, Yang-po-ho, Peparaminta (Hindi), Pudina (Telugu and Tamil).

Synonyms for Peppermint

Spiritus Peppermint oil, Oleum Menthae piperitae, Oil of peppermint, Pfefferminzol (German), Essence de Menthe poivree (French).

Synonyms for Menthol

Pipmenthol, Peppermint camphor, Alcool mentholique, Menthol gauche, Camphre de menthe (French), Mentholum, Pfefferminzkampfer, Mentha-kampfer (German).

Biological Source

Peppermint oil is obtained from dried leaves and flowering tops of *Mentha piperita* L. (=*M. balsamea* Willd.), (Family: Lamiaceae) in Northern India and Kashmir. *M. piperita* is a sterile hybrid mint, a cross between *M. aquatica* (Watermint) and *M. spicata* (Spearmint). This was first described by Linnaeus from the specimens in England where he treated it as a species. Now, it is universally agreed to be a hybrid. The name is derived from *Mintha* or *Minthe*, a Greek mythological 'nymph' and Latin *piper* meaning 'pepper'. Astrologically, mint is a herb of Venus. The original name mint was applied by Theophrastus. According to Greek mythology, the peppermint plant arose through a quarrel between two women, Mintha and Proserpine. Pluto, the God of the underworld fell in love with a beautiful nymph, Mintha. Because of this, his jealous wife, Proserpine, made a violent quarrel with the girl. Pluto did not succeed to soothe the quarrel.

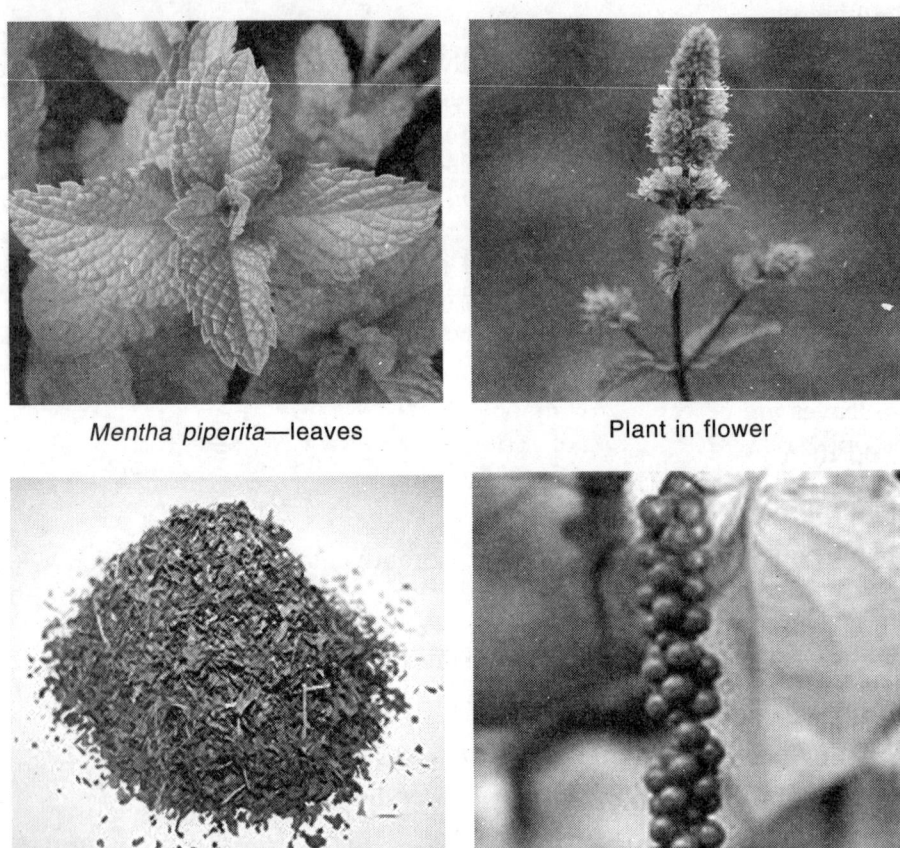

Mentha piperita—leaves | Plant in flower

Dry leaves | Fruits

Proserpine transformed the girl into a plant. Pluto did not succeed in his attempt to change her back. So, he gave her the fragrant aroma. Thus, the plant got the name of the girl.

Geographical Source

The plant is indigenous to and grows wild in Asia, Europe and North America. It is cultivated in Japan, Germany, England, France, Italy, Bulgaria, Russia, India and USA. The best peppermint comes from Michigan, Northern Indiana, New York, Oregon, Indiana of USA and Germany. Many mint species are native to North temperate regions of India, particularly Jammu and Kashmir, Punjab and Tamil Nadu. USA is a principal producer of peppermint.

Collection and Preparation

The harvesting of mint leaves can be done at anytime. The fresh leaves should be used immediately or stored up to a few days in plastic bags in a fridge. The leaves can also be frozen in ice cube trays. Dried leaves of mint should be stored in an air tight container placed in a cool, dark place. The harvest is usually made just before the flowers open and three successive yearly crops are usually taken, after which the field is cleared and new planting is made in a different place. For distillation of the oil, the crop is cut down and left for a day to partially dry in the shade. Fermentation should not take place during drying of the herb, as it adversely affects the quality of the oil. It is then rolled up in mats and is carried to the stills where the volatile oil is extracted by steam distillation.

Characters

Macroscopic Characters

The leaves are crumpled, ovate-oblong to oblong-lanceolate, dark green and opposite with a pubescent petiole. The lamina is 4–9 cm in length and up to 4 cm in breadth with an acute apex, rounded base and coarsely toothed margin. The colour is light-green to purplish brown and the upper surface is glabrous while the lower surface is hairy particularly on the midrib and veins. The inflorescence is verticillaster and compact terminal spike. The bracts are oblong-lanceolate up to 7 mm in length. The calyx is tubular, purplish, five-lobed, pubescent and glandular. The corolla is short, campanulate, light purple and four-lobed. The stamens are four in number, short and equal. The nutlets are four, ellipsoidal and blackish-brown in colour. Each nutlet is 0.5 mm in diameter with a characteristic aromatic odour and an aromatic taste followed by a cooling sensation on drawing in the breath. This sensation is due to menthol.

Microscopic Characters

A section of the lamina shows an upper epidermis made of large epidermal cells with few or no stomata. The palisade is a layer of columnar cells rich in their chloroplasts. Spongy parenchyma cells are irregular with intercellular spaces and chloroplasts. The lower epidermis shows numerous elliptic stomata. The regions of mid rib and the veins show glandular hairs with a stalk and a head. These hairs contain the peppermint oil.

Properties

Mentha oil is colourless to yellow viscid liquid becoming brown on exposure to air of a peculiar pungent odour and hot taste followed by cooling sensation. Menthol is colourless, crystalline (acicular or prismatic), brittle with a strong odour and aromatic taste. It has a melting point of 43°C and a boiling point of 212°C with a specific gravity of 0.890. It is insoluble in water and glycerine, but dissolves in alcohol, ether, chloroform, liquid paraffin, petroleum spirit, olive oil and ethereal oils. Menthol liquifies with camphor, carbolic acid, naphthol, resorcin, thymol, chloral hydrate or butyl-chloral hydrate.

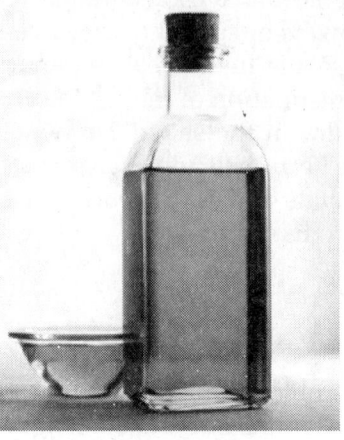

Peppermint oil

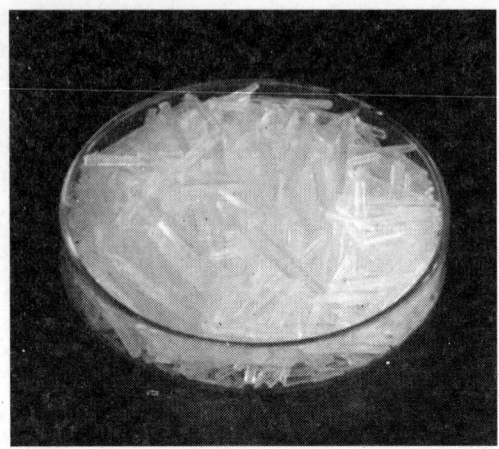

Menthol-crystals

Chemical Constituents

The oil contains chiefly a crystalline stearoptin called the menthol (a volatile secondary alcohol with a molecular formula $C_6H_{90}HCH_3C_3H_7$ or mint camphor (50–60%) and a liquid terpene in addition to glacial acetic acid and carbon disulphide. American peppermint oil contains 80% menthol while Japanese oil contains 70–90%. Other important constituents of the peppermint oil are menthone (a laevogyre ketone $C_{10}H_{18}O$), menthofuran ($C_{10}H_{14}O$), jasmone ($C_{14}H_{18}O$), menthyl isovalerate ($C_{15}H_{28}O_2$), menthyl acetate ($C_{12}H_{22}O_2$), limonene ($C_{10}H_{16}$), pulegone ($C_{10}H_{16}O$), cineol ($C_{10}H_{18}O$), cadinene ($C_{15}H_{24}$), azulene ($C_{10}H_8$) and several other terpene derivatives. It also contains flavonoids like methoside and rutin in addition to carotenes like betaine and choline. Jasmone and esters are responsible for the pleasant flavour. The leaves contain a volatile oil, menthol, resin, tannin and gum.

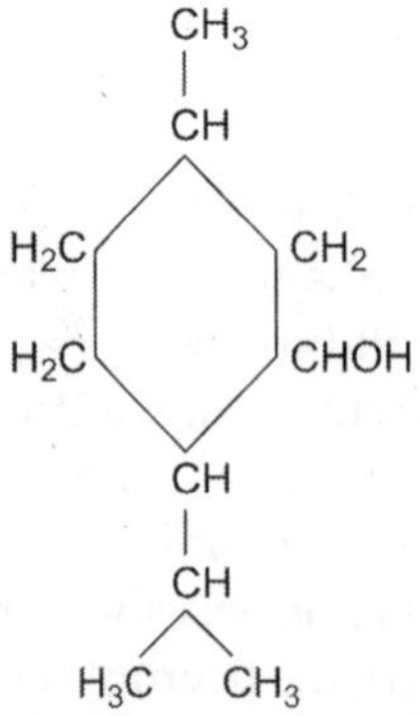

Menthol ($C_6H_{90}HCH_3C_3H_7$)

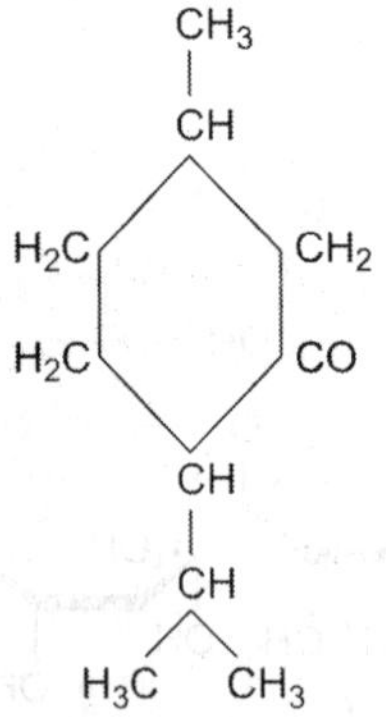

Menthone ($C_{10}H_{18}O$)

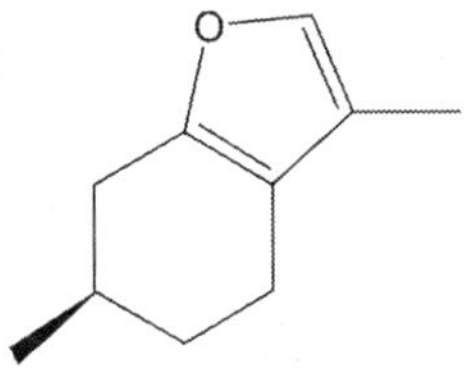

Menthofuran ($C_{10}H_{14}O$)

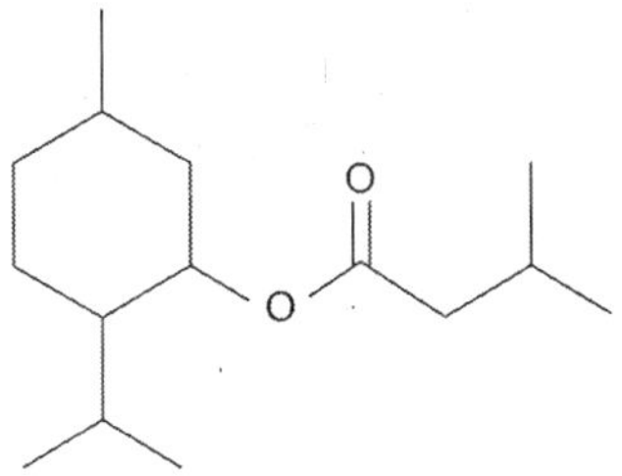

Menthyl isovalerate ($C_{15}H_{28}O_2$)

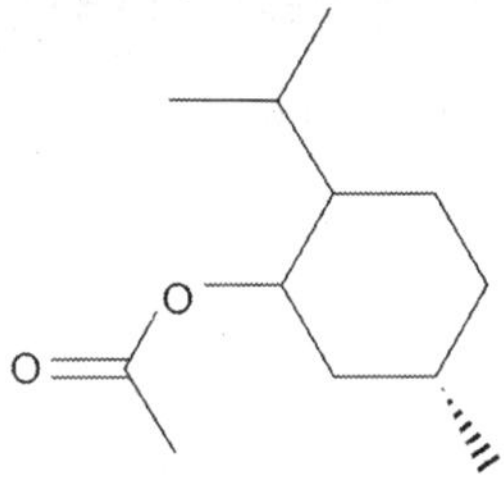

Menthyl acetate ($C_{12}H_{22}O_2$)

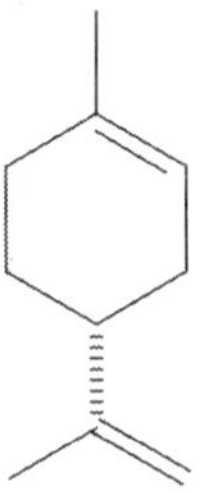

Limonene ($C_{10}H_{16}$)

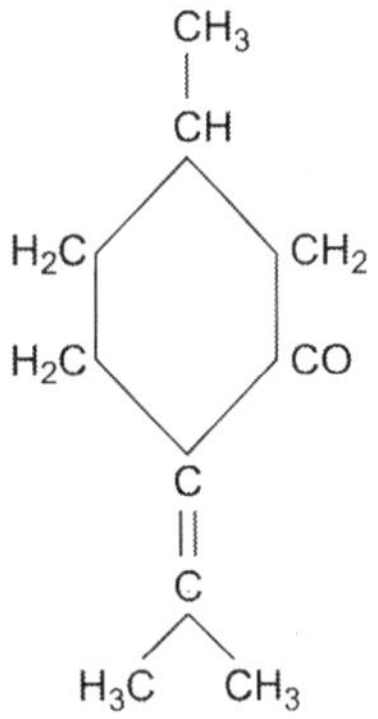

Pulegone ($C_{10}H_{16}O$)

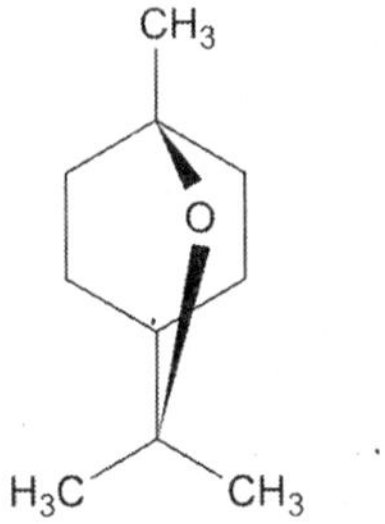

Cineol ($C_{10}H_{18}O$)

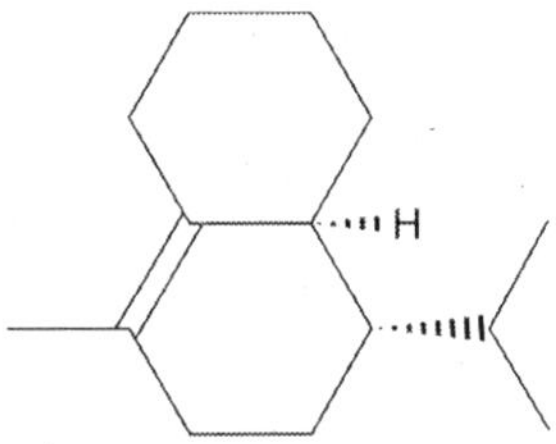

Cadinene ($C_{15}H_{24}$)

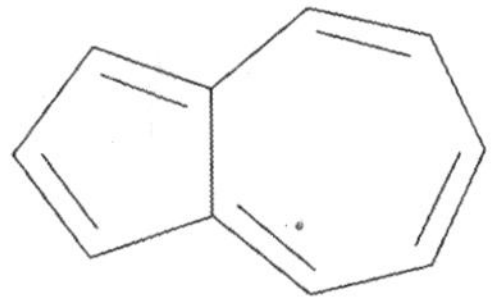

Azulene ($C_{10}H_8$)

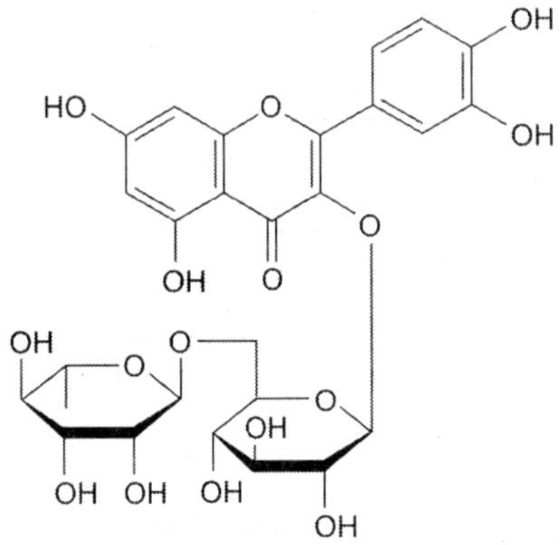

Rutin ($C_{27}H_{30}O_{16}$)

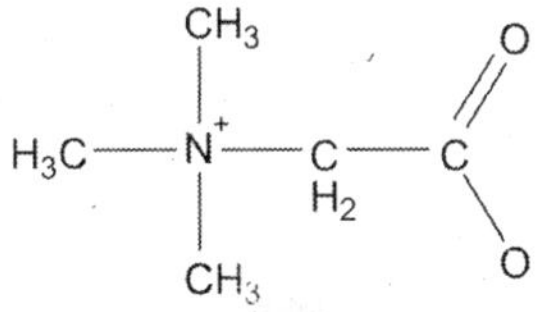

Betaine (C[N+](C)(C)CC([O-])=O)

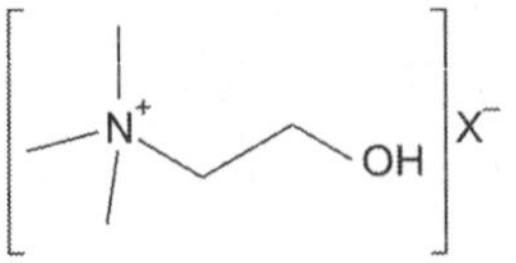

Choline ($C_5H_{14}NO^+$)

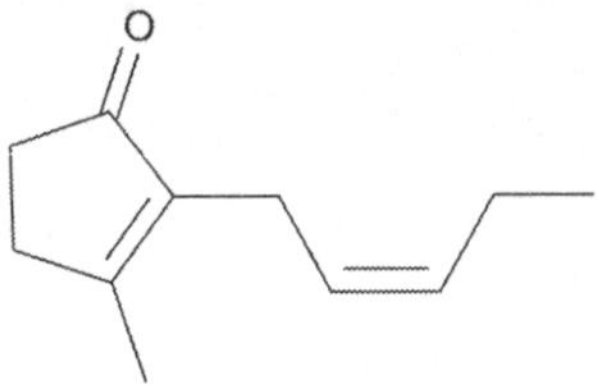

Jasmone ($C_{11}H_{16}O$)

History of Mint

Mint is a symbol of wisdom and hospitality. Peppermint is regarded as *'the world's oldest medicine'* with archaeological evidence at least as far back as 10 thousand years ago, dating back to ancient Egypt, Greece and Rome. Dioscorides described mint for the disorders of the stomach and Pliny recommended it for the abdominal pain and ailments of the gallbladder. Pliny also wrote that the Greeks and Romans crowned themselves with mint at their feasts and adorned their tables with its sprays and their cooks flavoured the sauces and wines with its essence. There is evidence that *M. piperita* was cultivated by the Egyptians. The ancient Assyrians used mint in their rituals to their fire God. The references related to the value of mint also appear in the bible. Pharisees collected mint along with dill and cumin and the Jews used it on the synagogue floor and called the herbs as *Erba Santa Maria* which has been followed over centuries in Italian churches. Mint was a symbol of hospitality for Romans. This has been used for centuries worldwide as a medicinal and culinary herb. The ancient Greeks and Egyptians used mint as a stimulant and nerve tonic because of its odour. In Ayurveda, it is used for treating mouth sores, nausea and impaired digestion. It is also used as an adjuvant in food for promoting digestion and as an expectorant in India. Mint is mentioned in the Icelandic Pharmacopoeias (13th century). The plant came into use in the Western European medicine in the middle of the 18th century and was first used in England. The great botanist of the 17th century, Ray, recognised the plant as a distinct species and published it in the second edition of his *Synopsis stirpium brittanarum* (1696) under the name *M. palustris* (Marsh mint) and this is the first documentation of mint. Sooner, its medicinal properties were recognised and the plant was admitted under the name *M. piperitis sapore* into the London Pharmacopoeia (1721). A. Vogel wrote that Missouri-Valley tribes used mint to lower flatulence and fever. The Japanese have used menthol in medicine as far back as 2000 years and mint was found in Egyptian graves from 1200 to 600 BC.

Medicinal Uses

It is an antiseptic, deodorant, stimulant, carminative, anti-inflammatory, anti-spasmodic, diaphoretic, anti-emetic, nervine, anti-microbial, stomachic, anaesthetic and rubefacient. Menthol is used as an ingredient in preparation for the nose and throat, in ointments to relieve local irritation. It is used as an external application in congestive headaches, rheumatism and neuralgia, etc. It is also applied on the skin or mucous membrane as a counter-irritant. It is used in throat lozenges, and also in colds and flu. Menthol is also used as topical antipruritic and local analgesic. *Linimentum Mentholis* (menthol ointment-menthol dissolved in chloroform) is used in neuralgia, sciatica and lumbago. Mentholeate (menthol dissolved in oleic acid) is used in neuralgia and pruritis. *Insufflatio Mentholis* (menthol mixed with camphor and eucalyptus oil) is inhaled from cotton wool or with hot water steam for the relief from catarrah. *Emplastrum Mentholis* (as plaster) is aplied in rheumatism and lumbago. The oil capsules if taken for four weeks reduce the irritable bowel syndrome. The oil can be aplied topically for soothing and cooling on irritant skin due to bees, poison ivy or poison oak. When applied to the forehead, it reduces the symptoms of headache. It helps to relieve the painful cramps in the muscles during menstrual period in women and relaxes the muscles in digestive gas. It also improves the flow of bile, reduces the swelling and inflammation from bruises, disorders of stomach and intestine and diseases of the gallbladder.

Non-medical Uses

Peppermint oil is used in toothpaste, tooth powders, shaving creams, and different pharmaceutical dosage forms. It is also consumed in the preparation of chewing gums, candies, jellies, perfumes and essences. It is also used as a flavouring agent in tea, ice cream, confectionery and tooth paste, mouthwash, cigarettes, dental creams in addition to shampoos and soaps.

Other Uses

The leaves and the volatile oil are aromatic, stimulant, carminative and antispasmodic. The leaf infusion and the oil are used in vomiting, gastric colic, cholera, diarrhoea, flatulence, etc. It is given in dysmenorrhoea, weak digestion, hiccups and palpitation. The oil is used locally as anodyne, anaesthetic, antiseptic and a germicide in herpes zoster and pruritis as a lotion. It is also used as an inhalation in diphtheria and relieves the tooth ache caused by caries. The oil is also used as a flavouring agent. The flowers produce large amount of nectar used in the production of a mild, pleasant variety of honey. The small amounts are safe but higher doses cause skin rash, necrosis of skin, interstitial nephritis (kidney damage), dizziness, confusion, muscle weakness, difficulty in breathing, asthma, purpura of skin, mouth sores, and irritation of eyes, headache, heartburn, slower heart rate, muscle tremor, nausea or double vision. The use of the oil and menthol should be avoided during pregnancy and breastfeeding.

Adulteration

The common adulterants are Spear mint (*Mentha viridis*) and the leaves of varieties of *Mentha piperita* like White mint (*M. piperita* var. *officinalis*) and Black mint (*M. piperita* var. *vulgaris*). The peppermint oil is adulterated with oil of erigeron, castor oil, turpentine oil, copaiba oil, camphor oil, sassafras oil, etc.

CORIANDER

Synonyms

Coriander seed, Coriandrum, Coliander (English), Koriandersamen or Koriander or Germeiner coriander (German), Coriandre or Coriander cultive, Fructus coriandri (French), Cilantro (Espanol), Culantro (Spanish), Coentro (Portuguese), Koriyun (Greek), Coriandolo comune (Italian), Kolendra (Polski), Koriander siaty (Slovencina), Chinese parsley, Dhanyaka and Kustumbari (Sanskrit), Kottimir or Dhania (Hindi), Hu sui, Dhana, Dhane (Bengali, Gujarati and Maharashtrian), Haveeja, Kishniz (Persian), Koriyun, Kotambri-beeja, Kothimbir, Kothimira (Telugu), Kottampalari (Malayalam), Kottumbari (Kannada and Konkani), Kottamalli (Tamil), Kushniz, Kusbara (Arabic).

Biological Source

Coriander is the dried ripe fruit of *Coriandrum sativum* L. (Family: Apiaceae) extensively cultivated in all parts of India for its fruits and seeds. The word is derived from Latin *coriandrum*. The Mycenean Greek form of the word *koriandnon* is similar to the name of Mino's daughter Ariadne which later evolved to *koriannon* or *koriandron*. The Greek name *koris* (meaning—a bug) is the root for the name coriander.

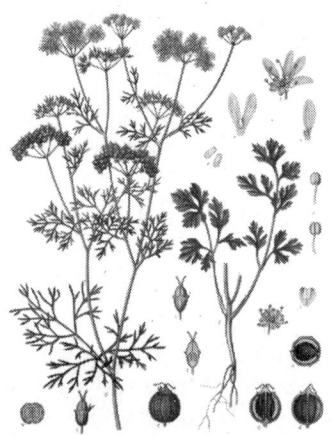

Coriandrum sativum

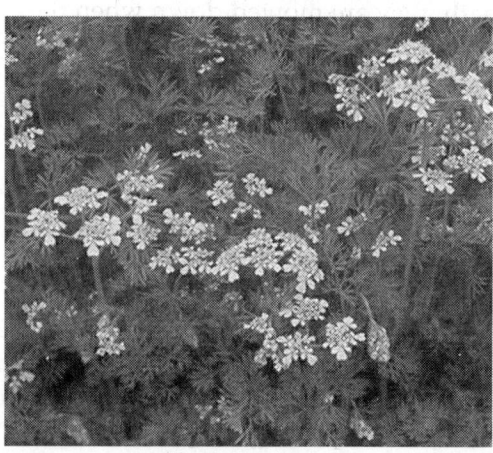

The plant in flower

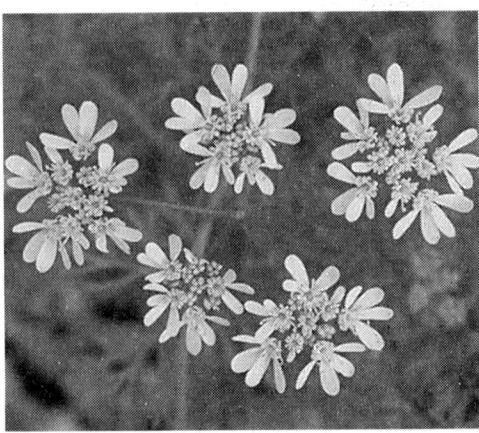

Coriander flowers

Geographical Source

The plant is indigenous to Italy and grows wild in Southern Europe and North Africa to South-western Asia. It is widely cultivated in The Netherlands, Central and Eastern Europe, the Mediterranean (Morocco, Malta, and Egypt), Northern Africa, USA, China, India and Bangladesh. Ukraine is the major producer of oil.

Collection and Preparation

The crop will be ready for harvest in about 90 to 110 days. The plants are pulled when the fruits are fully ripe, start changing from green to brown colour (drying). The plants are pooled into small stacks in the field, thrashed with sticks or rubbing with hands, winnowed and cleaned and dried in partial shade. The plants are pulled out when they are 30–40 days old for the leaves. When the plants are sufficiently strong and about 5 inches in length, they are mowed down when the fruits are ripe. They are partially cured in the field and dried under cover. The fruits are thrashed out and cleaned. The fresh coriander seeds should be dried in shade to retain the seed colour and quality. After drying, they are separated by light beating with sticks. Clean gunny bags lined with paper are used for packing the seeds and are stored in damp-free aerated rooms.

Characters

Macroscopic Characters

Morphologically, the fruits occur usually as entire cremocarps, which are subspherical, about 3 to 5 mm in diameter, brownish yellow, crowned by 5 small sepals and a stylopod. Each mericarp has five wavy rather inconspicuous primary ridges and four straight, more prominent secondary ridges. The seeds (dry fruits) have a warm, spicy, orange flavour.

Microscopic Characters

Microscopically, the epidermis of the pericarp is composed of polygonal tabular cells with occasional stomata. Several of the epidermal cells contain in each a single prism of calcium oxalate. The mesocarp is composed of an outer and an inner layer of parenchyma, between which is a layer of sclerenchyma consisting of fusiform, lignified sclerenchymatous cells in sinuous rows. The outer five or six rows of sclerenchyma run longitudinally while the inner one to three rows run tangentially, in the secondary ridges almost all the cells run tangentially. The inner epidermis of the pericarp is composed of parquetry cells.

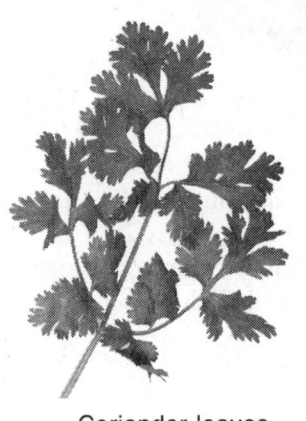

Coriander leaves

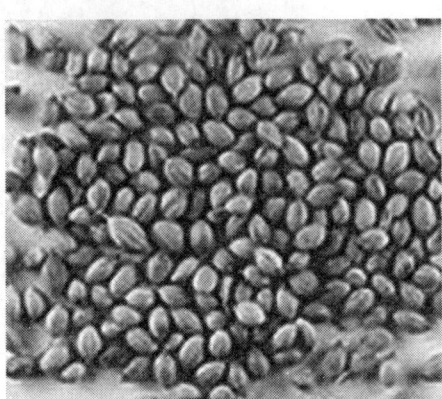

Coriander fruits

Coriander powder

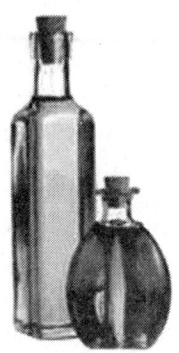

Coriander oil

Chemical Constituents

Coriander fruits contain about 1–1.8% of volatile oil (*Oleum coriandri*) in addition to fixed oil (13%), fatty matter (13%), mucilage, tannins, calcium oxalate, malic acid and ash (5%). The oil is colourless to pale-yellow with a watery viscosity. The chief constituents of the volatile oil are an alcohol called coriandrol or d-linalool ($C_{10}H_{18}$: 65–70%) and small quantities of

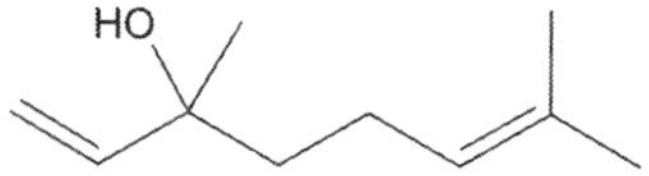

Coriandrol or d-linalool (C$_{10}$H$_{18}$)

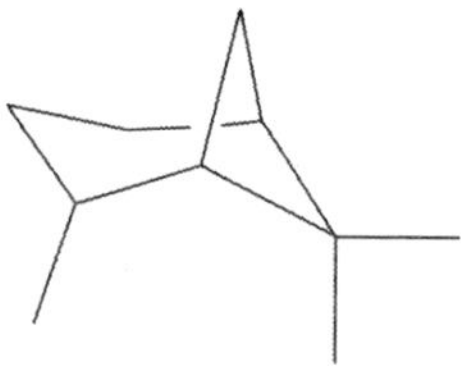

d-Pinene (C$_{10}$H$_{16}$)

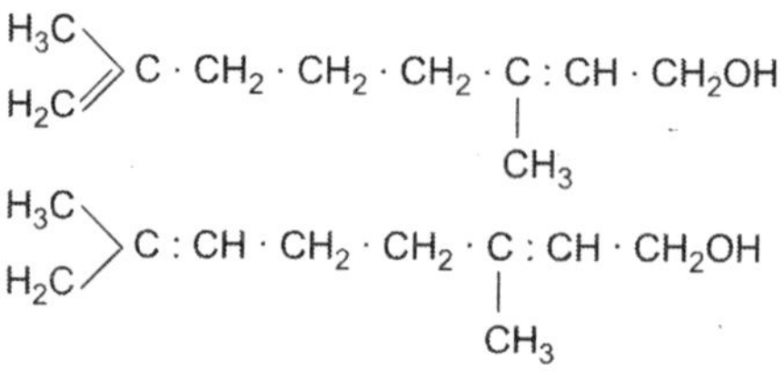

$$H_3C \\ H_2C {>} C \cdot CH_2 \cdot CH_2 \cdot CH_2 \cdot C : CH \cdot CH_2OH$$
$$\underset{CH_3}{|}$$

$$H_3C \\ H_2C {>} C : CH \cdot CH_2 \cdot CH_2 \cdot C : CH \cdot CH_2OH$$
$$\underset{CH_3}{|}$$

Geraniol or lemonol or rhodinol
(C$_{10}$H$_{18}$O)

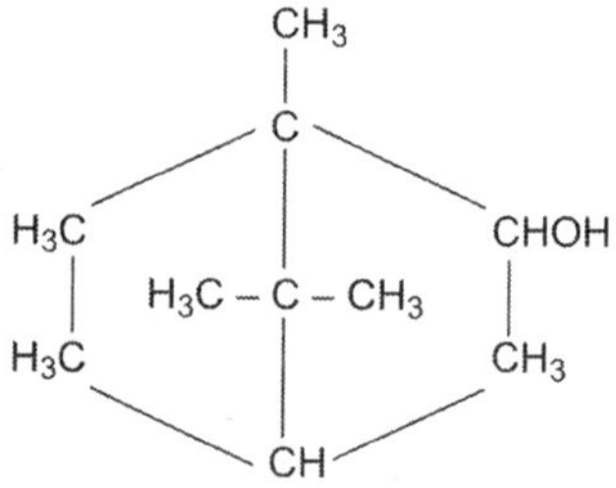

Borneol (C$_{10}$H$_{18}$O)

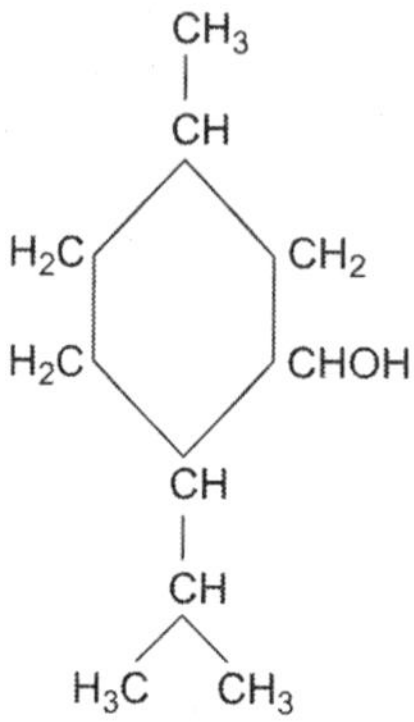

Camphor (C$_{10}$H$_{16}$O)

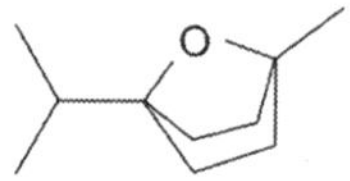

Cineole (C$_{10}$H$_{18}$O)

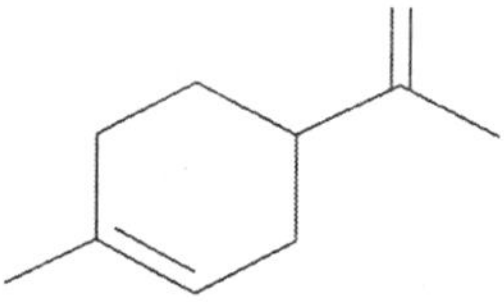

Dipentene (C$_{10}$H$_{16}$)

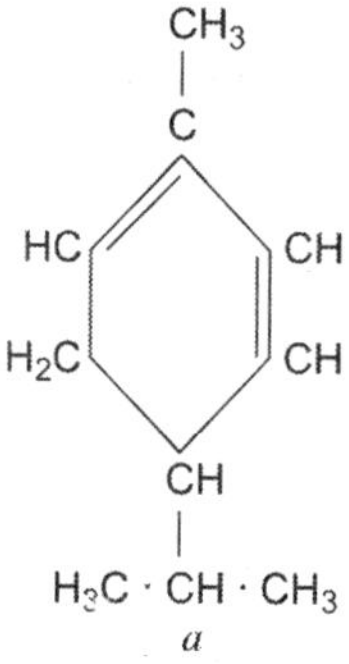

α-phellandrene (C$_{10}$H$_{16}$)

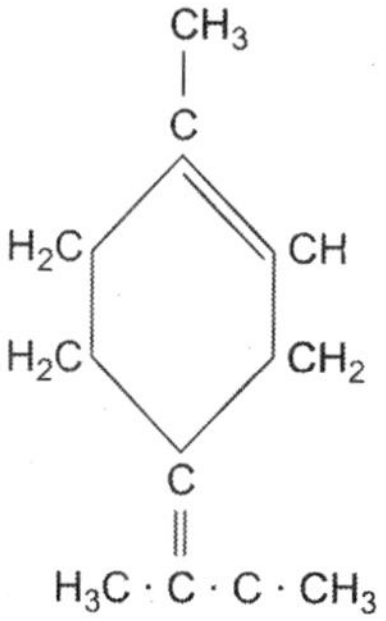

Terpinolene (C$_{10}$H$_{16}$)

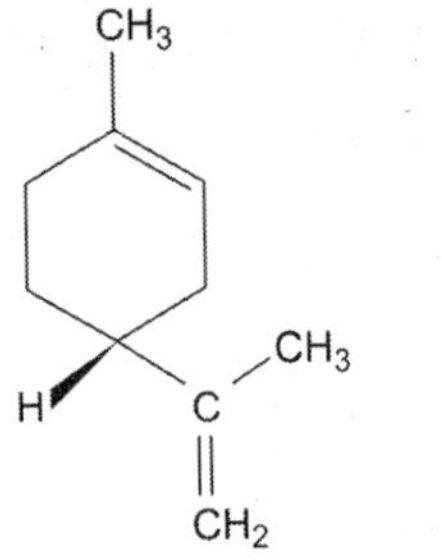

d-limonene ($C_{10}H_{16}$)

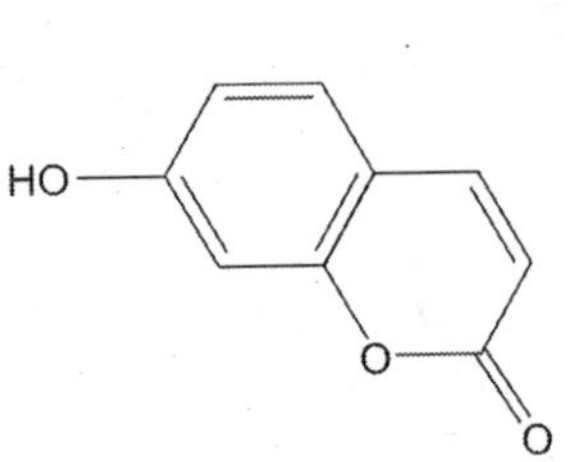

Scopoletine ($C_{10}H_8O_4$)

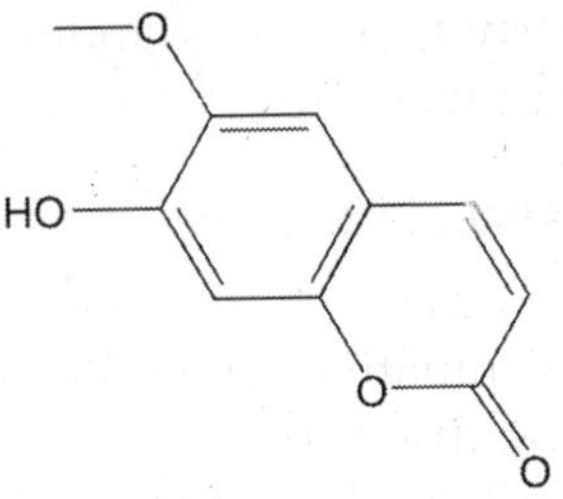

Umbelliferone ($C_9H_6O_3$)

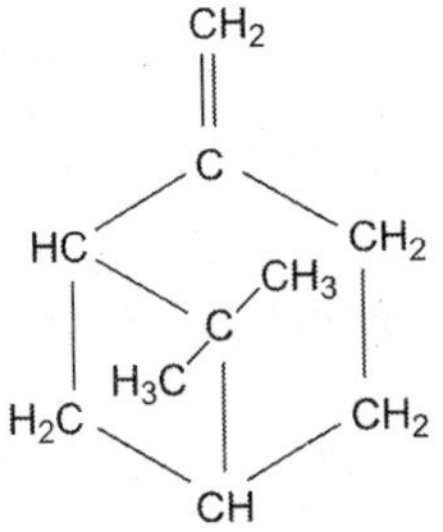

α-pinene ($C_{10}H_{16}$)

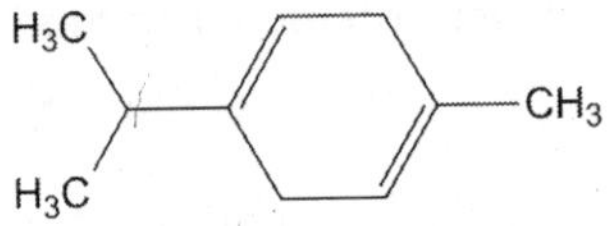

γ-terpinene ($C_{10}H_{16}$)

d-pinene ($C_{10}H_{16}$), 1-pinene, geraniol ($C_{10}H_{18}O$), borneol ($C_{10}H_{18}O$), γ-terpinene, camphor ($C_{10}H_{16}O$), cineole ($C_{10}H_{18}O$), dipentene ($C_{10}H_{16}$), α-phellandrene ($C_{10}H_{16}$), terpinolene ($C_{10}H_{16}$), alpha-pinenes, limonene ($C_{10}H_{16}$) and p-cymene together with various alcohols and esters. The fatty oil consists of petroselic acid, pleic acid and linolenic acid in addition to hydroxycoumarins like umbelliferone ($C_9H_6O_3$) and scopoletine ($C_{10}H_8O_4$).

History of Coriander

The oldest archaeological find of coriander is the pre-pottery neolithic B level of the Nahal Hemel Cave in Israel where 15 desiccated mericarps of the plant were found. Similarly, half a kg of mericarps of coriander were recovered from the tomb of Tutankhamun which is a proof that coriander was cultivated by the ancient Egyptians as it does not grow wild there (according to the interpretation of Zohary and Hopf). The use of coriander is also mentioned in Exodus 16 : 31 of the Bible – 'And the house of Israel began to call its name manna, and it was round like a coriander seed, and its taste was like that of flat cakes made with honey'. Coriander was cultivated in Greece in the 2nd millennium BC for the manufacture of perfumes, as a spice (seeds) and as an herb (flavour) evident from one of the Linear-B tablets recovered from Pylos. This has been confirmed by the archaeological evidence as large quantities of the plant was retrieved from Early Bronze Age layer at Sitagori in Macedonia which point out to the cultivation of the plant at that time. The plant was brought to the British colonies in

North America (1670) and was one of the first spices cultivated by the early settlers. Coriander seeds were mentioned in the early Sanskrit writings and were discovered in Egyptian tombs dating back to 960 BC.

Medicinal Uses

Pharmaceutically coriander and its oils are used as flavouring agents and carminative. The oil is useful in flatuent colic, rheumatism and neuralgia. The dried fruit is used in sore throat, catarrh and bilious complaints. The fruit is alterative, antibilious, antispasmodic, aphrodisiac, appetiser, carminative, diaphoretic, diuretic, antipyretic, antihistaminic, blood cleanser, refrigerant, stimulant, tonic and stomachic. It is used as an eye wash and in chronic conjunctivitis. The seeds are used in dyspepsia and as a paste in cephalgia, as a gargle in thrush and as a poultice in carbuncles and chronic ulcers. A strong decoction of the plant is used in dyspepsia, indigestion and flatulence. A cold infusion of seeds is useful in colic of children and relieves internal heat and thirst. Coriander water (*Aqua coriandir*) is useful in indigestion and bowel complaints. It is an aromatic stimulant and a corrective of purgative preparations. Coriander has been used in folk medicine to relieve anxiety and insomnia (anxiolytic) in Iran. The seeds are used in Indian traditional medicine as a diuretic. It is used as a carminative and a digestive in holistic and traditional medicine. It is also used as a toner for acne on the face. The essential oil is spasmolytic and has antibacterial and antifungal effects. The oil is analgesic, aphrodisiac, antispasmodic, depurative, deodorant, fungicidal and lipolytic. Chinese herbalists use the seeds to treat influenza, indigestion, anorexia and stomah ache. In Chinese folk medicine, the leaves and seeds are used to remove the unpleasant odour in the genital areas of men and women and bad breath. It is also an antidote to snake bite and scorpion sting and antiseptic and antitubercular.

Other Uses

All parts of the plant are edible and the fresh leaves and the dried seeds are commonly used in cooking as a spice. It is commonly used in Middle Eastern, Centra Asian, Mediterranean, Indian, South Asian, Mexican, Latin American, Chinese, African and South-East Asian cuisine. The fruit is used as a condiment and the leaves are used in the preparation of sauces, and are carminative and antibilious. In Belgium, it is used in their wheat beer called *witbier*. The fresh leaves are an ingredient in chutneys of South, in Chinese dishes and in Mexican salsas and guacamole. The leaves are chopped and are used as a garnish on cooked dal and curries, salads, soups and meat dishes. The seed is a spice in garam masala and curries in India. Roasted seeds, *dhania dal* are eaten as a snack. It is the main ingredient of two common South-Indian dishes, sambar and rasam. The seed is also used for pickling vegetables (outside Asia), for sausages (Germany and

South Africa) and an ingredient of rye bread (Russia and Central Europe) and stews, sweet bread and cakes. The roots have a more intense flavour and are common in Thai dishes, soups and curry pastes. The leaves (*cilantro*) are used extensively in Chinese, Indian, Middle Eastern, North African and Latin American cuisine, as a mince to salads, soups, sauces, fish and beans. In the form of a powder it is used to flavour sweet bread, cake and confectionery. The seeds are also used to flavour gin and liquor to disguise their taste. Commercially, a spice from the seeds is used for flavouring the meat products, bakery goods, tobacco, gin and other liquors, chilli and curry powder commonly used in the Middle East India, Mexico and China.

CINNAMON

Synonyms

Cinnamon bark, Ceylon cinnamon, Cinnamomum, True cinnamon, Ceylon bark (English), Cortex cinnamoni, Cinnam, Zeylan, Zeylonzimmt or Zimmt (German), Kinnamomon (Greek), Cannelle or Cannelle de Ceylon (French), Tvak (literally means the skin and refers to the bark) or Darusita (Sanskrit), Saila-myah or Darchin (Farsi or Persian), Qualami (Dukhhini), Darchini (Urdu, Hindi and Hindustani), Darasini or Qerfa (Arabic), Tarcin (Turkish), Yuh or Juh, Kevei (Chinese), Kayu manis (meaning sweet wood—Indonesian), Dalchin (Punjabi, Kashmiri and Maharashtrian), Chekke (Kannada), Dalchini (Marathi), Darchini (Bengali), Lavangampattai or Pattai or Karuvapattai (Tamil), Karugapatta (Malayalam), Dalchina chakka (Chakka meaning the bark or wood—Telugu), Kulit-manis (Malaysian), Kurunda or Kurundu (Sinhalese), Timbotik-yobo (Burmese), Alseni (Assamese), Taj (Gujarati).

Biological Source

Cinnamon is the dried inner bark (Cinnamomi cortex) of the shoots of coppiced (truncated) trees of *Cinnamomum verum* J. Presl. (= *C. zeylanicum*)

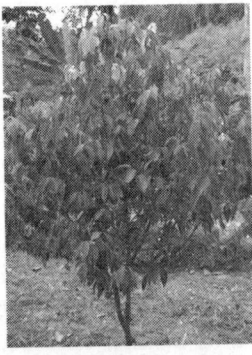

Cinnamomum verum

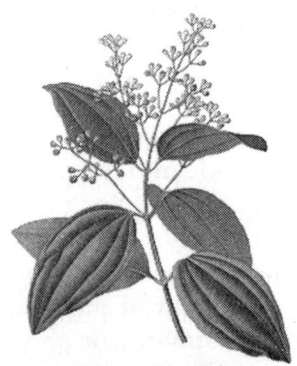

Flowering twig

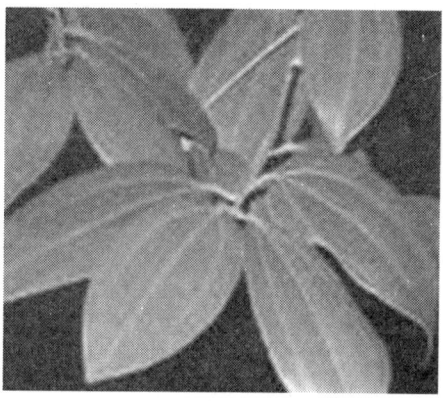

Leaves

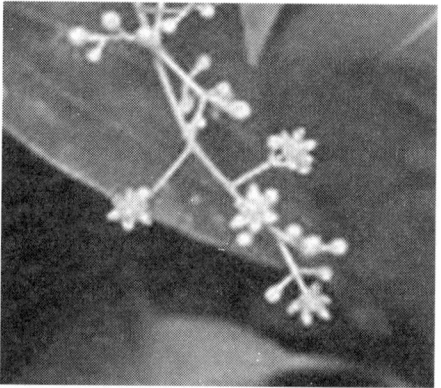

Flowers

of family Lauraceae, indigenous to Sri Lanka and Southern India. The name *cinnamon* comes from Greek word, *kinnamomon*, from Phoenician. The botanical name *Cinnamomum zeylanicum* is derived from Ceylon, the former name of Sri Lanka. The French word, *cannelle*, a diminutive of *canne* (meaning a reed or a cane) comes from its tube-like shape.

Geographical Source

Cinnamon is native to and has been cultivated from time immemorial in Sri Lanka. The tree is also grown in Myanmar and Kerala in South India. It is cultivated in Tropical Malaysia, Vietnam, Indonesia, China, Taiwan, Seychelles, Jamaica, Bangladesh, Java, Sumatra, West Indies, Madagascar, Zanzibar, Egypt, Caribbean and Brazil. Sri Lanka produces about 90% of world's supply.

Collection and Preparation

The shoots are cut from the trees when they are about 18 to 24 months old, and the tops and twigs are removed. The bark and cork are removed by peeling with a brass knife. The separated bark is wrapped in coir matting and allowed to 'ferment' overnight. The outer bark (cork and cortex) is scrapped off with the help of a curved steel scrapper. Many layers of the thin inner bark (0.5 mm) are rolled into one quill. The quills are dried by keeping them in shade for about 24 hours, and on the second day are placed in the open air on wooden frames. After drying, the quills are sorted into grades and made into compact bales. The quills are cut into 5–10 cm length for sale. The oil is distilled from the cortex. The oil is prepared by pounding the bark, macerating it in sea water and quick distillation.

Cinnamon oleoresin is prepared by extracting the bark with organic solvents. The yield of the oleoresin varies from 10 to 12%. The resin is dispersed on sugar, salt and used for flavouring the processed food. Cinnamon bark oil is a pale yellow liquid with a delicate aroma of the spice and this is obtained by the steam distillation of the quills (0.2–0.5%). Its major component is cinnamaldehyde (about 55%) which imparts a characteristic odour and flavour to the oil. The oil is used in flavouring bakery foods, sauces, pickles, confectionery, soft drinks, dental and pharmaceutical preparations and also in perfumery. Cinnamon leaf oil is produced by the steam distillation of the leaves (which yields 0.5 – 0.7% of oil). It is yellow to brownish-yellow and has a warm, spicy, harsh odour. The major component is eugenol (about 70–90%) while cinnamaldehyde is less than 5%. This is used in perfumery, flavouring, and is also a source of eugenol. Cinnamon root bark oil contains 1.0–2.8% oil and contains camphor as the main component. Cinnamaldehyde as well as the traces of eugenol are found in the oil with a less commercial value.

Characters

Macroscopic Characters

The outer surface is dull yellowish-brown, while the inner surface is dark yellowish-brown. The taste is warm, sweet and aromatic. The bark from Sri Lanka is smooth and very thin, light-yellowish brown and has highly

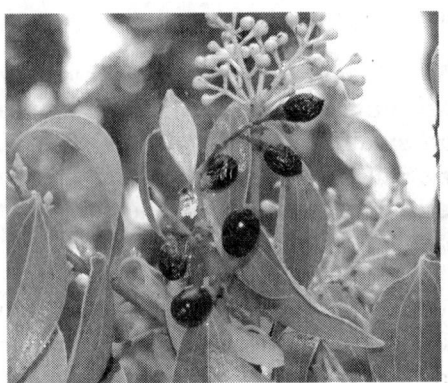

Fruits

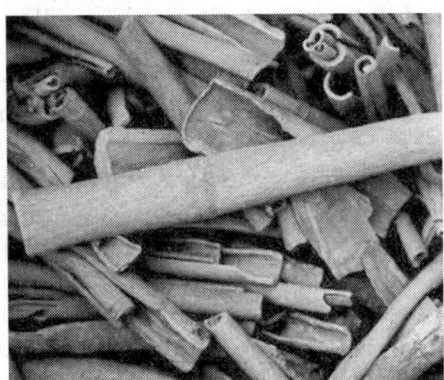

Bark—inner cortex

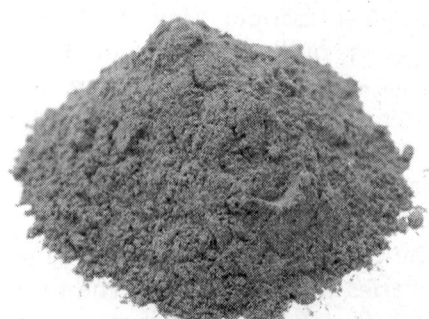

Cinnamon powder

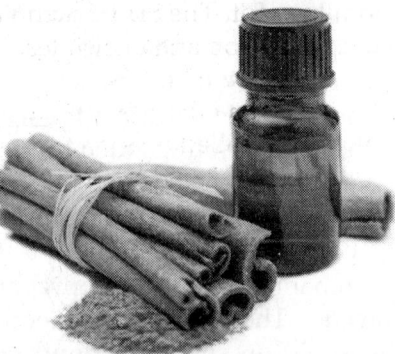

Cinnamon oil

fragrant aroma. It has a finer, less denser and more crumbly texture. The oil is of a golden-yellow colour (leaf oil) to reddish-brown (bark oil), with a characteristic odour (spicy musky smell) and a very hot aromatic taste and medium to watery viscosity.

Microscopic Characters

Microscopically excepting for occasional patches of cork and underlying parenchyma, cork and cortex are absent. The outermost layer consists of a continuous band, three or four cells wide, of pericyclic lignified sclerenchyma, on the outer margin of which small groups of about six to fifteen pericyclic fibres occur at intervals. The pitted scleroids are often more thickened upon the inner walls than upon the other three giving them characteristic appearance; they contain a few starch grains. The sieve tubes are arranged in tangential bands which are completely collapsed in the outer layers; the sieve plates are on the transverse walls. The phloem fibres of the vascular bundles occur either singly or in short tangential rows of two to five. Idioblasts are somewhat longitudinally elongated; contain volatile oil or more rarely mucilage. The medullary rays are usually two-seriate, widening slightly as they approach pericycle; many of these cells also contain minute needles of calcium oxalate or starch grains.

Chemical Constituents

Cinnamon bark (*Cortex cinnamoni*) contains about 1 to 2% of volatile oil, cinnamic acid ($C_9H_8O_2$), resin, tannin, lignin, sugar, mannitol, gum, coumarin, starch, mucilage, calcium oxalate and ash. Cinnamon oil (*Oleum cinnamomum*) contains cinnamaldehyde or cinnamic aldehyde (C_9H_8O: 60–75%), eugenol ($C_{10}H_{12}O_2$: 5–10%), cinnamyl acetate ($C_{11}H_{12}O_2$), pinene, ethyl cinnamate ($C_{11}H_{12}O_2$), phellandrene, linalool, methyl chavicol or estragole ($C_{10}H_{12}O$) and beta-caryophyllene ($C_{15}H_{24}$). It also contains calcium, chromium, copper, iodine, iron, manganese, phosphorus, potassium, zinc, vitamins – B, A and C. The oil from the leaves contains 70–80% of eugenol and the rest cinnamic aldehyde. The oil is also collected from the root. The Sri Lankan variety of oil is the best and contains more sugar and aromatic principles.

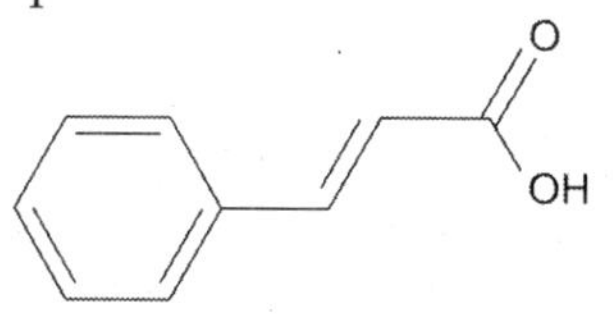

Cinnamic acid or phenylacrylic acid ($C_6H_5CHCHCOOH$)

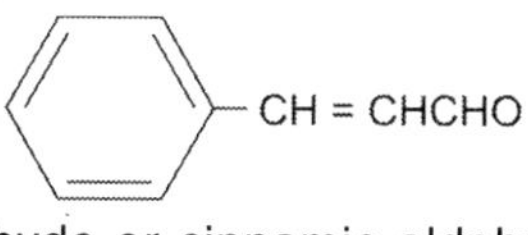

Cinnamaldehyde or cinnamic aldehyde (C_9H_8O)

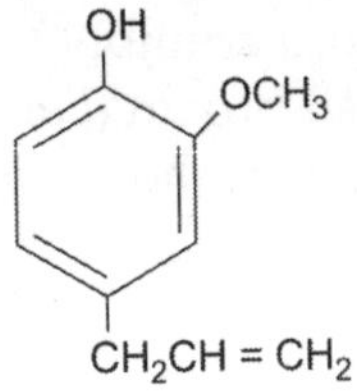

Eugenol ($C_{10}H_{12}O_2$)

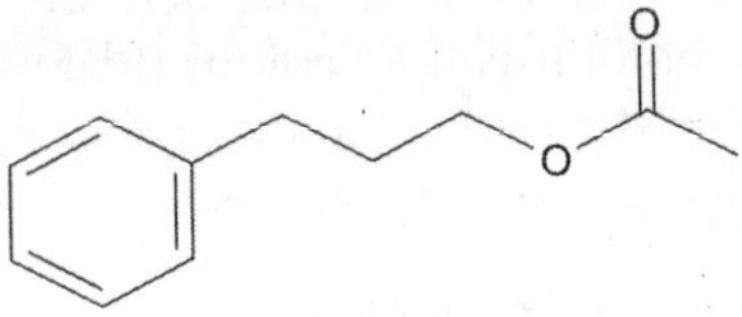

Cinnamyl acetate ($C_{11}H_{12}O_2$)

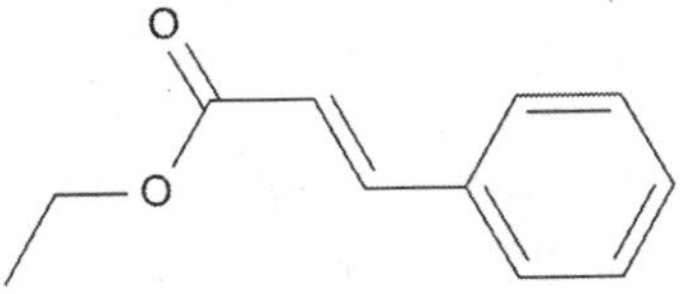

Ethyl cinnamate ($C_{11}H_{12}O_2$)

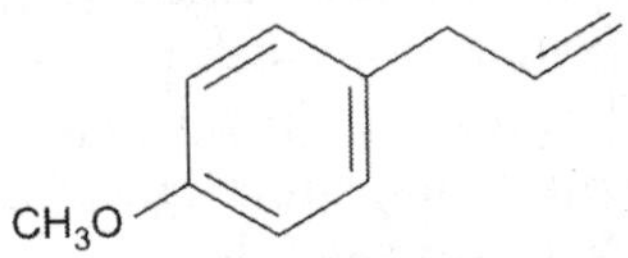

Estragole or methyl chavicol ($C_{10}H_{12}O$)

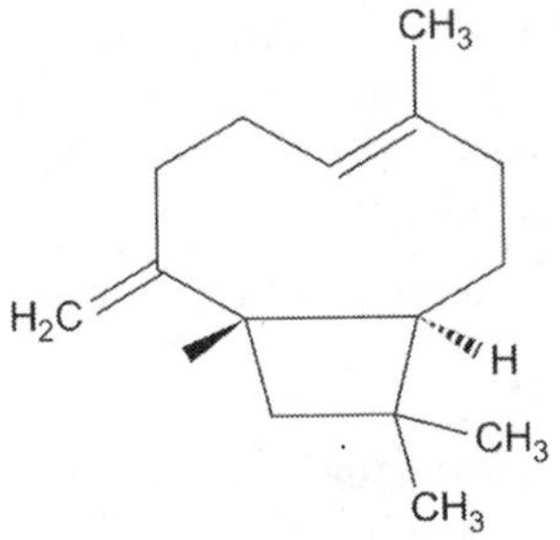

Beta-caryophyllene ($C_{15}H_{24}$)

History of Cinnamon

Cinnamon is known from antiquity and is the first spice to be mentioned in Old Testament where Moses is commanded to use both sweet cinnamon (*qinnamon* in Hebrew) and cassia in the holy anointing oil; in proverbs, where the lover's bed is perfumed with myrrh, aloe and cinnamon; and in the Song of Solomon, which describes the beauty of his beloved as: '*Cinnamon scents her garments like the smell of Lebanon*'. In ancient nations, it was regarded as a gift fit for monarchs and God and an inscription records the gift of cinnamon and cassia to the temple of Apollo at Miletus. It was imported to Egypt as early as 2000 BC. It was also mentioned by Herodotus and other authors. Emperor Nero of Rome is said to have burnt a large suply of cinnamon on the funeral pyre of his wife, Poppaea Sabina (65 AD). Pliny, the Elder also made a mention of the bark. The use of bark and the oil in Chinese herbal medicine was mentioned in Chinese texts as far back as 4000 years (2700 BC). In traditional Chinese medicine, this is one of the oldest remedies for everything from diarrhoea and chills to influenza and parasitic worms. It was also used for embalming in Egypt. A first mention of the plant growing in Sri Lanka appeared in Zakariya al-Qazwani's *Athar al-bilad wa-akhbar al-'ibad* (Monument of Places and History of God's Bondsmen) in 1270 and in a letter by John of Montecorvino (1292).

Medicinal Uses

Cinnamon bark is carminative, antispasmodic, stimulant, haemostatic, astringent, antiseptic and a germicide. It is used as a flavouring agent and stomachic. It is also a mild astringent. As an infusion, decoction or powder, the bark is used in flatulent dyspepsia, dyspepsia with nausea, intestinal colic, digestive atony, diarrhoea, vomiting and debilitated conditions. It is used as an adjunct in purgatives, astringents and bitter tonics. It is a stimulant of uterine muscular fibre and is used in menorrhagia and tedious labour. As a powder, it is used for diarrhoea and dysentery. Because it is a stimulant, it is used for the cramps of the stomach, enteralgia, toothache, and parpalysis of the tongue. *Bhavaprakash nighantu* mentions the use of the bark in diseases like pruritis, piles, worms, sinusitis, cough, asthma and urinary bladder. The bark is a distinct aphrodisiac in male sexual debility and in amenorrhoea and oligomenorrhoea. The oil is analgesic, antibiotic, aphrodisiac, and cardiac, emmenagogue, insecticidal, stomachic and vermifuge. The oil is used as a stimulant in amenorrhoea, nausea and vomiting. The oil is also locally applied in neuralgia and headache. It is used as an antiseptic in gonorrhoea and a germicide in malaria. In a massive dose, it can be used in the treatment of cancer and other microbial diseases. This can be used externally in rheumatic pains, arthritis, headaches and toothaches. It also strengthens the gums and relieves bad breath. The oil is a vascular and nervine stimulant but in larger doses, it is an irritant and a narcotic poison. The bark is highly antioxidant and the oil is antimicrobial and used in food preservation. Recent studies have determined that consumption of half of a teaspoon a day reduces blood sugar, cholesterol and triglyceride levels by 20% in patients of Type 2 diabetes without insulin.

Non-medical Uses

The bark is widely used as a spice. It is used as a condiment in cookery and a flavouring material. In Mexico, it is used in the preparation of chocolate. It is also used in desserts like apple pie, donuts, candies, tea, hot cocoa and liquors. In Middle East, it is used in chicken dishes, in the USA, to flavour bread-based dishes and apples and in Persia, to make thick soups, drinks and sweets. The oil is used in flavouring of sweets and confectionery. Cinnamon lowers the rate of respiration in the cells of yeast. The leaf is effective in killing the mosquito larvae mainly due to its components, cinnamaldehyde, cinnamyl acetate, eugenol and anethole. It is used as a hair rinse for dark hair, as a toothpaste for fresh breath, to prevent athlete's foot and to promote a rosy complexion. Overdose may result in increased pulse rate, dizziness, shorter breath, etc.

Adulteration

The cinnamon powder is adulterated with sugar, ground walnut shells, Galanga rhizome, powdered Cassia buds, etc.

LEMON OIL

Synonyms

Oleum limonis, Limonis cortex, Lemon peel, Ecorce de Limon (French), Limonenschale or Limonen (German), Limone (Italian), Limon agria or Limon real or Limon frances (Spanish), Citronnier (French), Citroen (Dutch), Limon France (Haiti), Limon amarillo (Puerto Rico), Lamoentsji or Lamubchi (Antilles, The Netherlands), Limpaka or Mahajambiram or Nimbaka or Vijapura (Sanskrit), Jambira or Paharikaghu or Pahadi-nimbu (Hindi and Dakkhini), Karnanebu or Gora-nebu (Bengali), Khuttia or Gulgul (Punjabi), Motunimbu (Gujarati), Thorla-limbu (Maharashtrian), Periya elimichcham (Tamil), Peddanimma (Telugu), Dodda nimbe hannu (Kannada).

Biological Source

Lemon oil is obtained from the fresh peel (rind or zest) of the ripe fruit of *Citrus limon* (L.) Burm. f. (=*Citrus limonum* Risso, *C. limonia* Osbek, *C. medica* var. *limonium* Brandis) (Family: Rutaceae), cultivated in India particularly Northern India. The name *lemon* is derived from the oval yellow fruit (derived from Middle English word *limon*; Old French word *limon*; Italian word *limone*; Arabic word *laymun* or *limun*; Persian word *limun*). The name *citrus* is derived from Greek *kedromelon*. The Romans shortened the Greek name to *citrus* derived from Latin. This is used in many European languages as Zitrone (German), Citron (French), Sitruuna (Finnish), Citrons (Latvian), Citron (Czech), Cytryna (Polish), Citrom (Hungarian), Gidron (Armenian), etc. all of which mean lemon.

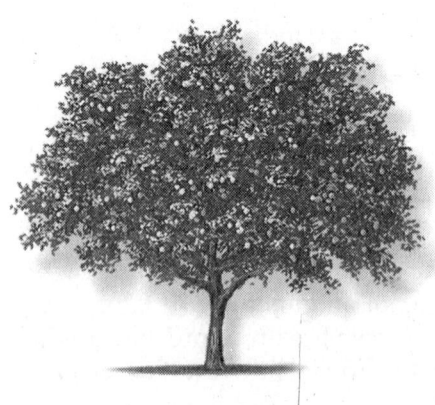

Citrus limon

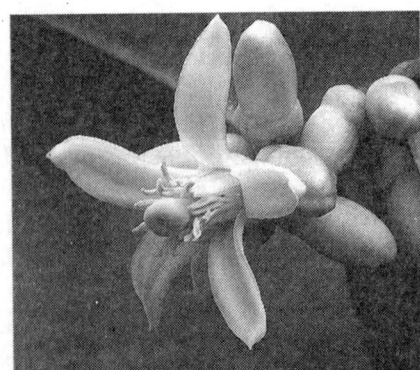

Flower of citrus

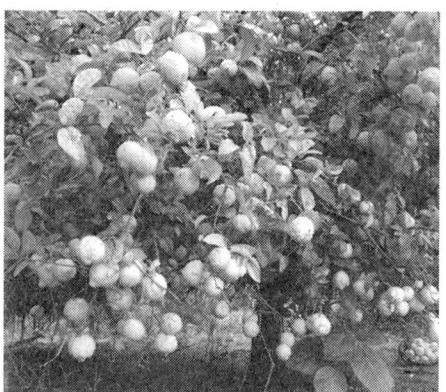

Plant with fruits

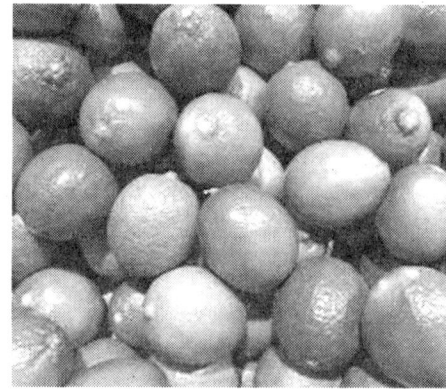

Ripe fruits

Geographical Source

The plant is a native to Asia. It is now cultivated in Spain, Italy, Socily, Portugal, Southern USA, Jamaica, and Australia. The largest producer of lemon is India (16%) followed by Mexico (14.5%), Argentina (10%), Brazil (8%) and Spain (7%).

Collection and Preparation

Mechanical picking is impossible and the fruits are to be hand-picked. They cannot be handled roughly and cannot be picked wet. Normally, they are picked from July to October, anytime after they reach the size with about 25% of juice. Manual hand picking is a common practice. The undersized fruits are to be discarded. After harvest, they are sorted according to their colour, washed, coated with a fungicide and cured (stored at 13–14°C and 85–90% of relative humidity) until they are lifted to the market.

The lemon oil comes from the peel of lemon and the manufacturers who want to extract the oil generally use a cold pressed method that involves the machinery which presses the oil from the rind. This generally takes some 101 lemons to get about an ounce of oil. There is yet another way to make the oil that is to infuse it with another oil (olive oil). The outside peel is zested by using a citrus zester and a small glass bottle is filled with lemon peels. The olive oil (or alcohol) is poured over the peels that they are completely covered in the oil and a lid is tightly placed over the bottle. The bottle is placed in window in sun and is allowed as such for several weeks. The contents are shaken once or twice a day to blend the mixture. The mixture is strained and the peels are thrown away. The mixture is taken in a shallow bowl and the alcohol is allowed to evaporate. The oil is stored in an amber-coloured bottle for use when needed. The orange oil may irritate the skin. Hence, gloves are used during the preparation of the oil and also avoid getting the oil into eyes and open wounds.

Characters

Macroscopic Characters

Externally, fresh outer lemon peel or rind of the ripe fruit (*Limonis cortex*) is lemon-yellow or dark yellow, smooth, gland-dotted with numerous small elevations over the large oil-glands embedded in the hypodermal tissue. The rind is 6–10 mm thick. Internally, the peel is white pithy. It has a fragrant odour and somewhat a bitter, pungent and aromatic tart taste.

Microscopic Characters

The epidermis is made of small tabular cells. The hypodermal parenchyma is colourless, thin walled with granular parietal protoplasm rich in yellow chromoplasts and crystals of calcium oxalate. It has many large elliptic cavities with globules of volatile oil. The oil has a fragrant distinctive taste and pungent aromatic odour.

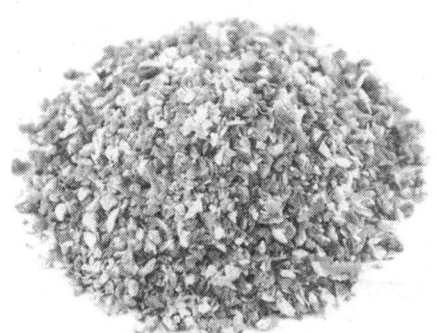

Pieces of rind

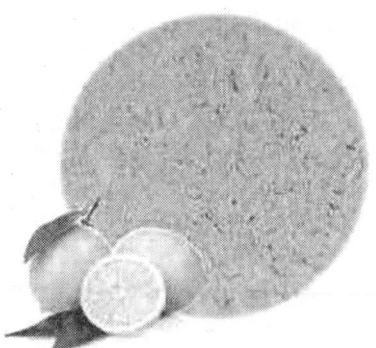

Powdered peel

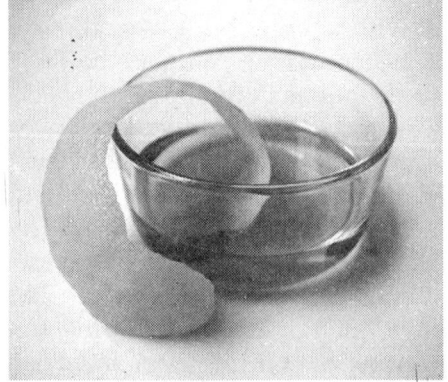

Lemon oil

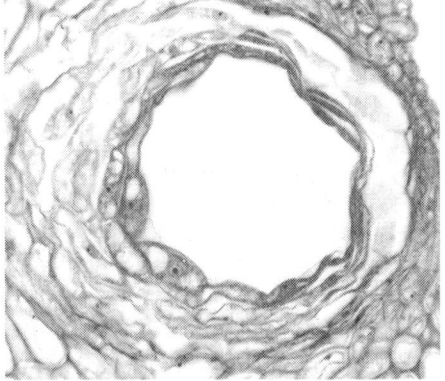

Oil cavity in section

Chemical Constituents

Oil of the lemon peel (*Oleum limonis*) consists of 2–4% volatile oil. The other constituents of the peels are hesperidin, pectin, calcium oxalate and bitter substances. Oil of lemon is a pale yellow liquid and contains terpenes (about 90% mainly limonene and gamma-terpinene and beta-phellandrene), sesquiterpenes, aldehyde (citral, about 5% and citronellol; in addition to citronellol, alpha-terpineol, n-octyl aldehyde and n-nonyl aldehyde) and esters (about 1% geranyl acetate). The inner layer is without essential oil but contains bitter flavone glycosides and coumarin derivatives. It is obtained by either distillation or by simple expression of the finely grated rind. The juice of the fruit contains about 5% citric acid.

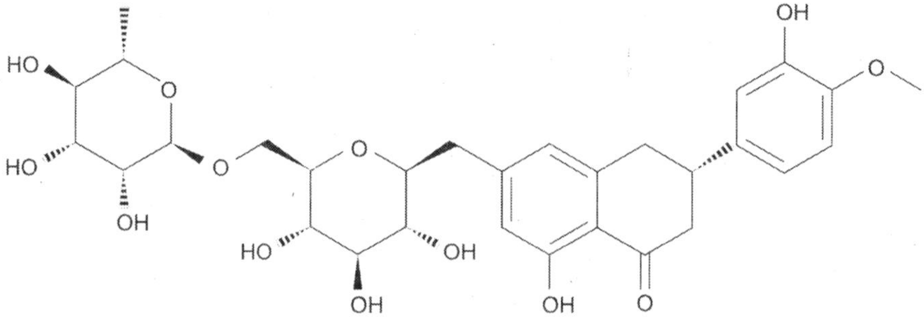

Hesperedin ($C_{28}H_{34}O_{15}$)

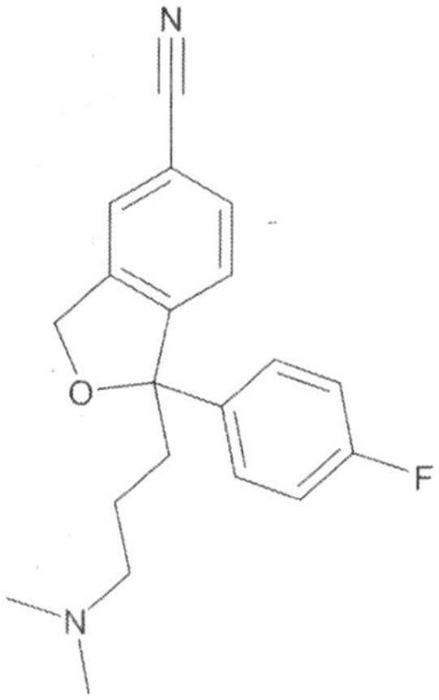

Citrol ($C_{20}H_{21}FN_{20}$)

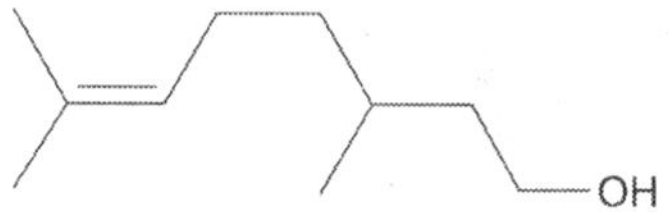

Citronellol or rhodinol ($C_{10}H_{20}O$)

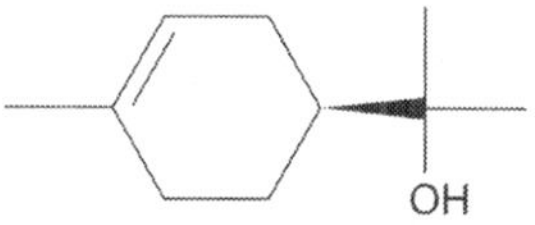

Alpha-terpineol ($C_{10}H_{18}O$)

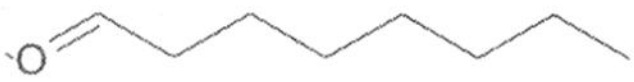

n-octyl aldehyde or octanol ($C_8H_{16}O$)

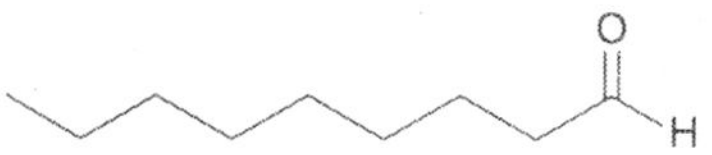

n-nonyl aldehyde or 1-nonanal ($C_9H_{18}O$)

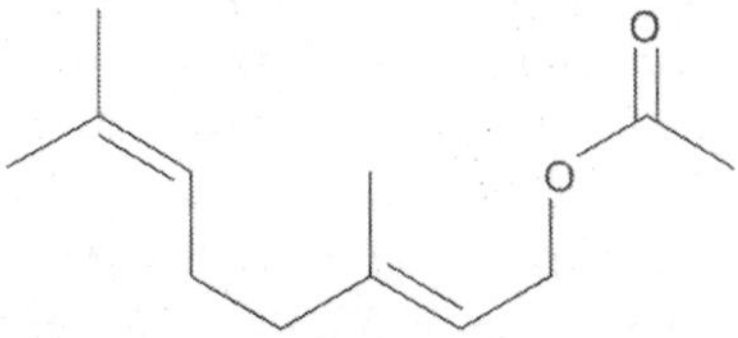

Geranyl acetate $(C_{12}H_{20}O_2)$

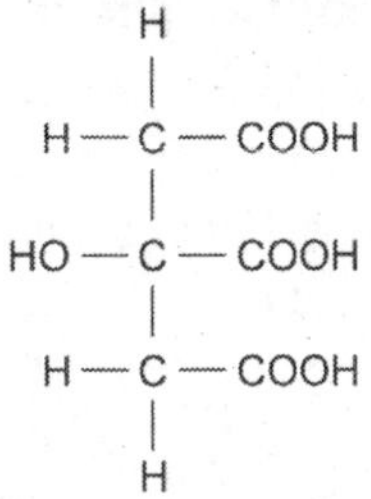

Citric acid $(C_6H_8O_7)$

History of Lemon

It is presumed that lemons were first grown in India, Northern Burma and China; its exact origin has remained a mystery and probably it is in 1350–1400. It was known for its antiseptic properties and was used as an antidote for various poisons in South and South-East Asia. It was introduced to Persia to Iraq and Egypt around 700 AD. The first record of lemon was in a 10th century Arabic treatise and it was an ornamental plant in the early Islamic gardens. Between 1000 and 1150 AD, the plant was distributed in the Arab world and the Mediterranean region. The fruit entered Europe in the 1st century AD and the cultivation began only in the middle of the 15th century. It was Christopher Columbus who brought the seeds to Hispanola through his voyages and introduced it to America (1493). Lemon juice and sometimes lemon peel is the important ingredient of the famous Greek yolk-lemon sauce, *avgolemono* prepared from fish or meat broth, lemon juice, egg-yolk and a pinch of black pepper.

Medicinal Uses

Oil of lemon is used for flavouring and in perfumery. The oil is carminative. The oil is used as a local aplication in ophthalmia, with doubtful results. Mixed with glycerine, the oil is applied to the eruption of acne, to pruritis of the vulva and scrotum, to sun burns, etc. The oil is also applied to check the postpartum haemorrhage. The rind is stomachic and carminative. Lemon juice (*Succus limonis*) of the ripe fruit is antiscorbutic and refrigerant, primarily anti-alkaline and secondarily antacid. The bark can be used as a febrifuge and the seeds as a vermifuge. The juice is a diuretic, antiscorbutic, astringent and febrifuge. The sweet juice is used to relieve gingivitis, stomatitis and tongue inflammation. Given with warm water, it is used as a daily laxative and to prevent common cold. The oil from the seeds is medicinal. The decoction of the root is used for fever in Cuba, for gonorrhoea in West Africa and bark or peel infusion relieves colic.

Other Uses

The juice, the pulp and the rind are used in cooking and baking. The fruits are used in lemonades, marmalades and garnishes. The fruit is used as a sauce by Indians, and the pickle is a popular remedy for indigestion. The rind is used as a flavouring agent in soft drinks, baked goods, puddings, mixed drinks and iced tea. The rind is used in the preparation of liquor called *limoncello* in Southern Italy. *Sarangadhara* recommended lemon juice with impure carbonate of potash and honey in rheumatic affections such as pleurodynia, sciatica, lumbago and pain in the hip joints. Lemon juice and gun powder is a topical application for scabies. The juice of the baked lemon with equal quantity of sugar or honey is a best remedy for cough. Fresh lemon juice taken in the evening relieves dyspepsia with vomiting and bilious headaches. The juice is also used to neutralise the odour of fish meat (marination). The juice is used for pies, cakes, cookies, puddings, confectionery, preservatives, etc. as a flavouring agent. The juice is a stain remover at home and for bleaching. The oil is used in furniture polish, detergents, soaps and shampoos as well as perfumes and colognes. The peel is dehydrated and used as a cattle feed. Lemonade is applied to potted plants to keep the flowers fresh for a longer time. The wood is carved into chess men, toys, spoons, etc. Lemons are served with sugar or honey is useful in sore throat and also act as detergent prior to the administration of the purgatives. Lemon is the commercial source of citric acid, lemon oil, pectin, lemon batteries in science experiments, kitchen deodouriser and nontoxic insecticides. The fruit is rich in vitamin C and helps the body to fight infections and also to prevent scurvy. Locally, it is a good astringent and gargle for sore throat. It is antibacterial and antiperiodic. The ripe skin is carminative and stomachic. The oil from the skin is rubefacient. The bark of the stem is a bitter stomachic and tonic. The oil from the seed is used in making soaps. The dry rind is an insect repellant.

NUTMEG

Synonyms

Myristica, Oleum myristicae, Semen Myristicae, Round nutmeg, Common nutmeg, Fragrant nutmeg, Nutmeg (English), True mace, Fleur de muscade, Muscadier, Musque, Muscade (French), Muskatbluthe, Myristicasamen, Muscatbaum, Achter muscatnussbaum (German). Jatiphalam (Sanskrit), Jaephal (Hindi and Bengali), Zafal (Kashmiri), Jayiphal, Javantri (Punjabi, Gujarati and Maharastrian), Jajikaya (Telugu), Jadikay (Tamil), Jajikai (Kannada), Jatika (Malayalam), Jadika (Sinhalese), Zadi-phu (Burmese), Bush-pala (Malaysian), Zauz-bawwa (Persian), Jawzt-at-Tiyb (Arabic), Musky nut or moschokarydo (Greek), Nootmuskaatboom (Dutch), Noce moscata (Italian), Moscadeira (Portuguese), Nuez moscada (Spanish).

Synonyms for Mace

Jatipatri (Sanskrit), Mace (English), Macis (French), Jaepatri (Hindi, Kannada, Telugu and Maharashtrian), Jauntari (Punjabi), Jadi-pattiri (Tamil and Malayalam), Vasavasi (Sinhalese), Zadi-phu-apoen (Burmese), Bunga-pala (Malaysian), Bazabaza (Persian and Arabic).

Biological Source

The plant is a source of two important spices, the nutmeg and the mace. This is the only tropical fruit that yields two different spices. Nutmegs are the dried kernels of the seeds of *Myristica fragrans* Houttuyn (Family: Myristicaceae), which is the most important commercial species. Other species include *M. argentea* (Papuan nutmeg or Macassar nutmeg from New Guinea) and *M. malabarica* (Bombay nutmeg or Wild nutmeg from South India). The seeds are the nutmeg of commerce and the aril (arillus or arillode) around the seed when dried is the mace. It is also a source of other commercial products like essential oils, oleoresins. The word *'nutmeg'* in English has been derived from *'notemugge'* of Middle English. The term *'mace'* in English might have been derived from *'magha'* from Sanskrit meaning a kind of herbal drug. The name *'Myristica'* is derived from the Greek *'myron'* meaning *'bitter'* (taste) and *'fragrans'* from Latin meaning *'smell'*.

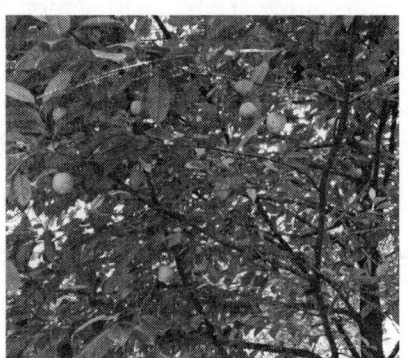

Myristica fragrans

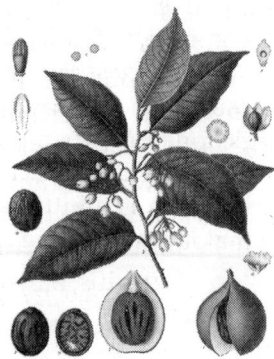

Nutmeg

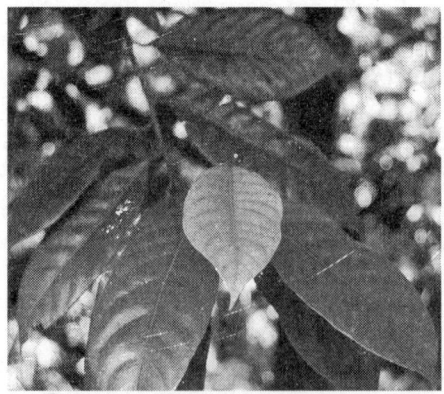

Leaves

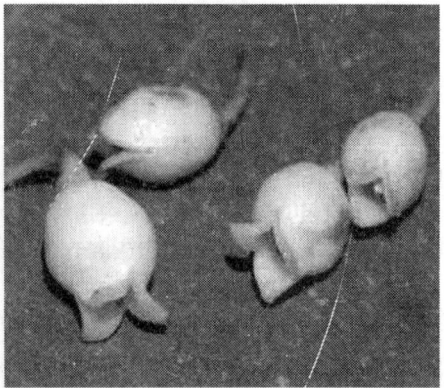

Flowers

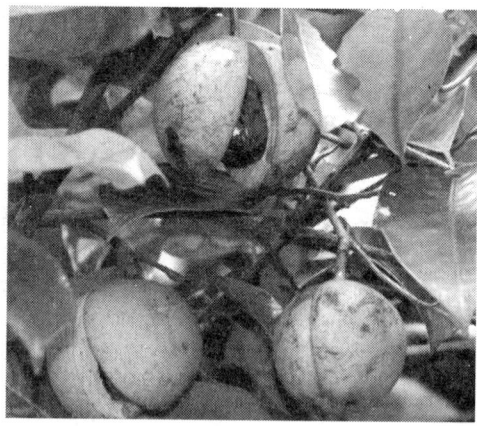

Mature fruit

Geographical Source

The plant is indigenous and a native to the Banda Islands (popular as Spice Islands, the largest of the islands and a tiny archipelago in Eastern Indonesia) in the Moluccas of Malay Peninsula and Penang Island, Indonesia (East Indian Nutmeg). The plant is now widely cultivated not only in Indonesia but also in Malaysia (Molucca Islands), Sumatra, Java and Penang), and in Sri Lanka, the Caribbean (Grenada-West Indian Nutmeg), South Africa and the West Indies and other tropical islands. In India, it is cultivated in Tamil Nadu and Kerala. Indonesia and Grenada (75% and 20%) dominate the world production and export of nutmeg and mace. Other producers of nutmeg are India, Malaysia (Penang), Papua New Guinea, Mauritius, Singapore, USA, Sri Lanka and St. Vincent Islands (Caribbean).

Collection and Preparation

The nutmeg tree bears the fruit when it is 5–8 years old (West Indian Mace and East Indian Mace). The fruit turns yellow when it is ripe, and the pulpy outer pericarp (the husk) splits into 2 halves and exposes a purplish-brown shiny seed that is surrounded by a red-coloured aril. The fruits are usually allowed to split and fall to the ground before harvest, and they are collected as soon as possible (before it bcomes discoloured). The fruits are collected by hand and sometimes, a long pole (hooked stick) is used to take the opened pods directly from the tree, which ensures a better quality harvest (but this can also result in damage to flowers and the younger fruits).

The fruits are opened by hand (orange-yellow pericarp is removed) and the arillode (mace-scarlet in colour) is removed when dried by cutting with a small pointed knife. A different option is to soak the nuts in water for 4–12 hours and then squeeze between the thumb and the forefinger until the nut pops out. The mace is flattened by hand and dried on mats in the sun (2–4 hours). After grading, the mace can be fumigated, classified and bagged.

The seeds (nutmegs) are dried in their shells in the sun which take about 3 to 6 weeks, after which the testa is cracked off (by the machine). The sound kernels are removed (by floatation), sorted on the basis of their quality and size, and the best ones are often coated with milk of lime or powdered slaked lime to prevent the attack of insects. Inferior kernels are used for expression of oil. Finally, the sorted kernels are bagged and labelled. The bagged nutmeg is fumigated with methyl bromide.

Characters

Macroscopic Characters

The seeds (nutmegs) are globular, ovoid or ellipsoidal, 20–30 mm in length and 15–18 mm wide and weigh between 5–10 gm when dry. The colour is light to dark brown. The testa is reticulately furrowed and deeply grooved on one side which indicates the position of the raphe. At one end is a white projection in the centre of which is the micropyle. The albumen is ruminate and the odour is strong and aromatic and the taste aromatic. The mace is the dried lacy covering (arillus) of the seed, buff, reddish or brownish-orange in colour, oily, 25 mm or more in length, branched and lobed above and united below. It has a fragrant odour and aromatic taste.

Microscopic Characters

Anatomically, the seed shows perisperm of small, thin walled parenchyma with brown pigment. It contains few spiral ducts in which large reservoirs of volatile oil are imbedded. The endosprem is made of large polygonal parenchyma filled with starch and aleurone grains. The starch grains are simple or compound (2–20), spheroidal or polygonal with a distinct hilum.

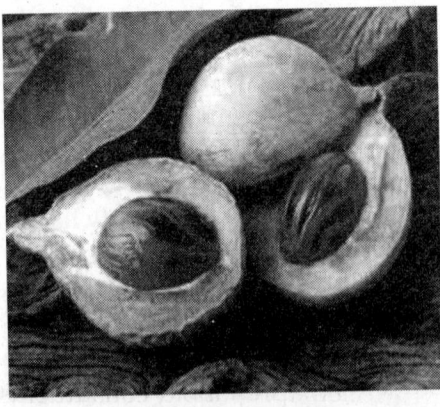

Fruit split open

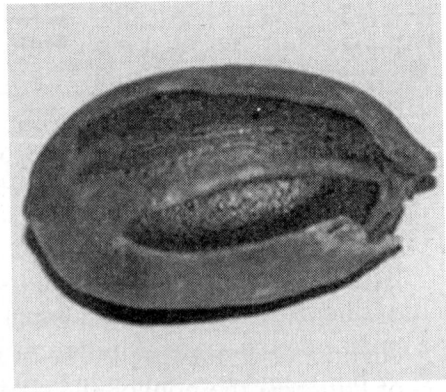

Seed with aril

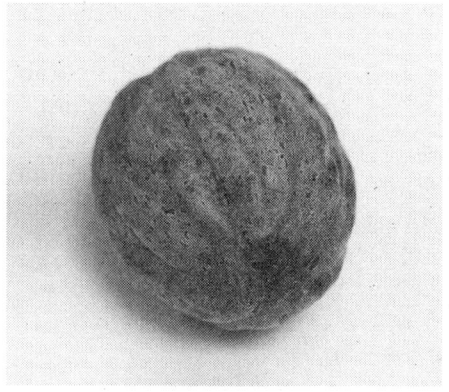

Nutmeg—the seed

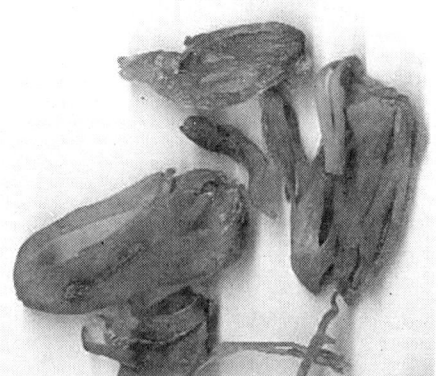

Mace—the aril

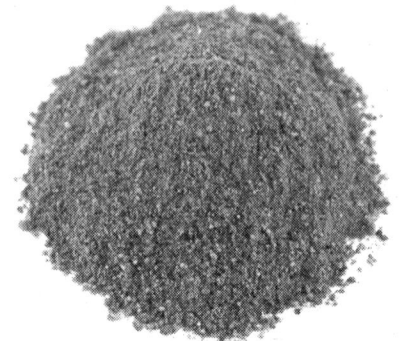

Nutmeg powder

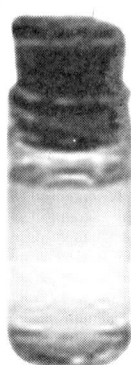

Nutmeg oil

Chemical Constituents

The kernel (nutmeg) contains a volatile oil (5–16%), a fixed oil, proteins, fat (30%), starch mucilage and ash. The mace contains a yellowish volatile oil (8–17%), a fixed oil, resin, fat, sugar, dextrin and mucilage. The fixed oil called 'butter of nutmeg' consists of myristin (*Oleum myristicae*— methoxy-safrole, about 4 to 8% which is a weak monoamine oxidase inhibitor), myristic acid ($C_{14}H_{28}O_2$), elemicin and safrole. The essential oil contains myristicin and myristicol. The essential oil of mace consists of macene. The oil is mostly composed of terpene hydrocarbons like sabinene, pinene, camphene, phellandrene, terpinene, limonene of about 60–80%, terpene derivatives such as linalool, geraniol, terpineol of about 5–15% and phenylpropanoids like myristicin, elemicin, safrol, and eugenol of about 15–20%. Both the nutmeg and mace contain about 2% of lignanes, the nonvolatile dimers of phenylpropanoid constituents of the oil such as dehydrodiisoeugenol.

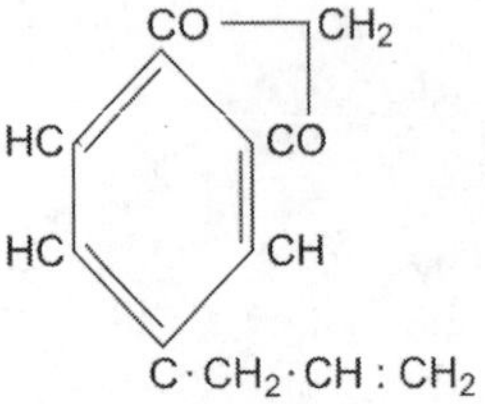

Safrole ($C_{10}H_{10}O_2$)

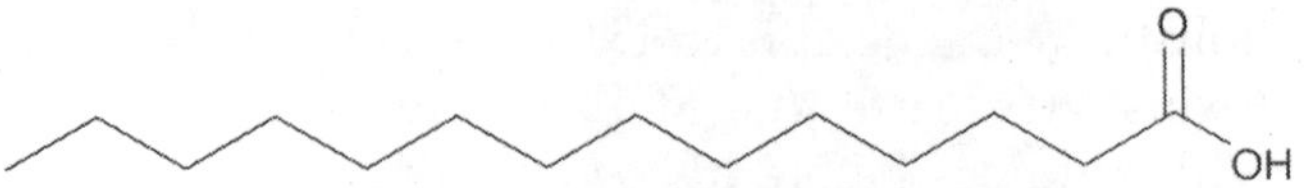

Myristic acid ($CH_3(CH_2)_{12}COOH$)

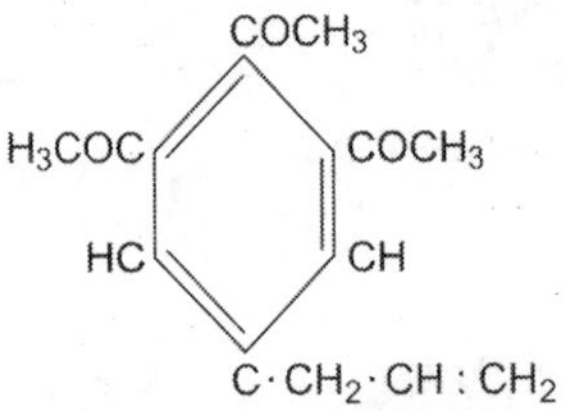

Elemicin ($C_{12}H_{16}O_3$)

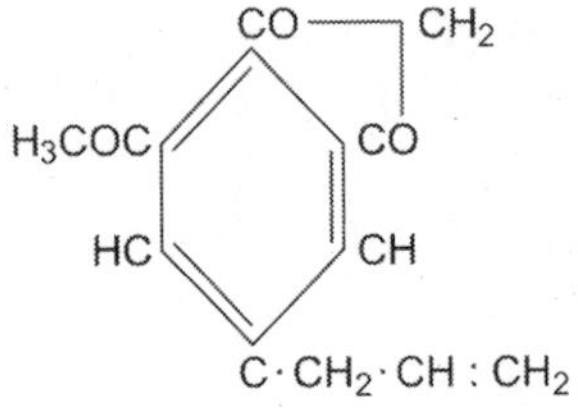

Myristicin ($C_{11}H_{12}O_3$)

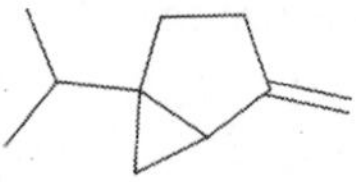

Sabinene ($C_{10}H_{16}$)

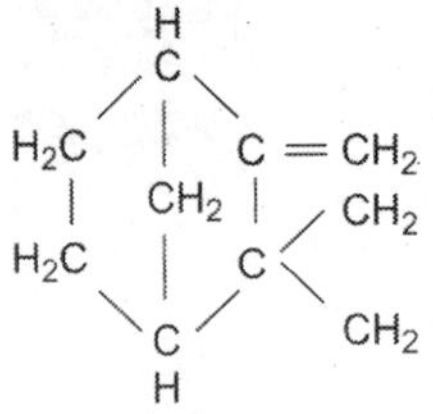

Camphene ($C_{10}H_{16}$)

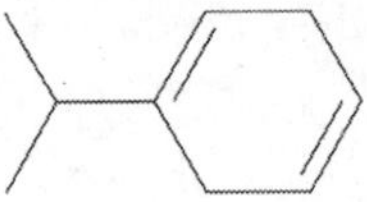

Terpinene ($C_{10}H_{16}$)

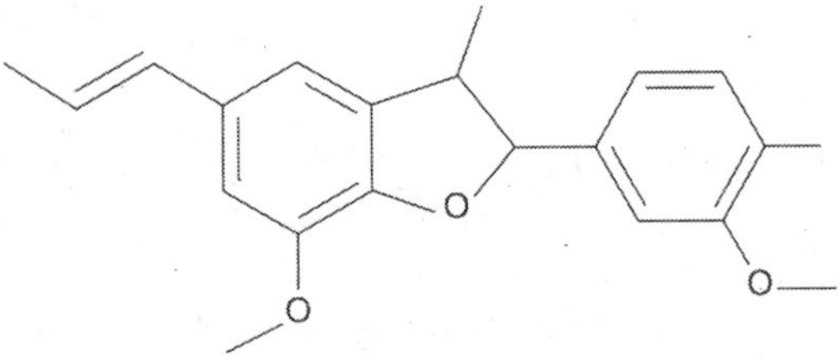

Dehydrodiisoeugenol ($C_{20}H_{22}O_4$)

History of Nutmeg

The early history of nutmeg dates back to the 1st century A.D., and this is evident in the writings of Pliny, the Roman philosopher, who spoke of a tree bearing nuts with two flavours (the nutmeg and the mace) and it is believed that Roman priests have burnt nutmeg as incense but this is disputed. In Vedic writings (India), it was recommended for headache, fever and bad breath. The Arabian writings refer it to be good for stomach ailments and also as an aphrodisiac. The ancient Greeks and Romans used it as a brain tonic though it was rare and costly. It is an integral drug in Chinese medicine and was used for stomach pain and inflammation. In holistic medicine, it is an excellent liver tonic which helped to remove the toxins. It is learnt that Emperor Henry VI fumigated the streets of Rome with nutmegs before his coronation. Nutmeg has also been found in the Egyptian tombs. In middle ages it was brought to Europe by the Arabs through the Venetians. It was in the 6th century that Arab merchants brought the nutmeg to Constantinople. It was traded by Arabs and was sold to the Venetians for high prices. In the 14th century, half a kilogram of nutmeg costed as much as three sheep or a cow. The trade of nutmeg was taken over by the Dutch (1600) followed by the English after a war. The Dutch explorers in particular, Van den Broeke and Jan Pieterscoon took away the first batch of nutmegs from Banda islands, Indonesia (the first specific place of origin of nutmeg) in 1608, followed by its meteoric spread in Europe. The British East India Company brought it to Penang, Singapore, Sri Lanka and the West Indies. Nutmeg has been used since 7th century in China. The Chinese are responsible for our current knowledge of the medicinal properties of nutmeg. The nutmeg was also popular with Byzantine traders who purchased it from Arabs. It is believed that here the plant got its name from 'mesk' in Arabian, translated into French, as 'noix nuguette' and then it became 'nutmeg' in English. Earlier, it has been used for everything from the cramps in the stomach to plague. Nutmeg is known to have been used as a spice of high value in medieval cuisine and in the European markets in the preparation of flavourings, medicines and preservatives. In Elizabethan times, it was very popular as it was believed that nutmeg could ward off the plague. The national flag of Grenada bears a split-open nutmeg fruit on it. Connecticut of USA has a nickname as the Nutmeg state or Nutmegger as its traders carved out nutmeg from wood and sold. Arabs used nutmeg as an aid for digestion and also as an aphrodisiac. In Indonesia the pulp is used to prepare a jam, 'selei buah pala'. It was believed that nutmeg possessed magical powers and it was recorded by a 16th century monk who advised young men to carry the vials of nutmeg oil to anoint their genitals for increased virility. It was also believed that inserting a nutmeg into the left armpit helps in attracting the admirers in social events. The nutmegs were also used as amulets to be protected against many dangers and evils, from boils to rheumatism to broken bones and misfortunes. According to European folklore, Pagans used nutmegs as a symbol of luck, money, health and fidelity.

Medicinal Uses

Both nutmeg and the mace have a similar taste; nutmeg is slightly sweeter while the mace has a delicate flavour. Nutmeg is an aromatic, stimulant and carminative and in larger doses it is narcotic. The concrete oil is a rubefacient while the volatile oil is a stimulant and carminative. Mace is carminative and aphrodisiac while the wood is astringent. Nutmegs, maces and their oils are largely used for flavouring, condiments and as carminatives. It can be administered in delirium tremens and in insomnia. The pills are used as anodyne and astringent in dysentery. The churna is used as a sedative and antispasmodic in asthma, colic, neuralgia, menorrhagia, dysmenorrhoea, spasmodic cough and lumbago. The confection is a useful tonic for the heart, brain and sexual debility, incontinence of urine and general weakness. The ointment is a topical application for itching and irritable haemorrhoids. The concrete oil is used in ringworm infections and stimulates the growth of the hair. It is a good liniment for chronic rheumatism, paralysis and sprains. Mace is used in low fevers, humoral asthma and bowel complaints. The roasted mace and nutmeg are useful in chronic diarrhoea, flatulent colic and some forms of dyspepsia and obstructions of liver and spleen. Nutmeg has narcotic and anaesthetic action and peripherally has an irritant action which is due to myristicin. The hallucinogenic activity of the drug is due to myristicin and elemecin which are transmitted in human body to amphetamines. It is used as a spice.

Non-medical Uses

The pericarp of the fruit is used to make a jam, 'Morne Delice', in Grenada. The fruit is a source of a jam, 'selei buah pala' in Indonesia and is also used in the preparation of fragrant candies called 'manisan pala' (nutmeg sweets). It is a common constituent of cuisine all over the world. In Penang, it is made into pickles, 'Ais Kacang' and it is also blended or boiled to prepare iced nutmeg juice, 'Lau Hau Peng' in Penang Hokkien. In Indian cuisine, it is used in many sweet and savoury dishes, in particular the Mughalai cuisine, and in small quantities used in garam masala (North Indian spice mixture) and also sometimes smoked. It is used as a spice in savoury dishes in Middle Eastern cuisine, in cooking and the preparation of savoury dishes in Greece and Cyprus, in the preparation of potato and meat dishes along with soups, sauces and baked goods in European cuisine, is added to the vegetables like Brussels sprouts, Cauliflower and String beans in Dutch cuisine, an ingredient of curry powders in Japanese cuisine and in the production of drinks like Bushwacker, Painkiller and Barbados rum in the Caribbean.

Other Uses

The essential oil is used in perfumery and pharmaceutical industry as an oleochemical. It is a natural food flavouring substance in baked goods, syrups, beverages and sweets. It is also used in the cosmetic industry, such as in toothpastes and tobacco. In medicine, it is used in diseases related to the nervous and digestive systems as it is an analgesic, antiseptic, carminative, stimulant, etc. The oil is a powerful tonic, stimulates the orgasm and dissolves the muscular fatigue in addition to reviving the vital functions. Nutmeg butter which is expressed from the nut is a semisolid and reddish brown with a taste and the smell of nutmeg. About 75% of it is trimyristin which can be converted into myristic acid (14-carbon fatty acid) which can be used as a replacement for cocoa butter and can be mixed with cotton seed oil or palm oil and is used as an industrial lubricant. The butter can also be used to make candles. Myristicin poisoning induces convulsions, palpitations, nausea, dehydration and body pain and it is also a strong deliriant. Fatal poisoning in humans is very rare but it is deadly to pets and livestock even in small quantities. Nutmeg inhibits prostaglandin production and it may affect the foetus in large quantitites. Though it was considered to be an abortifacient, it is safe for culinary use.

Adulteration

The powder is often adulterated with exhausted nutmeg, corn meal, curcuma, powdered beans, ground olive pits and coconut shells. This is often substituted with Macassar nutmegs or Papuan nutmegs of *Myristica argentea* Warburg and/or with Bombay nutmegs or wild nutmegs of *Myristica malabarica* Lamarck. The mace is often adulterated with Bombay mace.

EUCALYPTUS

Synonyms

Eucalyptus tree, Blue gum Eucalyptus, Australian Fever Tree leaf, Tasmanian blue gum tree, Southern blue gum tree, Silver Mountain Gum tree, Iron Bark Tree, Bloodwood tree, Fuzzy box tree, Stubborn wood tree, Wooly-butt tree, Stringy bark tree (English), Folium Eucalypti, Feuilles d' Eucalyptus or Gommier bleu (French), Eucalyptus Blatter (German), Blauwe gomboom (the Netherlands), Eulaliptus galkowy (Polski), Blauer Eukalyptus (Deutsch), Eucalipto (Espanol), Eucalitto (Italian), Ocalittu or Ocaritti (Sardu), Tailapatra or Tailaparna or Nilanirgasa (Sanskrit), Sugandhapatra, Nilgiri taila, Nilagiri tailam (Telugu), Yukeliptas (Hindi), Yukkali (Malayalam), Karpoor maram (Tamil).

Biological Source

Oil of Eucalyptus is distilled from the fresh or dry sickle-shaped leaves of various species of *Eucalyptus* particularly *E. globulus* Labillardiere (Family: Myrtaceae). The gum (Eucalyptus kino) is collected as an exudation from the stem and the oil is distilled from the leaves. There are more than 700 species, mostly native to Australia and a small number are found in New Guinea and Indonesia and Philippine archipelago. Outside Australia, only 15 species occur and 9 do not occur in Australia. The name *'Eucalyptus'* comes from the Greek, *'eucalyptos'* (*eu* and *kaluptos*) meaning *'well-covered'* (describe the operculum) or *'beautiful bark'*. Other species used for the commercial production of the oil include *E. cineorifolia, E. dives, E. dumosa,*

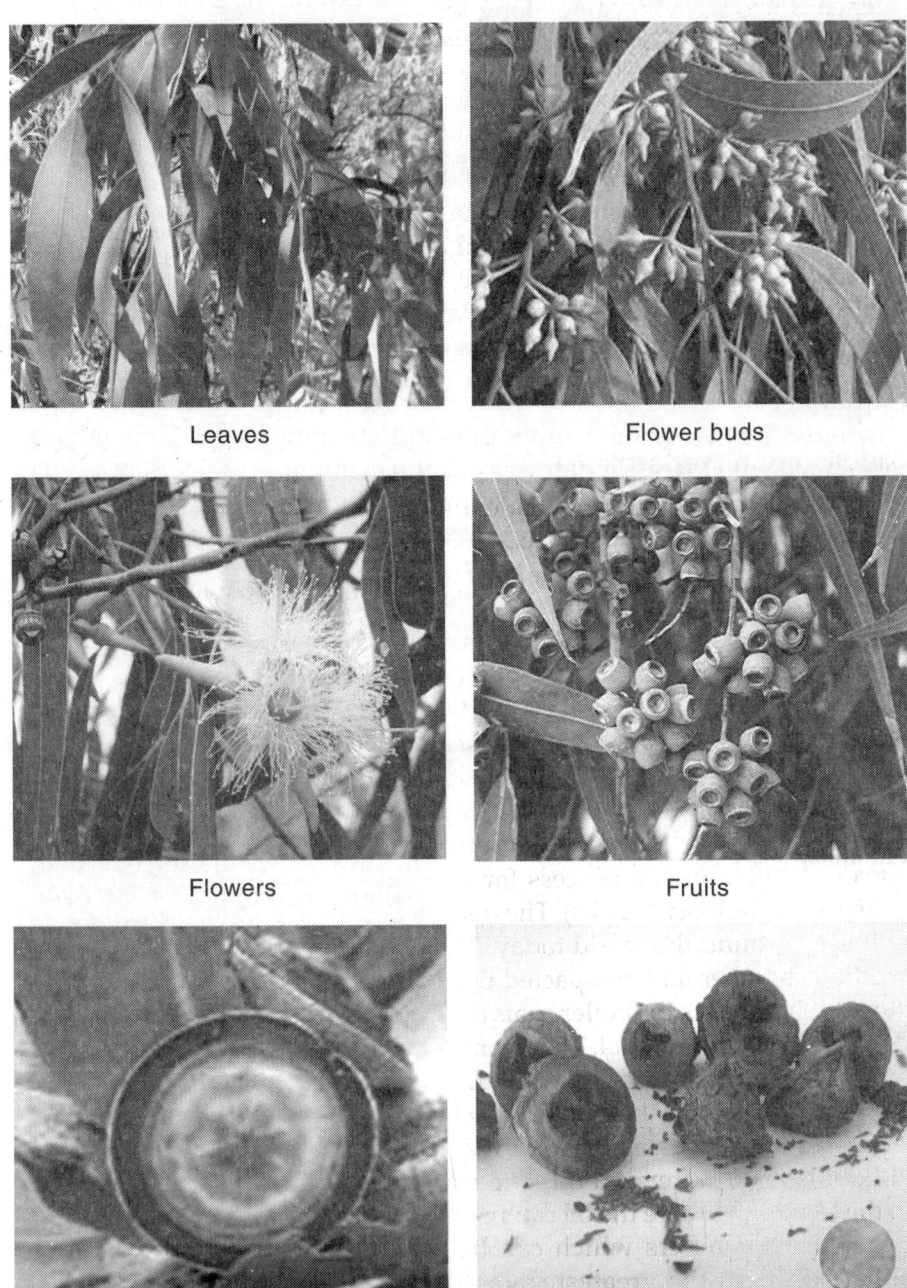

Leaves

Flower buds

Flowers

Fruits

Mature capsule

Dry capsules

E. goniocalyx, E. horistes, E. kochii, E. leucoxylon, E. oleosa, E. polybractea, E. radiata, E. sideroxylon, E. smithii, E. tereticornis, and *E. viridis. E. globulus* was first collected by Jacques-Julien Houton de Labillardiere (1755–1834), a French Botanist, who came along with the French Expedition, on the South-East coast of Tasmania in 1792–1793 and was described by him in 1791–1794.

Geographical Source

The main habitat is Australia and Tasmania. The species which is indigenous to Australia is cultivated in the high lands of India, chiefly on the Nilgiris. The species are cultivated throughout tropics and subtropics including America, Southern Europe, Africa, the Mediterranean basin, the Middle East, Argentina, Brazil, Paraguay, China, Indonesia and the Indian subcontinent. Eucalyptus oils are produced in Portugal, South Africa, Spain, China, Brazil, Australia, California, Southern Europe, India and Paraguay.

Collection and Preparation

The leaves are collected from the older parts of the trees and dried to express the oil. There are two types of steam distillation, water/steam distillation and direct steam distillation. The former is an improved method in which the still contains a grid which keeps the plant material above the water level. The water is boiled below the charge and wet steam passes through the plant material. During the process of distillation, only very tiny molecules can evaporate, so they are the only one which leave the plant. These extremely small molecules make up the essential oil. This proccess involves the use of steam to percolate and vapourise out the essential oils fom the plant material, with the subsequent condensation of steam and the essential oil prior to the separation.

Steam distillation is a process for the materials that are temperature-sensitive (like the essential oils). The traditional method of steam distillation is still used around the world today. The plant material is loaded into the extraction chamber and compacted tightly. The steam is released into the bottom of chamber as the boiler heats the water, and starts to travel upward, thus, saturating the material. The steam impregnates the plant fibre causing it to release the oil molecules as a gas from the molecule channel. Then, the steam carries the gas to the condenser where it goes through a phase change condensation as it passes through the cooling process in the swan neck and liquifies into water and oil. The mixture of oil and water then flows into the separator where the oil can rise to the top of the water to be poured off into the containers which can be drained off. The vertical steam distillation offers the greatest potential for protecting the therapeutic benefits and the quality of the essential oils. Similarly, the temperature also has a distinct effect.

Characters

Macroscopic Characters

The leaf stalk or the petiole is twisted and the lamina is sickle-shaped. It measures 8–30 cm in length and 2–7 cm in breadth, coriaceous, bifacial with an acute or acuminate tip. The base is unequal, obtuse to round with an uneven or revolute margin. The colour is greyish-green to pale yellowish-green and glaucous, glabrous or glandular punctate. The venation is pinnate reticulate. The veins of the first order run to margin and anastamose parallel to the margin. The leaves are evergreen and covered with oil glands. It has an aromatic odour and bitter cooling taste.

Microscopic Characters

Anatomically, the upper and lower epidermis of the leaf is made of polygonal cells with thick cutinised outer walls and both the layers possess sunken stomata. The mesophyll is differentiated into palisade and spongy parenchyma. Within these tissues occur large, subglobular internal glands lined with secretory epithelium containing yellow eucalyptus oil. Some of the cells of spongy parenchyma contain rosette like aggregates of calcium oxalate. Fibrous pericycle occurs outside the vascular bundles in the region of the midrib and the petiole.

Chemical Constituents

The fresh leaves contain about 0.4–1.6% of volatile oil (the dried leaves about 1–3%) of which 54–90% is eucalyptol ($C_{10}H_{18}O$ – 1,8-cineol, 1,8-Epoxy-p-menthane, 1,3,3-Trimethyl-2-oxanicyclo(2,2,2)octane, Cajeputol) and balance being composed of eudesmol, alpha-pinene (2.8%), p-cymene (2.7%), aromadendrene ($C_{15}H_{24}$), cuminaldehyde, globulol, pinocarveol, d-pinene and other terpenes in addition to crystallizable resin, a bitter principle, tannin, cerylic alcohol, butyric aldehyde (C_4H_8O), valerianic aldehyde ($C_5H_{10}O$), phellandrine, eucalyptic acid and calcium oxalate. 48 components out of 70 of the oil have been identified. Eucalyptol which

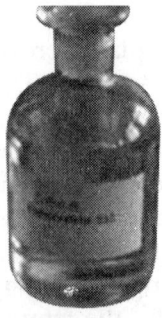

Eucalyptus oil

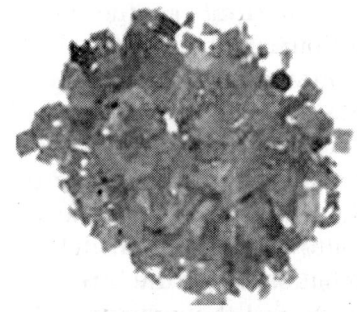

Crystals of eucalyptol

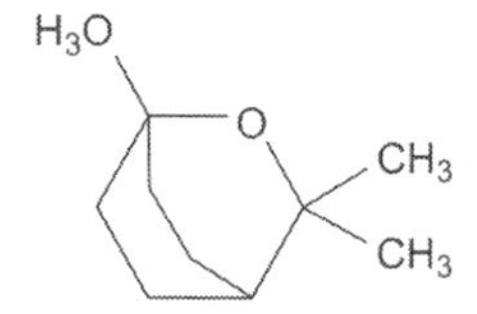

Eucalyptol ($C_{10}H_{18}O$)

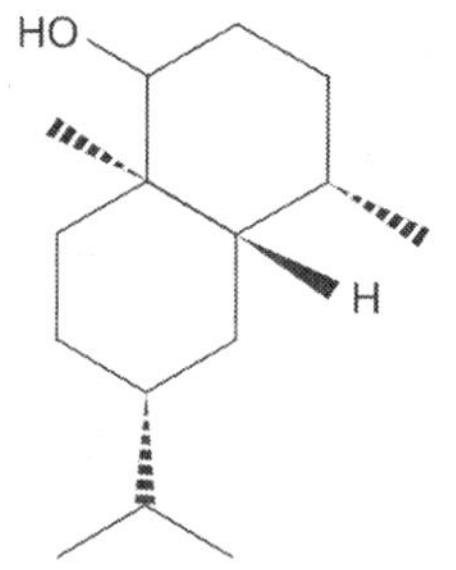

Eudesmol ($C_{15}H_{26}O$)

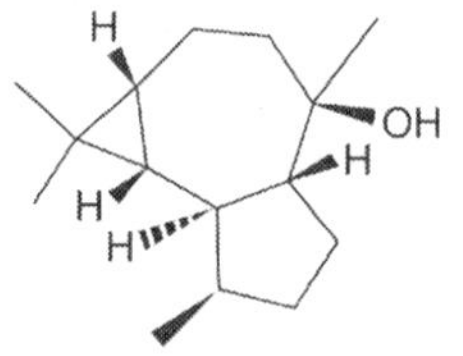

Globulol ($C_{15}H_{26}O$)

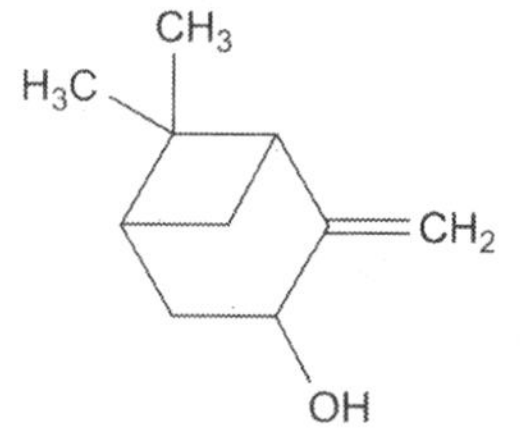

Pinocarveol ($C_{10}H_{16}O$)

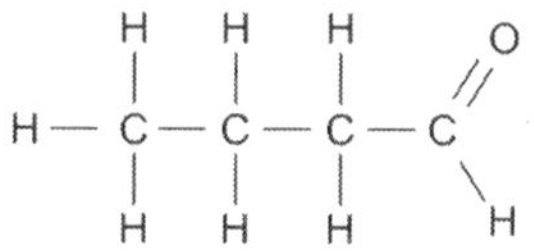

Butyricaldehyde ($CH_3(CH_2)_2CHO$)

comprises up to 90% of the essential oil is colourless liquid, cyclic ether and a monoterpenoid which has a density of 0.9225 g/cm^2, a melting point of 1.5°C and a boiling point of 176–177°C. Eucalyptus oil is a collective generic name for the oils from the genus. The gum contains kino-tannic acid, catechin and pyrocatechin.

History of *Eucalyptus*

The Australian aboriginals use the infusion of eucalyptus leaves as a traditional medicine for body pains, sinus congestion, fever and colds. The botanical collections of *Eucalyptus* species have been made in 1770 by Joseph Banks and Daniel Soalnder with Captain James Cook at Botany Bay near the Endeavour River in Northern Queensland, Australia, though they have been seen by the European explorers. They have collected *E. gummifera* and *E. platyphylla*. David Nelson (1777) on Cook's third expedition collected *E. obliqua* (the French Botanist, L'Heritier coined the generic name, *Eucalyptus*, from the Greek roots *eu* (well) and *kaluptos* (covered), in reference to the operculum of the flower bud which protects the developing parts of the flower and is shed at flowering; and the species *obliqua* from

Latin, *obliquus* referring to the unequal leaf base) on Brunny island in Southern Tasmania and took the specimen to the British Museum in London. The surgeons on the First Fleet, Dennis Considen and John White (1788) distilled eucalyptus oil from the leaves of *E. piperita* growing on the shores of Port Jackson to treat the convicts and marines. Subsequently, the oil was extracted by the early colonialists. Several more species were collected, named and published in the 19th century by James Edward Smith, an English Botanist, from the regions of Sydney like *E. pilularis*, *E. saligna* and *E. tereticornis*. The French Botanist, Jacques Labillardiere, collected the first endemic Western Australian species, *E. cornuta* from Esperance area in 1792. The first comprehensive account of the genus *Eucalyptus* was due to the work of Baron Ferdinand von Mueller, the German Botanist and explorer (the Director of the Botanical Garden, Melbourne, Australia, from 1857 to 1873), who made known the qualities of *Eucalyptus* all over the world and led to its introduction into Europe, North and South Africa, California and the nontropical *South America*. He was the first to suggest that the leaves might be of use as a disinfectant in malarial fever. He also promoted the disinfectant qualities of *Eucalyptus* and also encouraged Joseph Bosisto, a pharmacist from Melbourne, Australia, to investigate the commercial potential of the oil. In 1852, Bosisto set up a distillation plant to start the industry near Dandenong, Victoria, and extracted the oil from *E. radiata*. This later became the generic 'oil of eucalyptus' or 'Bosisto's Eucalyptus Oil' and this brand still survives in the market. The details of Mueller's work appears in *Flora Australiensis* of George Bentham (1867) and this remains the only complete Australian flora even today and is the most important early systematic treatment of the genus. In India, the plantations were made in 1863 in the Nilgiris at Ootacamund (Ooty). In 1870, F. S. Cloez, the French Chemist, identified and ascribed the name eucalyptol to the dominant portion of *E. globulus* (Tasmanian blue gum) oil, now referred to as cineole. By 1880s, the surgeons began using the oil as an antiseptic during surgeries. Bentham's work was later elaborated by Joseph Henry Maiden (1903–1933) and by William Faris Blakely (1934). *Eucalyptus* has a long history in India. Around 1790, it was first planted by the ruler of Mysore, Tippu Sultan, in his palace garden on Nandi hills, near Bangalore, Karnataka. Subsequently, it was introduced in the Nilgiri hills, Ootacamund, Tamil Nadu, in 1843. From 1856, regular plantations were raised to meet the demand for firewood. The first plantation was raised at Malabavi (Devarayanadurga), Tumkur district by the Forest Department in 1877.

Medicinal Uses

Eucalyptus oil is a stomachic, carminative, expectorant, rubefacient, antiseptic, febrifuge, stimulant, diaphoretic, antimalarial and antiperiodic. It is much used for alleviating the symptoms of nasopharyngeal infections, for treating coughs and as a decongestant. It is taken internally in the form of mixtures, inhalations, lozenges and pastilles and applied externally as ointments and liniments. The oil increases the flow of saliva, gastric and intestinal juices thus aiding in appetite and digestion. It is used in the treatments of catarrh of the bronchopulmonary mucous membranes, intermittent and septic fevers, croup, diphtheria, whooping cough, purulent catarrh of genitourinary organs, surgical wounds, ulcers, etc. The leaves are chewed to clean the breath and harden the spongy and bleeding gums. The leaf infusion checks the secretions in bronchitis and coryza. The tincture is used in croup and in pulmonary gangrene. It is also useful in purulent catarrhal affections of the bladder, urethra and vagina, and in chronic cystitis with haematuria. The extract of the leaf is also used as a local application in erysipelas of the face, legs and scrotum. It also increases the heart beat, lowers the arterial tension and speeds up respiration. It is eliminated through perspiration (skin), urine (kidneys), bronchi (lungs) and milk. In higher doses, it is an irritant of the alimentary canal and produces eructation, indigestion, nausea, vomiting and purging. It is also a narcotic poison in toxic doses, which paralyses the respiratory centre in the medulla of the brain. It controls asthma and is used in mouthwashes and in rhinosinusitis. Topical application reduces inflammation and pain in headaches on bending, frontal headache, nasal obstruction, etc. The oil is an ingredient of 'cathedral oil' that is used for sterilising and lubricating urethral catheters.

Culinary and Other Uses

Eucalyptol is used as a flavouring agent, for fragrance and in cosmetics. It is used in baking goods, confectionery, meat, cigarettes and beverages. The oil is a natural insecticide and sometimes used to clean the swamps for reducing the risk of malaria. The oil is antibacterial and is used for cleansing, deodourising the respiratory tract, and in very small quantities in dental care, soaps, detergents, lotions, cough drops and decongestants. It also stimulates the immune system. The oil possesses insect repellant (disinfectant) properties which destroys the lower forms of life, and used as an ingredient in commercial mosquito repellants and also as a biopesticide. The plant is also used as an ornamental tree, for timber, firewood and pulpwood. It is used in industries like fence posts, charcoal, cellulose and biofuel. The plant shows a very fast growth and is suitable for windbreaks and to reduce erosion. It is also used for lowering the water table and thus reduces soil salination (as it draws large amounts of water by transpiration). The nectar is the source of high quality monofloral honey. The wood is used in the manufacture of a traditional Australian aboriginal wind instrument, *digeridoos*. All parts of the plant are used to make coloured dyes ranging from yellow and orange through green, tan, chocolate and deep rust red. In veterinary medicine, the oil is administered in influenza in horses, in distemper in dogs and in septicaemia in all animals in addition to its use for parasitic skin affections. The plant is also used in the manufacture of paper, in the production of poles for huts and houses, in making plywood, etc.

Adulteration

The older leaves are often adulterated with the leaves from younger branches (ovate-oblong and opposite) and the leaves of allied species (less leathery and less fragrant).

GINGER

Synonyms

Zingiber, Rhizoma zingiberis, Ginger rhizome, Ingwer (German), Gingembre (French). Zangebilarataba (Persian), Sheng-jiang or Gan-jiang—dried (Chinese), Shringavera or Adrakam—dried or Sunta or Mahaushada (Sanskrit), Aadrak or adrak (Bengali, Punjabi, Hindi and Urdu), Adhu (Gujarati), Sho-ont (Kashmiri), Sunt (Konkani and Maharastrian), Zanjabil (Arabic), Vona Shunti or Hashi sonti—dried (Kannada), Allam or Sonti—dried (Telugu), Shuku or Inji—dried (Tamil), Chukka (Malayalam), Alay (Marathi), Inguru (Sinhalese), Aduwa (Nepali), Sinjibil (Somaliland), Aadha (Bangladesh), Gyin or Ginsi-khiav or Gin-sin—dried (Burmese).

Biological Source

Ginger is the scraped or unscraped fresh or dried rhizome of *Zingiber officinale* Roscoe (Family: Zingiberaceae). The English name *ginger* comes from the French, *gingimbre*, from medieval Latin, *gingiber*, from Greek, *zingiberis*, from Pali, *sringivera*, finally of Dravidian origin from Tamil, *inji ver* (meaning *root of inji*). The word *Zingiber* is thought to have come from the Sanskrit word, *shringavera* (horn-root) derived from Arabic and Greek

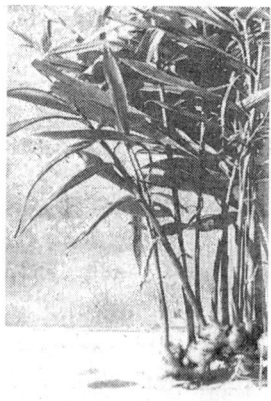

Zingiber officinale

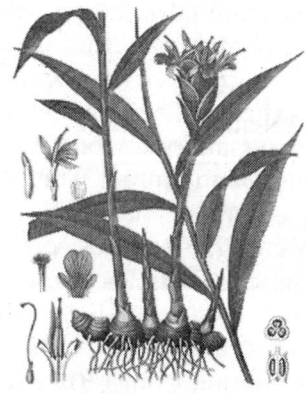

Ginger plant

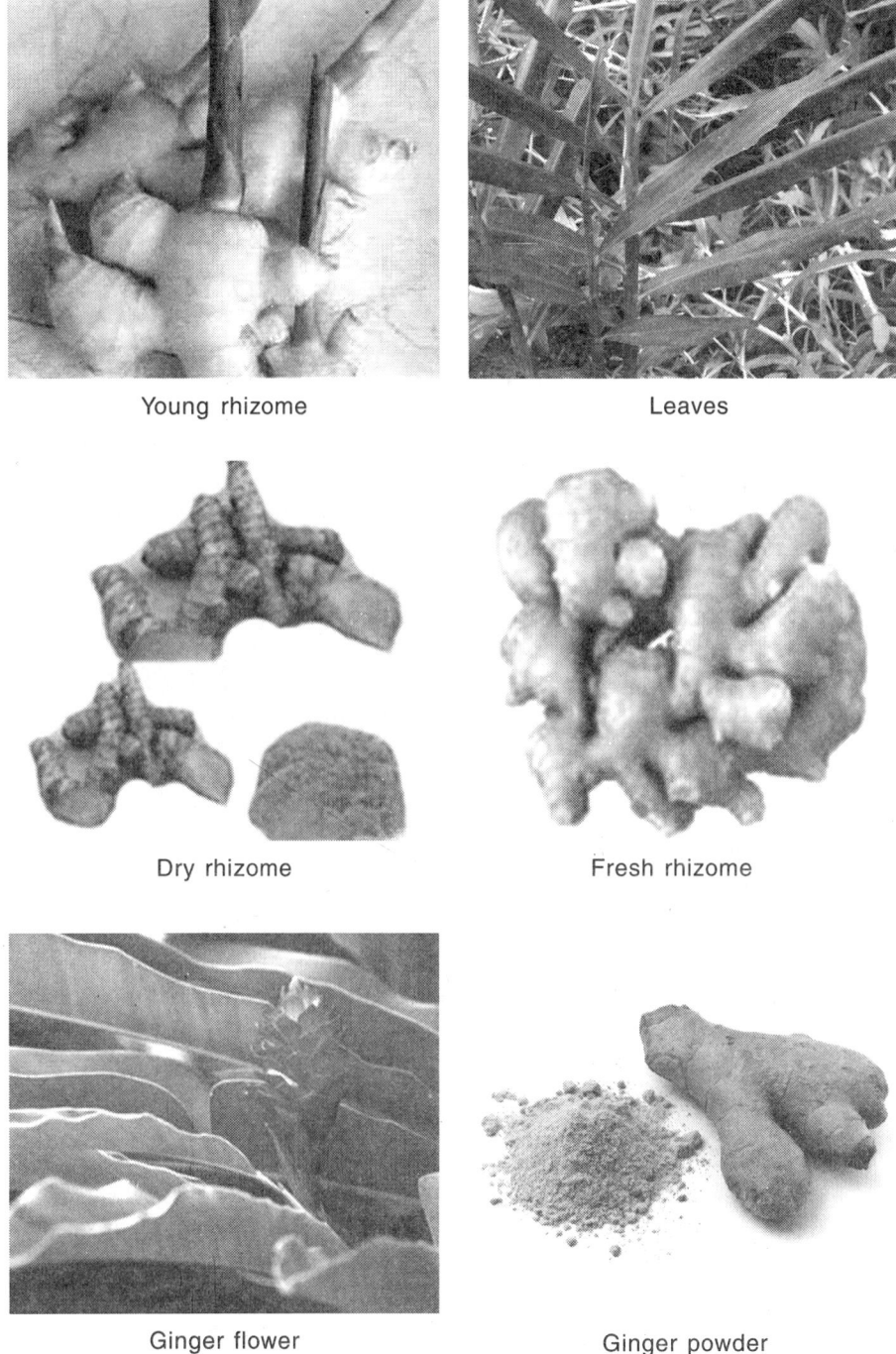

Young rhizome

Leaves

Dry rhizome

Fresh rhizome

Ginger flower

Ginger powder

words meaning *'shaped like a horn'* as the rhizomes often look like the antlers of a deer.

Geographical Source

The habitat of the plant is South Asia and ginger has been cultivated in India from the earliest times; the plant is unknown in the wild state. It is also grown in many parts of the world, the chief countries producing it are West Indies, Africa, India, Japan, Jamaica, China and Africa, and extensively cultivated in tropical and subtropical areas of both the Eastern and Western Hemisphere. In India, it is cultivated on a large scale in Tamil Nadu, Kerala, and Karnataka and also in West Bengal and Punjab.

Collection and Preparation

The plants of ginger emit their aerial shoots that dry up after flowering and fruiting in about 8 to 10 months time. The rhizomes are dug upon the death of the older portions and washed. Abundant rainfall is necessary during the growing season and at no time water logging should be permitted. They are peeled and washed in clean water with lime juice and dried in the sun. Sometimes, they are washed in boiling water and dried (African and Indian varieties) in the sun for 5–6 days. They are then bleached by washing and dried again for 2 days (Jamaica ginger). In Indian and African varieties, the rhizome is peeled on the flat sides, and then treated with boiling water and dried in the sun. Sometimes, the rhizomes are washed with carbonate or sulphate of lime to prevent the insect larval attack. The rhizomes are also bleached with sulphurous acid or chloride of lime (Bleached ginger). The oil is extracted by distillation. The important commercial varieties include ginger from Jamaica, Kerala and Africa.

Characters

Macroscopic Characters

It occurs in branched pieces called races or hands. These are 8–14 cm long and 2–3 cm thick. Each hand or finger has a depressed scar or bud capable of giving birth to a new plant. Externally, the drug is pale yellowish buff with longitudinally striated surfaces. Fracture is short with projecting fibres, hard and resinous. Odour is agreeable and aromatic. Taste is pungent, aromatic and spicy.

Microscopic Characters

A cross section of unpeeled rhizome shows a zone of cork tissue and inner cortex. The outer zone of cork consists of irregularly arranged cells and an inner zone consists of cells arranged in radial rows. However, the cork is absent in Jamaica Ginger. Cork cambium is indistinct. Cortex is differentiated into an outer zone of flattened parenchyma and an inner zone of normal parenchyma. Cortical cells contain simple, ovate or sack-shaped starch grains within hilum at the pointed end. The inner cortical zone usually contains about three rings of collateral, closed vascular bundles. The inner limit of the cortex is marked by a single-layered endodermis free from starch. The outermost layer of the stele is marked by a single-layered pericycle. The stele consists of scattered vascular bundles.

Ginger is mainly of three types, namely, Jamaica ginger (uncoated and unbleached ginger—Jamaica is the major exporter to all parts of the world), Cochin ginger (cultivated in South India—coated and bleached ginger—less aromatic than Jamaica ginger) and African ginger (darker and smaller than Cochin ginger—more pungent but lacks the aroma of the Jamaica ginger).

Chemical Constituents

Ginger contains about 1–3% volatile oil and 5–8% of resinous matter (gingerin–oleoresin which is yellow and pungent), starch and mucilage. The principal constituents of volatile oil are a small fraction of monoterpenes (β-phellandrene, dextro-camphene, cineol, citral and borneol), sesquiterpene hydrocarbons (zingiberene as the main component, smaller amounts of β-bisabolene, farnesene, β-sesquiphellandrene and curcumene) and sesquiterpene alcohol zingiberol. The characteristic odour of ginger is due to a mixture of zingerone, shogaol and gingerol, a yellowish oily mixture of homologous phenols. This gives hot pungent taste to the drug.

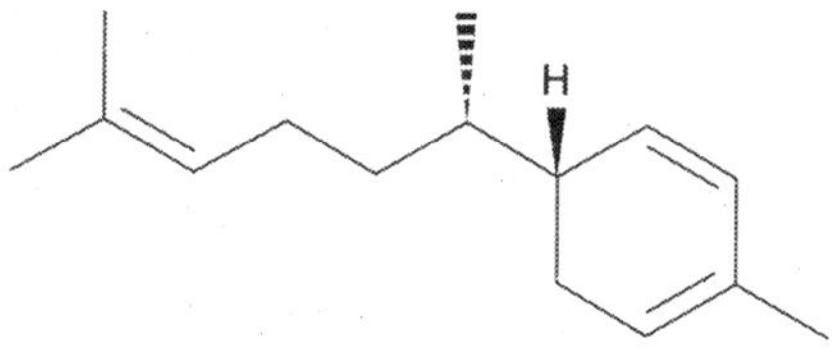

Zingiberene ($C_{15}H_{24}$)

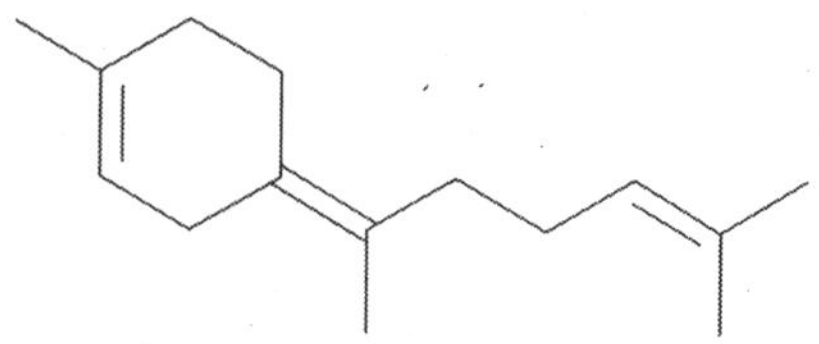

Beta-bisabolene ($C_{15}H_{26}$)

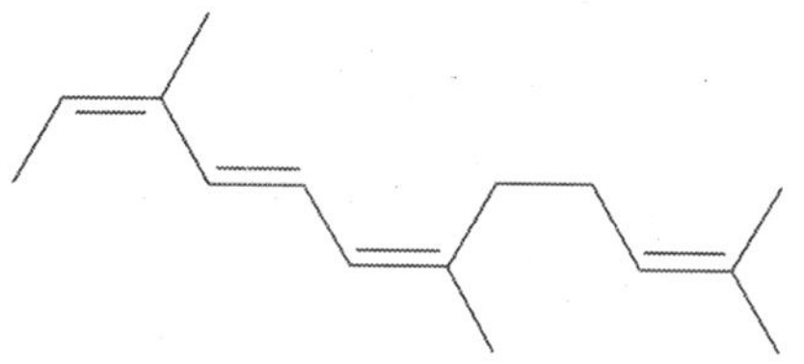

Farnesene ($C_{15}H_{24}$)

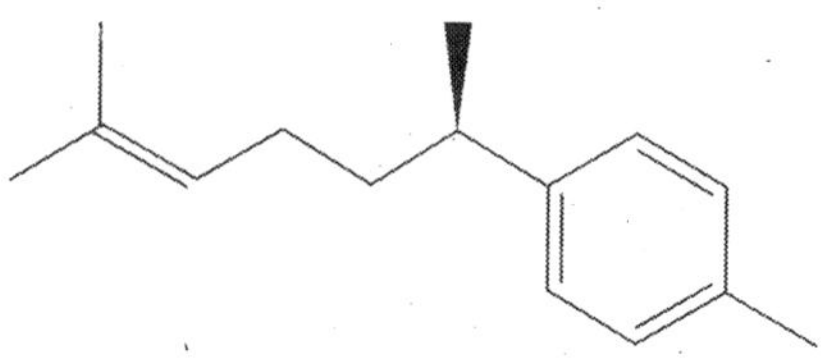

Curcumene ($C_{15}H_{22}$)

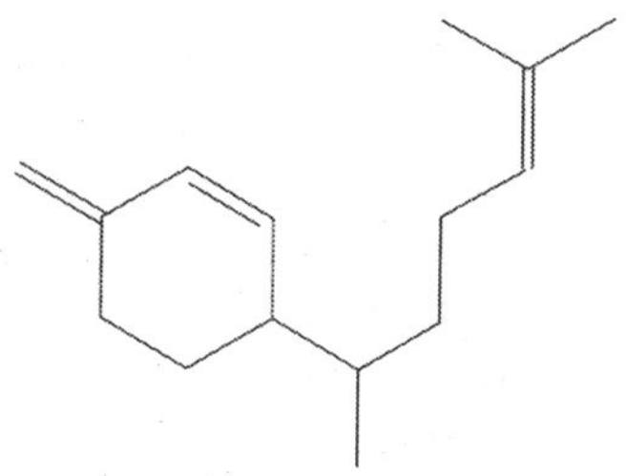

Beta-sesquiphellandrene ($C_{15}H_{24}$)

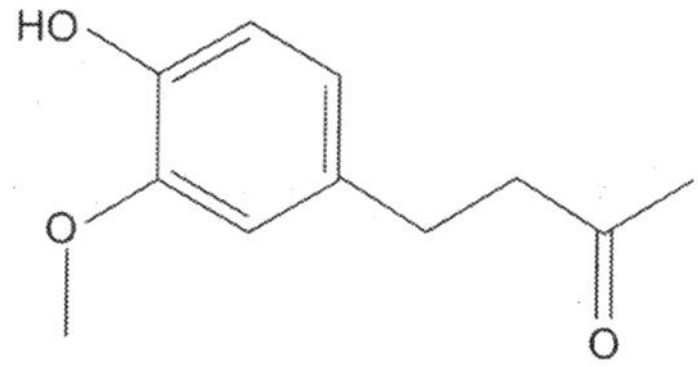

Zingerone ($C_{11}H_{14}O_2$)

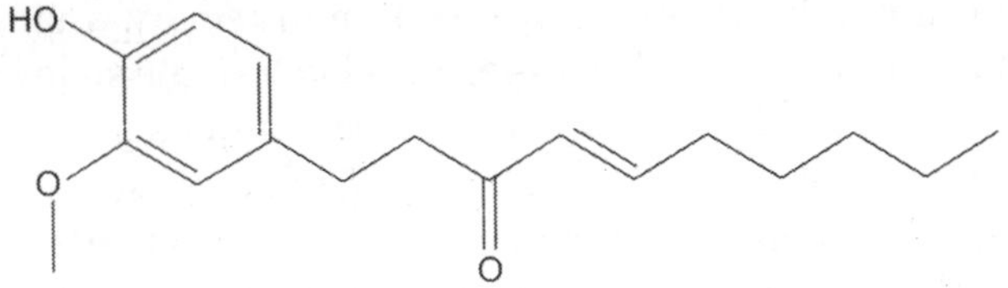

Shogaol ($C_{17}H_{24}O_3$)

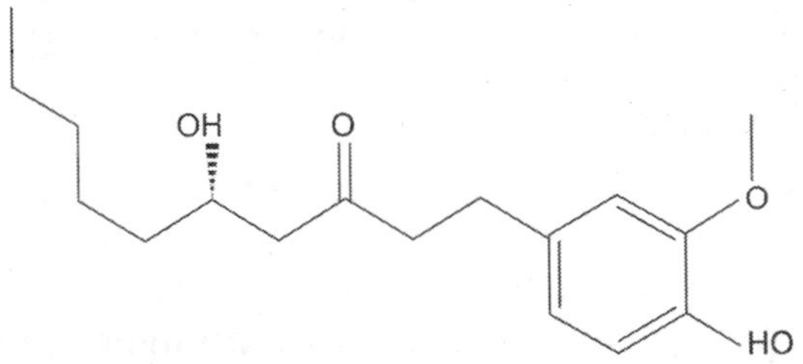

Gingerol ($C_{17}H_{26}O_4$)

History of Ginger

Ginger cultivation began in tropical Asia and spread to West Africa and the Caribbean in the 16th century. Ginger is an ancient spice which was exported as dried powder from India to Roman empire 2000 years ago, mainly as a medicine. Arabs traded in ginger for centuries and carried the rhizomes to East Africa to plant them on the coasts of Zanzibar. People have valued the qualities of ginger for more than 5000 years. The earliest use as a flavouring agent pre-dates the historical records but its origin is uncertain, though it is believed to have originated in Southern China. In the 5th century AD and before the potted plants were carried along the maritime trade routes of Indian Ocean and South China Sea. In South Asia it has a long history of use. The Hindu epic, *Mahabharata*, describes a meal where meat is stewed with ginger and other spices. Ginger was also a plant of immense importance in Ayurveda. It was mentioned as a flavouring agent for buttermilk drinks in the *Manasollasa* literature in the 11th century AD. With the advent of the Muslim rule in the 13th century AD its use in food became widespread. The culinary use of ginger in Asia dates back to 4400 years. In France, it was used around 1200. It was known that in Senegal, West Africa, it has been used in love rituals and women wore belts of ginger rhizomes to arouse their partner's desire. In 1800s, the Eclectics used the powder for relief from many digestive complaints like indigestion, gas, nausea and infant diarrhoea. In Africa, this was used to treat yellow fever and malaria.

Medicinal Uses

Ginger is used as a carminative, stomachic, sialagogue, digestive, rubefacient and stimulant. It is also useful in cold, cough and asthma, sore throat, dyspepsia and colic. It is used as a good stomachic also. Ginger promotes the secretion of bile, decreases pains from arthritis, thins blood and lowers cholesterol. It has proven effective for nausea caused by sea sickness, morning sickness, pregnancy and chemotherapy. Ginger is useful in flu, common cold, headache, fatigue, rheumatoid arthritis, migraine, sore throat, dyspepsia, flatulence, colic, vomiting, spasms, etc. and also to improve circulation and reduce the blood cholesterol, minimise the risk of thrombosis and also help in preventing cancer (due to its antioxidant properties). In Ayurveda, it is used as a cure for cholera, anorexia and inflammed liver. Ginger oil is used in various beverages and liquors, mouth washes, gargles, etc. The ginger is also used as a condiment in culinary preparations. In laboratory animals, gingerols increase the motility of the gastrointestinal tract and are analgesic, sedative, antipyretic and antibacterial properties. The oil has been shown to prevent skin cancer in mice and can kill the cells of ovarian cancer. Ginger is also an irritant and was used as a horse suppository by the mounted regiments of pre-World War I. It also possesses a sialagogue action and stimulates the production of saliva and makes swallowing easier.

Ginger is of immense importance in alternative medicine. In Ayurveda, Herbal medicine and Naturopathy, it is said that ginger clears congestion and helps detoxification by eliminating the wastes by sweating through the skin. The recent research shows that the ginger essence can be used to treat allergy, asthma, colds, infection, inflammation, nausea, internal parasites and controls the cholesterol. Some species of ginger are anti-bacterial, anti-inflammatory and anti-parasitic. The chemical constituents of ginger act as blood thinners, and thus reduce the risk of cardiovascular diseases. Ginger helps alleviate hypertension, colic, cough, flu, headache and muscle ache and also increases the energy and vitality. The practitioners of Naturopathy advocate the use of ginger to treat gallstones, sinus problems, toothache, motion sickness, abdominal cramps, stiffness of joints, skin burns, gout, spinal pain, swollen glands, menstrual cramps, etc.

Culinary and Other Uses

Ginger is commonly used as a spice and in the preparation of condiments. Young rhizomes are juicy and fleshy with a mild taste and are pickled in vinegar, used to make ginger tea with added honey or sliced orange and lemon. Mature ginger is fibrous and the juice is used as a spice in Indian recipes and Chinese cuisine to flavour seafood, goat meat or vegetarian dishes. It is also a food preservative and is known to kill *Salmonella*. As a dry powder it is used to flavour cookies, cakes, ginger ale and ginger beer. The powdered ginger is used in the food preparations for pregnant or nursing women. In South India, it is used in the preparation of a candy called *Inji-murappa* (Tamil) or *Allam-murappa* (Telugu) and is sold in bus stops and in tea stalls. In siddha medicine, ginger is used in coffee or tea.

In Bangladesh, ginger is used as a base for chicken and meat dishes. In Myanmar, it is used in cooking and is also a main ingredient of traditional medicines. In Indonesia, with palm sugar a beverage called *Wedang Jahe* is prepared. In Vietnam, the fresh ginger leaves are added to a soup called *canh khoai mo*. In China, whole/sliced ginger is used in savoury dishes of fish. In Japan, it is pickled to produce *beni shoga* and *gari* and raw ginger is used on *tofu* (noodles). In Western cuisine, ginger is used in ginger ale, ginger bread, ginger snaps, ginger biscuits, etc. Liquor called *Canton* is made in France and *green ginger wine* is produced in United Kingdom. In the Caribbean, a seasonal drink called *sorrel* is made during Christmas season, in Greece, a traditional drink, *tsitsimpira* (beer) is made and in Ivory Coast, a juice called *Nyamanku* is made along with orange, pineapple and lemon. In Tamil Nadu, South India, this is used as a folk medicine to treat cattle suffering from gastric upset, as a herbal paste mixed with black pepper (*Piper nigrum*), asafoetida (*Ferula asafoetida*) and sweet flag (*Acorus calamus*). If consumed as a powder, ginger can cause heartburn, bloating, gas, belching and nausea.

Adulteration

The ginger powder is adulterated with exhausted ginger. In addition, wheat middslings, wheat flour and ground turmeric are also often added.

CARDAMOM

Synonyms

Cardamom seeds, True cardamom, Cardamon, Lesser cardamom (English), Cardamomi Semen, Cardamom Elattarie (Greek), Kardamomen (German), Cardamome (French), Cardamomo (Italian and Portuguese), Kardamon (Russian), Karudamon (Japanese), Pai-tou-k'ou (Chinese), Ela or Ellka or Truti or Varni or Karangi (Sanskrit), Hal (Arabic), Palah or Bala (Burmese), Raputage pinvar (Malaysian), Chhoti elaechi (Hindi), Garate or Ghota elaichi (Bengali), Illychi (Urdu), Elachi (Gujarati and Punjabi), Elakki (Kannada), Elakkay (Malayalam), Aa'lbuduaa'l (Kashmiri), Elakkai or Elakaya (Tamil), Valdode or Elachi (Maharashtrian), Yelakkaya or Yelakulu (Telugu).

Biological Source

Cardamom consists of the dried seeds recently removed from the nearly ripe fruits of *Elettaria cardamomum* White *et* Mason var. *miniscula* (Syn: *Amomum cardamomum*: Family: Zingiberaceae). *A. subulatum* (Syn: *Elettaria major*: Black Cardamom) is the best known related species.

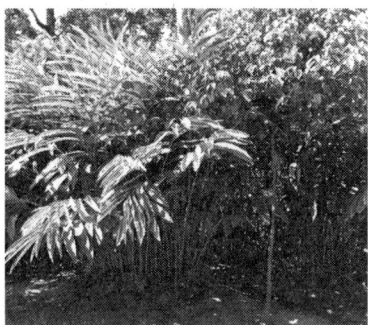

Elettaria cardamomum

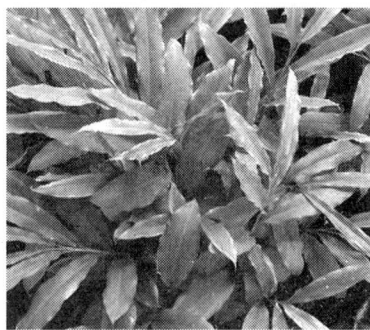

Leaves

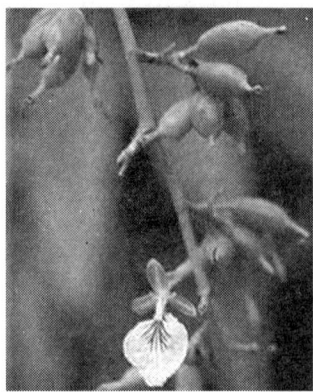

Inflorescence

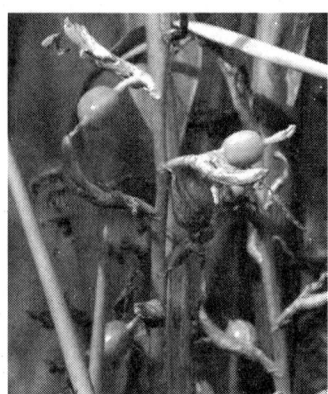

Unripe fruits

Geographical Source

The plant is native to India and Sri Lanka and occurs wild and introduced all over tropical Asia where it is cultivated. The habitat of the plant is Indo-China where it occurs in mountainous districts. It also occurs wild in Myanmar (earlier Burma) and Malaysia and grows wild in Kerala. In India it is cultivated in Karnataka, Kerala coast and Tamil Nadu. Guatemala is the largest producer of cardamom in the world. It is also grown on a small scale in Tanzania, Sri Lanka, El Salvador, Vietnam, Laos, Thailand, Cambodia, Honduras, Malaysia, Sumatra, Nepal and Papua & New Guinea.

Collection and Preparation

The cardamom fruits are in racemes and ripen at different times. It is important to collect the fruits when they are nearly ripe and before they split. Either the racemes or each fruit is cut off with a pair of short-bladed scissors. The fruits are dried slowly as rapid drying may cause splitting of the fruits. Sometimes, the fruits are bleached by exposing them to sun or by placing trays of the fruit over burning sulphur. The fruits may have remains of the calyx at the apex and a stalk at the base. These are removed by hand-clipping or by machines. On the basis of the size, the cardamoms are classified into three categories namely, 'shorts' (which are 12 mm long and 6 mm broad and plump), 'short-longs' (18–25 mm long and 6 mm broad, finely ribbed and lighter than shorts) and 'longs' (25–30 mm long and 4 mm broad). According to the commercial source, there are four varieties namely, Malabar (finest grade), Mangalore, Mysore (second best grade) and Guatemala varieties. The inferior varieties of cardamom come from *E. cardamomum* var. *major* Smith (Ceylon cardamom—the source of oil), *Amomum cardamomum* L. of Siam and Java and *A. globosum* Loureiro of China (Round cardamom—with a taste of camphor), *A. aromaticum* Roxb. (Bengal Cardamom—a taste of camphor) and *A. maximum* Roxb. (Winged Java Cardamom). In general, two varieties of Indian cardamom are recognized, *viz.* Malabar cardamom and Mysore cardamom.

Characters

Macroscopic Characters

The cardamom fruit is an inferior, oblong or ovoid capsule, 1–2 cm long, greenish to pale buff or yellowish in colour. The apex is shortly beaked and the base is round with remains of the stalk. The capsule is 3-celled. In each cell there is a double row of seeds attached to axial placenta. The colour of the seeds is dark reddish-brown when fully ripe. The seeds are covered externally by a colourless, membranous arillus which becomes thicker and oily in the fully ripened seeds. The seeds have a powerful aromatic odour and an agreeable, pungent aromatic taste but the pericarp possesses neither aroma nor taste. The proportion by weight of pericarp to seeds of cardamom fruits is about 1 to 3.

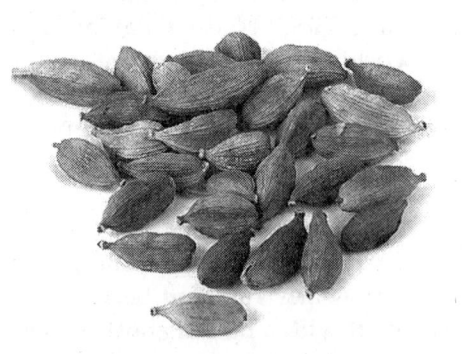
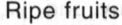

Ripe fruits

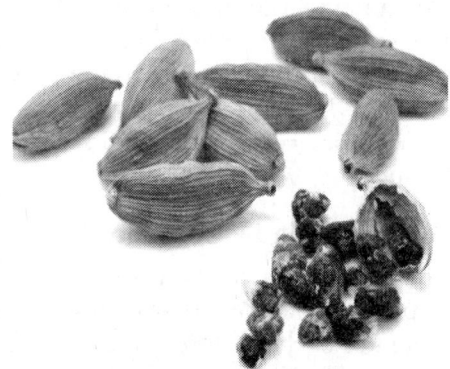

Dry fruits and seeds

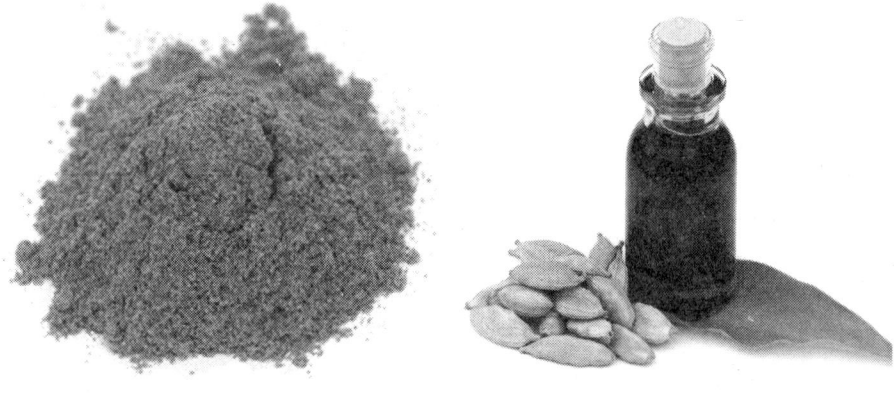

Seed powder   Cardamom oil

Microscopic Characters

The pericarp has an outer epidermis of small, polygonal, tabular cells and a mesocarp of thin-walled parenchyma in which are a few scattered cells with brown resinous contents. Some of the cells contain calcium oxalate in small or almost needle-shaped prisms and often radiating groups. The mesocarp is traversed longitudinally by vascular bundles, each of which is partially surrounded by a sheath of sclerenchymatous fibres, which are lignified. Transverse section of seed shows the presence of outermost layer of arillus, followed by two layers of testa which contain highly aromatic volatile oil. Perisperm, endosperm and embryo characteristic to the seed are observed in the section. Calcium oxalate crystals and starch grains are present in the perisperm.

Chemical Constituents

The principal constituent of the seeds is the volatile oil, the yield of which varies from 4 to 5% and may be as high as 8%. The active constituent of the volatile oil is 1, 8–cineole (2%). Other aromatic compounds present are palmitic acid, oleic acid, linoleic acid, borneol, pinene, humulene, limonene

Humulene ($C_{14}H_{22}$)   Caryophyllene ($C_{15}H_{24}$)

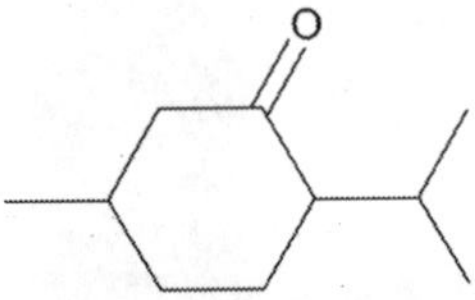

Menthone ($C_{10}H_{18}O$)

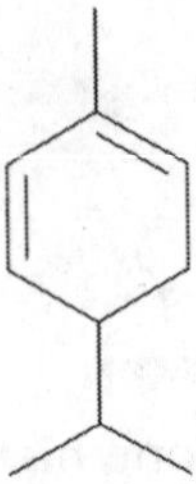

Phellandrene ($C_{10}H_{16}$)

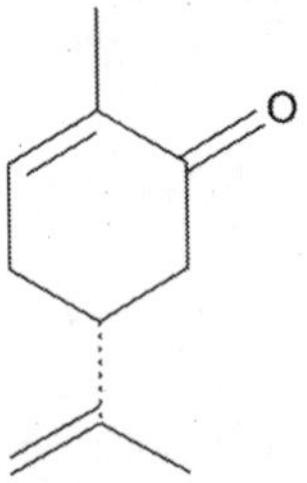

Carvone ($C_{10}H_{14}O$)

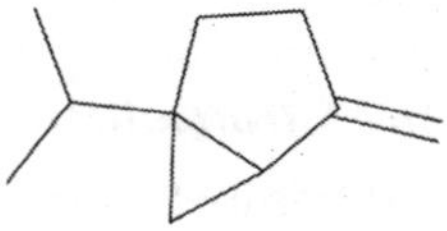

Sabinene ($C_{10}H_{16}$)

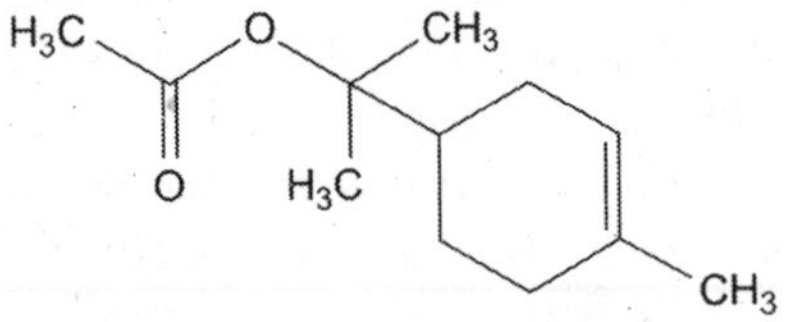

Terpinyl acetate ($C_{12}H_{20}O_2$)

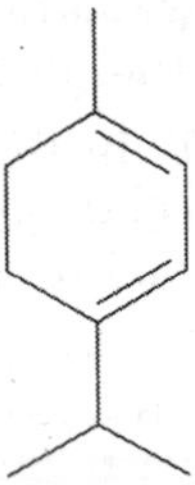

Terpinene ($C_{10}H_{16}$)

$$CH_2$$
$$\|$$
$$H_2C = CH - C - CH_2 - CH_2 - CH = CMe_2$$

Myrcene ($C_{10}H_{16}$)

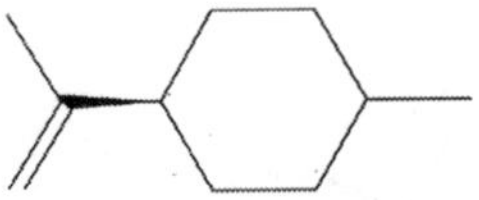

Limonene ($C_{10}H_{16}$)

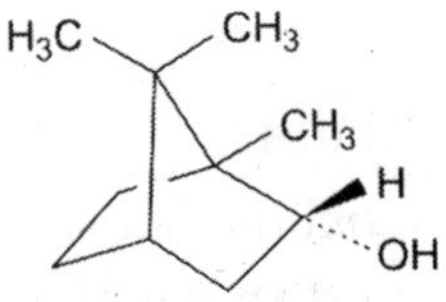

Borneol ($C_{10}H_{18}O$)

(8%), caryophyllene, menthone (6%), phellandrene (3%), carvone, eucalyptole, sabinene (2%), terpinyl acetate (30%), heptane (2%), terpineol

(45%), myrcene (27%), terpinene, etc. The other constituents of the cardamom seeds are fixed oil, starch, calcium oxalate, potassium salts, starch, mucilage, ligneous fiber, manganese and protein. The taste is warm and spicy.

History of Cardamom

Cardamom has a long history of use and trade in India and it is believed that it was brought to India in 1214 and until 19th century it was supplied to the world. The plant grows wild in the monsoon forests of the Western Ghats in Southern India and it has become popular as the Cardamom hills until 200 years ago. The fruits have been traded for at least 1000 years in India, and it was known as the 'Queen of Spices' while the black pepper was referred to as the 'King of Spices'. *Charaka Samhita*, the medical compendium written in 2nd century BC refers to cardamom as an ingredient in some medicinal preparations. Its use during the ceremonies as an offering is also mentioned in *Arthashastra* of Kautilya and *Taitirriya Samhita* of 4th century BC. At this time, Greeks were importing spices from the East and they called it as Amomon and Kardamomon and Roman writers distinguished two varieties but the descriptions were not clear. It is thought that the Vikings spread it in Scandinavia. The Egyptians chewed the seeds to use it as a tooth cleaner. The Greeks used it as a perfume. In India (11th century), cardamom was included as an ingredient in the preparation of *'panchasugandha-thambula'* (five-fragrance betel chew) in the 'Book of Splendor' or *Manasollasa*. It was also included in the recipes (sherbet and rice dishes) from the court of the Sultan of Mandu (1500). The Portuguese traveller, Barbosa (1524) described the export of cardamom from the Malabar Coast, and an international trade in cardamom was well- developed by the time of Garcia da Orta (1563). Until colonial times, Kerala continued to monopolise the trade of cardamom until 19th century when the British colonies established this as a secondary crop in coffee plantations in other parts of India. Indian cardamom is preferred in the Middle East, Japan and Russia and 'Alleppey Green Extra Bold' (AGEB), 'Alleppey Green Bold' (AGB) and 'Alleppey Green Superior' (AGS) varieties of Kerala have an instant appeal throughout the world.

Medicinal Uses

In traditional medicine, the fruit and the seed extract is used to treat the conditions of skin and also to aid in digestion. It is also used in cases of food poisoning. To treat nausea and indigestion, the seeds are roasted and boiled with betel nut to make a drink. The tea with added cardamom makes a tonic which relieves stress symptoms due to depression or overwork and seeds with honey are known to improve the eyesight. In Ayurveda, cardamom is used to treat the disorders of the stomach and the urinary system, asthma, bronchitis and cardiac problems. It is used to treat colds mixed with neem and camphor and as an infusion used as a gargle in sore throat. Seeds are used as drug and flavour. The drug has stimulant, carminative, stomachic, diuretic, anti-inflammatory and digestive properties. The drug has also cholagogue and virus-static properties. It is also used to treat the problems of throat, pulmonary tuberculosis, inflammation of the eyelids, congestion of the lungs, and also an antidote for snake venom and scorpion bite.

Non-medicinal Uses

It is widely used as a flavouring agent for sweet and savoury dishes like rice, meat and vegetables in South Asia and it is also used as a food preservative because of its antibacterial properties. The seeds are also added to coffee, tea, confectionery and baked goods as a flavouring agent. It is an essential ingredient of the drink, *Kashmiri kahwa* and *Kashmiri black tea*. The oil is used to flavour the processed foods and drinks as cordials, bitters, liqueurs and perfumery in addition to chewing gum. It is also used in the manufacture of soaps and creams to treat the areas of the skin with red pigmentation, and in tooth pastes. No toxicity has been reported. In Scandinavia, it is used in baked goods and confectioneries. In Europe and North America, it is a component of curry powder and sausages. Cardamom is used in Oriental rice and meat dishes like *pilav* (Turkish), *kabsah* or *majboos* (Arabic) and *plov* (Uzbekistan). Cardamom is popular in Northern Africa and Eastern Africa where *ras el hanout* (Moroccan mixture) or *berbere* (Ethiopian spice) preparations are made.

Adulteration

The fruits are mainly adulterated with immature fruits, mold and insect infested fruits, cardamom splits (partially opened fruits). The seeds are adultered with small pebbles and aromatic seeds of *Amomum, Aframomum* and *Alpinia* species.

TULSI

Synonyms

Holy basil, Sacred basil, Mosquito plant of South Africa, St. Josephwort, (English), Vishnupriya, Tulasi, Divya, Bharati, Manjari, Arjaka, Bahupatri, Krishnamul, Krishna tulasi, Vishnu priya (Sanskrit), Basilic Saint (French), Kala-tulasi, Baranda (Hindi), Krishna-tulasi, Kala tulsi, Kural (Bengali), Tulasi or Tulsi (Telugu, Tamil, Konkani and Maharashtrian), Kari-tulasi (Kannada), Shiva-tulasi or Trittavu (Malayalam), Tulshi (Marathi), Maduru-talla (Ceylonese).

Biological Source

Tulsi or Tulasi consists of fresh and dried leaves and seeds (sometimes the dried whole plant) of *Ocimum tenuiflorum* L. (=*Ocimum sanctum* L.) (Family: Lamiaceae).

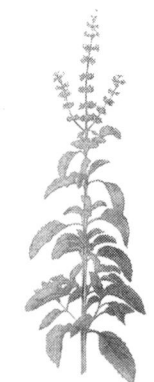

Ocimum tenuiflorum

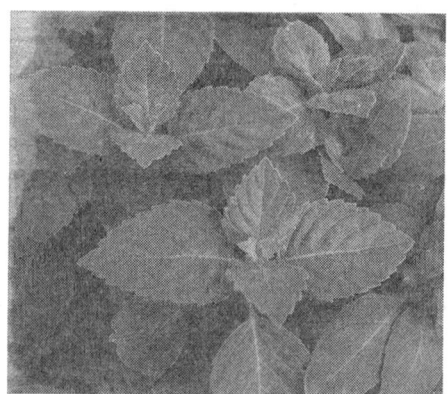

Leaves

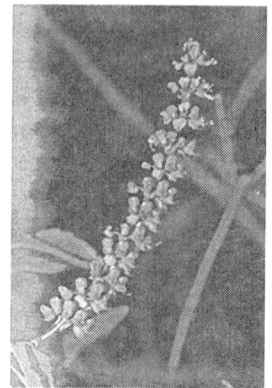

Inflorescence

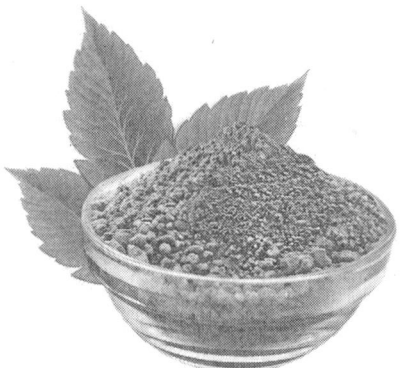

Powder

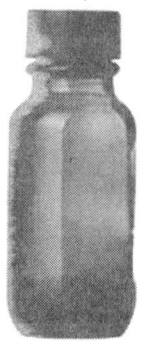

Tulsi Oil

Geographical Source

Tulasi is a native throughout the Old World tropics and it is cultivated in pots or on pedestals in Hindu houses and is also grown in temple gardens in India for religious, ceremonial and medicinal purpose. It is also cultivated for its volatile oil. The plant grows in Asia, and mainly there are two morpho-types cultivated in India, the green-leaved Sri Tulasi or Lakshmi tulasi and the purple-leaved Krishna tulasi. The plant has an important role with in the Vaishnavite tradition of Hinduism where the devotees worship the plant.

Collection and Preparation

The leaves of the plant on steam distillation yield a bright yellow coloured volatile oil with a pleasant odour with an appreciable note of the clove oil. The crop is harvested at full bloom stage to obtain maximum essential oil yield and a better quality oil. The first harvest is obtained at 90–95 days of planting, and thereafter, it may be harvested at every 65–75 day's interval. The harvesting should be done on bright sunny days, for high and good quality oil. The crop should be cut at 15–20 cm above the level of the ground. It is not desirable to harvest the crop if there was a rain in the previous day.

The oil is collected by steam distillation method from the leaves and flowering tops. The produce after harvest may be allowed to wilt in the field for 4–5 hours to reduce the moisture and the bulkiness. The oil quality and its yield do not diminish up to 6–8 hours after the harvest, but any further dealy may cause considerable loss in the yield and the quality of the oil. Steam distillation is superior to hydro-distillation and hydro-cum-steam distillation. The distillation unit should be clean, rust-free and free of any other odour. The oil obtained is decanted and filtered. The distilled oil is treated with anhydrous sodium sulphate or common salt at the rate of 20 gm per litre to remove the moisture, and stored in sealed, amber-coloured glass bottles (or containers) made of stainless steel, glavanised tanks, and aluminium containers and stored in a cool and dry place. All the activities are to be recorded.

Characters

Macroscopic Characters

It is an erect, much branched, softly pubescent, aromatic annual herb, 30–75 cm tall. The root is thin and wiry. The stem is herbaceous, branched and hairy with simple opposite leaves that are strongly scented with a characteristic taste. The leaves are elliptic-oblong, with petioles, 5 cm long and slightly toothed. The flowers are white to purplish in terminal elongate racemes. The fruits are groups of four ellipsoid nutlets, pale brown or red in colour and the seeds are subglobose and reddish-black.

Microscopic Characters

Under the microscope, the transverse section of the leaf through its mid rib shows two epidermal layers, an upper and a lower epidermis made of small quadrangular cells with thin walls and a thin smooth cuticle. The epidermal trichomes are bent made of 2–6 cells and are glandular with a single-celled stalk cell ending with round heads made of 2–4 cells. The palisade tissue consists of long cylindrical cells with chloroplasts and spongy parenchyma is made of polygonal cells with thin, straight or slightly wavy side walls. The vascular bundles are collateral with collenchyma. The stomata are diacytic and occur on both the upper and lower epidermis.

Chemical Constituents

Tulsi leaves contain bright, yellowish-green and pleasant volatile oil (0.1–0.9%). Eugenol (1-hydroxy-2-methoxy-4-allylbenzene) is the predominant (70%) component of the volatile oil. The oil if kept for sometime crystallises and is known as basil-camphor. The oil contains terpinen (0.4). Other components are oleanolic acid, ursolic acid, rosmarinic acid, nerol (6.4), carvacol, methylchavicol, selinene (0.4), pinene (0.4),

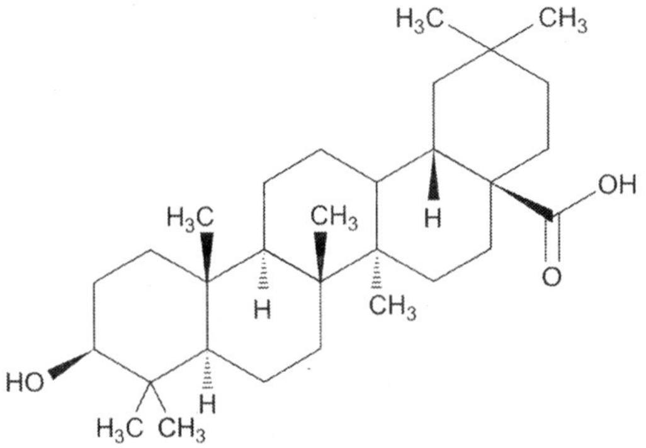

Oleanolic acid ($C_{30}H_{48}O_3$)

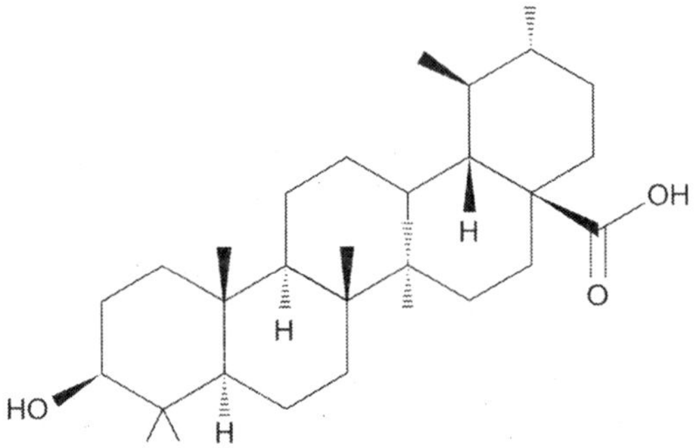

Ursolic acid ($C_{30}H_{48}O_3$)

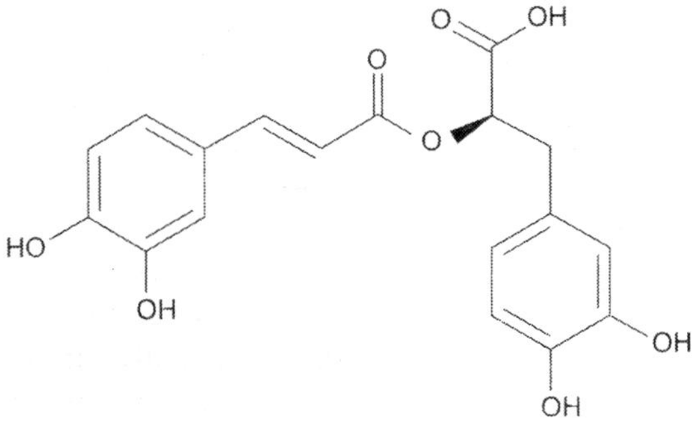

Rosmarinic acid ($C_{18}H_{16}O_8$)

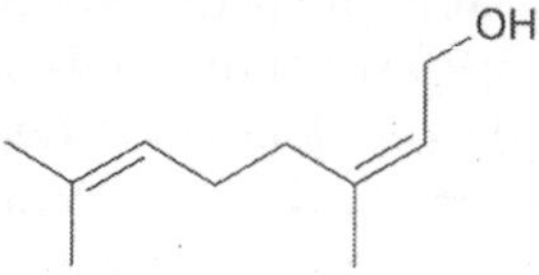

Nerol ($C_{10}H_{18}O$)

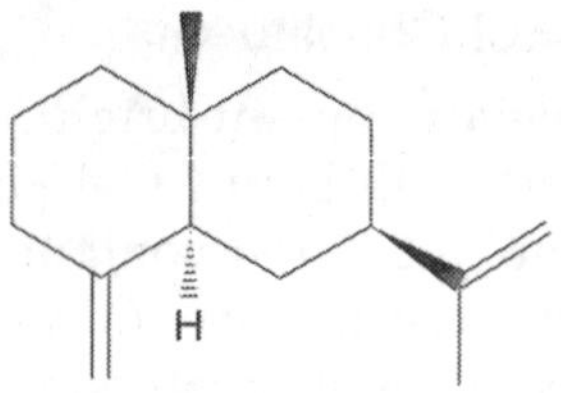

Decylaldehyde ($C_{10}H_{20}O$)

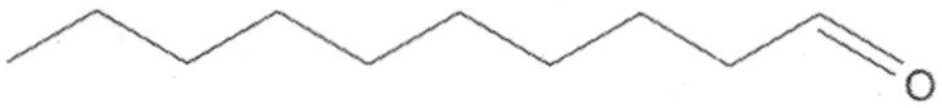

Selinene ($C_{15}H_{24}$)

camphene (2.0), decylaldehyde (0.2), limatrol, linalool and caryophyllene (7.5). It is pungent and bitter in taste.

History of *Ocimum*

In Sanskrit, *'tulsi'* means 'the incomparable one' and is worshipped throughout India (for more than five millennia) and is regarded as a consort of Lord Vishnu of Hindu trinity and considered to be an incarnation of Tulasi or Vrindavani (Goddess, Mahalakshmi). It is also considered as a symbol of fidelity and helps in the attainment of spiritual enlightenment. The plant is the most sacred for Hindus being devoted to Lord Vishnu. Hindus grow the plants in front of or near their homes in pots. A Hindu household is considered incomplete without a tulsi plant in the courtyard. In Varanasi (Banaras), it is grown next to Vishnu temples and in Tulsi Manas Mandir, tulsi is worshipped along with other Hindu Gods and Goddesses. Vaishnavites worship tulsi because of their belief that it is one that pleases Vishnu the most, and they also wear beaded necklaces which are used as rosaries during chanting made of the stems of the plant. The tulsi plant occupies the sixth place among the eight objects of worship in the ritual of the consecration of the kalasha, which contains holy water. The legend says that in 'Sri Krishna Tulabharam', Rukmini, wife of Lord Krishna could weigh him by placing a single leaf of tulsi on the balancing pan when Satyabhama failed to do so with all her wealth. The two types are commonly worshipped, 'Rama tulasi' with light green leaves and 'Krishna tulasi' with dark green leaves. Vaishnavites use japa malas made from the stems and roots and these are considered auspicious for the wearer. Tulsi has a rich and fanciful history. It had been a 'herb royale' to the French, a sign of love to Italians and a sacred herb to Indians. Pliny, the Roman naturalist (1st century AD) reported that *Ocimum* relieves flatulence. In the Far East, plant had been used as a remedy for cough, in Africa to expel the worms and American colonists used it as a component of a snuff to ease headaches. *Ocimum* has been used for thousands of years in Ayurveda because of its healing properties. Charaka mentioned tulasi in his *Charaka Samhita* around 1000 BC. It is considered as an adaptogen which helps in adapting for stress. In Ayurveda, it is considered as an 'elixir of life' as it is believed to promote longevity. At present, it has been claimed to possess an ability to keep at bay the deadly swine flu and help in the immediate recovery of the afflicted persons.

Medicinal Uses

In traditional medicine, *Ocimum* is used as an expectorant, analgesic, demulcent, anticancer, antiasthmatic, antiemetic, diaphoretic, antidiabetic, antiperiodic, antifertility, hepatoprotective, hypotensive and antistress agent. Tulsi is a mild analgesic and antiseptic. The leaf is demulcent, expectorant, anticatarrhal and antiperiodic. The extract of leaves is used in cough, colds, headache and disorders of stomach, inflammation, bronchitis, catarrh, halitosis, food poisoning, malaria, heart disease, bacterial and viral infections, foul ulcers, wounds, anorexia and ophthalmopathy. In traditional medicine, it is used as an anthelmintic, stomachic, expectorant, antipyretic, galactogogue, insecticidal and in a variety of skin diseases and genitourinary system. In malaria, gastric diseases and hepatic affections of children the leaf infusion is administered. Mixed with lime juice, the juice of the leaf is a cure for ringworm. The leaf juice is a good remedy for earache. The juice taken in the morning is said to cure chronic fever, haemorrhage, dysentery and diarrhoea. The fresh juice checks vomiting and destroys intestinal worms. The pulp of the leaves used as a dressing controls the infection and hastens the process of wound healing. The leaves are chewed to control the infections of the gums. The juice is added into the ears to relieve the earache. The dried powder of the leaf is inhaled like a snuff to relieve sinusitis. Tulsi is also a mild laxative and vermicidal. It is a good blood purifier. It is an excellent remedy for cough, allergic bronchitis, asthma and eosinophilia. The seeds are beneficial in dysuria. Therapeutically, *Ocimum* is analgesic, antispasmodic, anthelmintic, anti-bacterial, anticataract, antifertility, antihyperlipidaemic, anti-inflammatory, antilipidperoxidative, antioxidant, antistress, antithyroid, antitoxic, antitussive, antiulcer, cardiovascular, hypoglycemic, hypotensive, hepato-protective, immunomodulatory, radioprotective, wound healing and chemoprotective in action. Research studies suggest that tulasi is a COX-2 inhibitor and can be used as a painkiller due to its high concentration of eugenol. It is also effective in reducing the blood glucose levels and total cholesterol level due to its antioxidant property. It also protects from radiation poisoning and cataracts. In ethnoveterinary medicine, the whole plant is used in glossitis, ulcers, anthrax, pneumonia, tympanitis, constipation, liverfluke, stomach pain, dog bite, cannabis poisoning, opacity of cornea, tachycardia, maggots in the wounds, pain in the abdomen, stoppage of nutrition, loss of appetite, sore eyes, bleeding, cough and cold, eye diseases, udder infection and wound healing in ruminants. In Ayurveda, the juice is recommended for snake bites, chills, rheumatoid arthritis, anorexia, amenorrhoea, dysmenorrhoea etc. It is also used for stomach cramps, gastric catarrh, vomiting, intestinal catarrh, constipation and enteritis.

Other Uses

It possesses antibacterial properties and acts as an insecticide and is known to drive away the mosquitoes. In ringworm infection and other skin infections it is used locally. The root is febrifuge. The seeds are mucilaginous and demulcent and are used in urinary problems. The powder of the root with ghee is an aphrodisiac. The dried plant is stomachic and expectorant. The decoction of the dried plant is a domestic remedy for croup, catarrah, bronchitis and diarrhoea. The snuff made from the dry leaves is used in myiosis and ozaena. The basil is useful in *Ancylostoma* because of thymol. The fresh leaf juice, the juice of flower tops and slender roots is used as an antidote for snake bite. The decoction of the root is useful in febrile infections. The dried leaves are mixed with the stored grains for centuries to repel insects. In Thai cuisine, the leaves are used in the preparation of *phad kaphrao*. The root is a febrifuge while the seeds are demulcent.

LEMONGRASS

Synonyms

Indian Molissa oil, East Indian Lemongrass oil, Oil of Verbena, Barbed wire grass, Citronella grass, Geranium grass, Cochin grass, Fever grass (English), Hierba luisa, Citronnelle or Herbe de citron (French), Zitron-engras (German), Erba di limone (Italian), Hierba di limon (Spanish), Sera (Sinhalese), Takrai (Thai), Bhustrana and Takratrani (Sanskrit), Lemon grass, Sweet rush, Ginger grass (English), Gandhatrana or Hareechaha (Hindi), Gandha-bena, Lilicha (Bengali), Sugandhi chaha, Gavatichaha, Patichahaha (Maharashtrian), Nimmagaddi, Chippagaddi (Telugu), Karpoorpul (Tamil), Majjige-hullu (Kannada), Chayapul (Malayalam), Mikkotiu (Burmese), Serai (Malaysian), Sereh (Indonesian), Gavat grass or Gavati chaha (Marathi).

Biological Source

Lemongrass oil is the volatile oil distilled from the leaves and aerial parts of the plants, *Cymbopogon citratus* (DC) Stapf. (=*Andropogon citratus, A. schoenanthus*: Guatemala Lemongrass, West Indian Lemongrass, Madagascar Lemongrass) and *C. flexuosus* Nees ex Stapf. (East Indian Lemongrass, Cochin Lemongrass, British Indian Lemongrass, French Indian Verbena or Malabar Grass: Family: Poaceae). The genus has about 55 species at present.

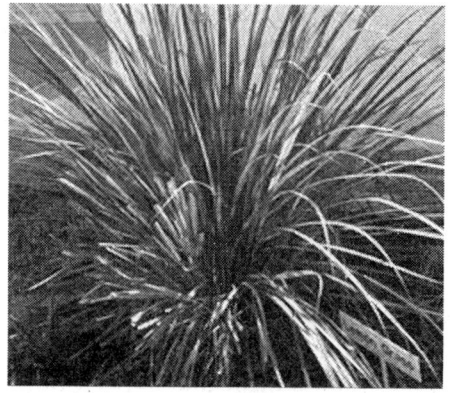

Cymbopogon citratus

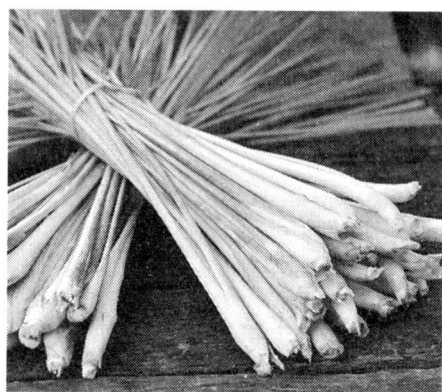

Plant with rooted ends

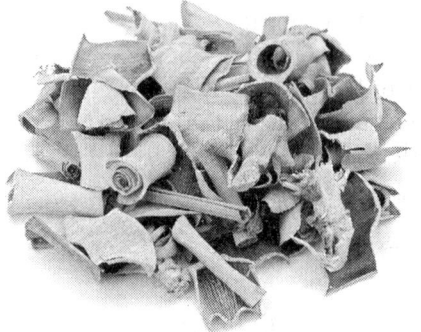

Dried Lemongrass

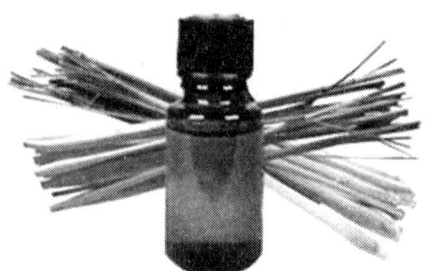

Lemongrass oil

Geographical Source

The plant is a native to India (old world) and is cultivated in the gardens. It is also cultivated in South-east Asia, Southern India, Sri Lanka, Central Africa, Brazil, Madagascar, Vietnam, Malaysia, China, Paraguay, England, Guatemala, Central America, South America, USA and West Indies.

Collection and Preparation

Lemongrass comes to harvest 90 days after planting and it is harvested at 50–55 days interval. The grass is cut 10 cm above the level of the ground and 5–6 cuttings can be taken in a year subject to the conditions of the climate. The crop can be retained in the field for 5–6 years depending on the soil and climatic conditions. On the basis of the planting period, 1 or 2 cuttings are taken in the first year, and from the second year onwards, 3–4 cuttings are available. The harvesting consists of fresh leaves and also the dry or semidried leaves at intervals of 60 days. The crop should not be allowed to flower profusely as it reduces the overall yield.

The harvested leaves can be stored under shade for three days without much adverse effect to the oil yield or quality of oil. They are then chopped into smaller pieces before distillation. The volatile oil is obtained by steam distillation of the fresh herb or dried leaves which takes about 2–3 hours. The plant is pulled close to the root and the lower bulb and the tough and outer leaves are snapped off just before use. The dried slices are soaked in water for 2 hours before use. The oil is popular as 'Cochin oil'. India annually produces nearly 1000 MT per year. In the international market, our country is facing a critical competition from Guatemala.

Characters

Macroscopic Characters

This is a perennial thick grass which grows up to 2 m in height and 1.3 m in width under ideal conditions. The strap-like, evergreen leaves with sharp-edged blades are 1–2.5 cm in wide and about 1 m long with drooping tips. These are located at the top of a solid root end. It propagates by the division of the root end. The plant lasts 3–4 years and is harvested every 3–5 months. It tolerates many types of soils but a fertile loamy soil is preferred.

Microscopic Characters

Anatomically, the characters of diagnostic importance are the micro-hairs which are sparsely distributed in the adaxial epidermis and the prickle hairs which occur in both the adaxial and abaxial epidermis. The papillae are absent. The stomata are abundant on the adaxial epidermis and sparse on the abaxial side. The mesophyll is distinct and the bulliform cells can be seen only on the adaxial surface.

Properties

Lemongrass oil is a pale yellow or light brown or a tinge of red volatile oil. It has fresh, strong, lemon-like pungent odour. The oil contains citral. It is almost entirely soluble in 70% alcohol; the solubility gradually decreases on storage. The oil is watery and thin in its viscosity.

Chemical Constituents

The fresh grass has 0.4% of volatile oil. The chief constituent of lemongrass oil is a terpene aldehyde, citral (65–85%) which is a mixture of geraniol (50%) and nerol. Other compounds are geranic acid, nerolic acid, myrcene (12–25%), diterpenes, methylheptenone, citronellol, linalool, farnesol, aldehydes, terpineol and other minor components. The nonvolatile components include luteolin, homo-orientin, chlorogenic acid, caffeic acid, p-coumaric acid, fructose, sucrose, octacosanol, etc.

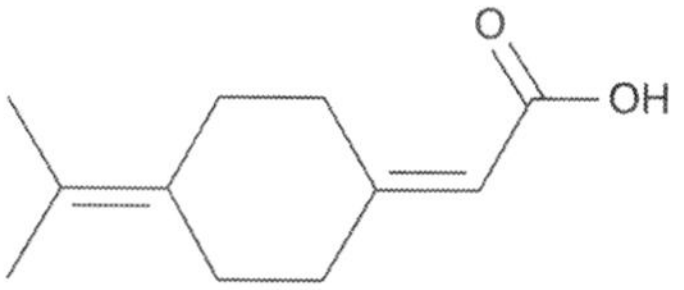

Geranic acid ($C_{10}H_{16}O_2$)

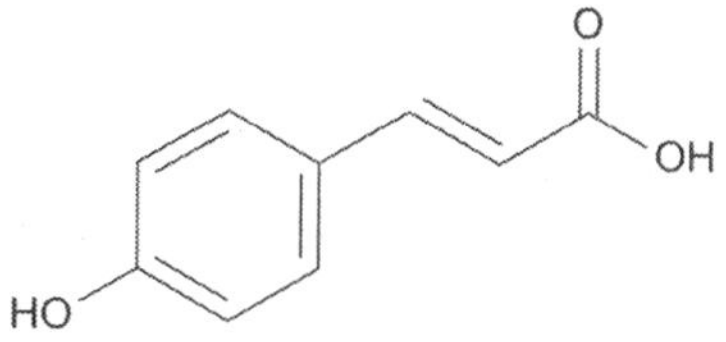

p-coumaric acid ($C_9H_8O_3$)

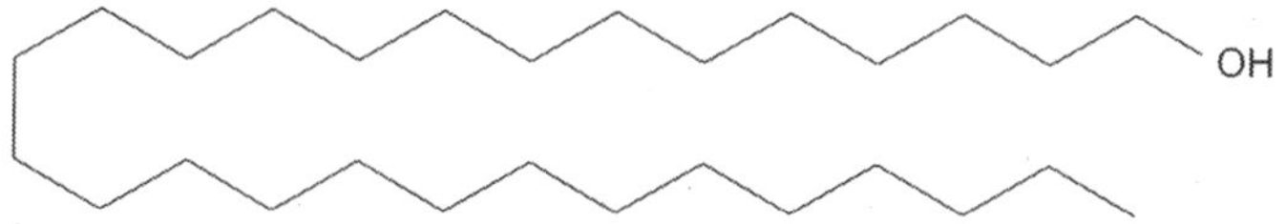

Octacosanol ($C_{28}H_{58}O$)

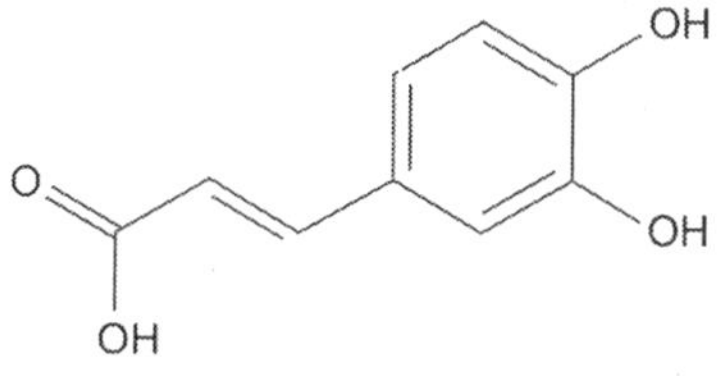

Caffeic acid ($C_9H_8O_4$)

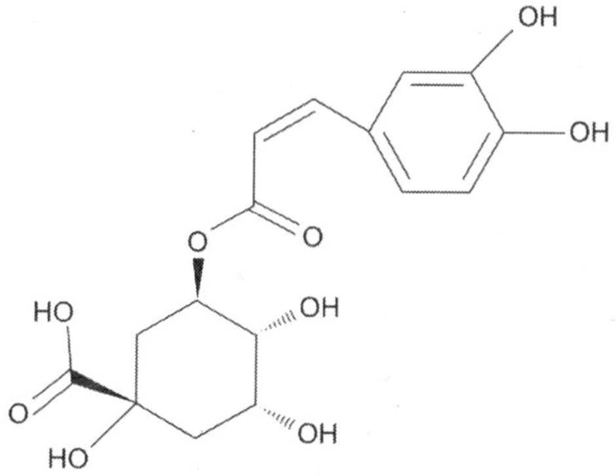

Chlorogenic acid ($C_{16}H_{18}O_9$)

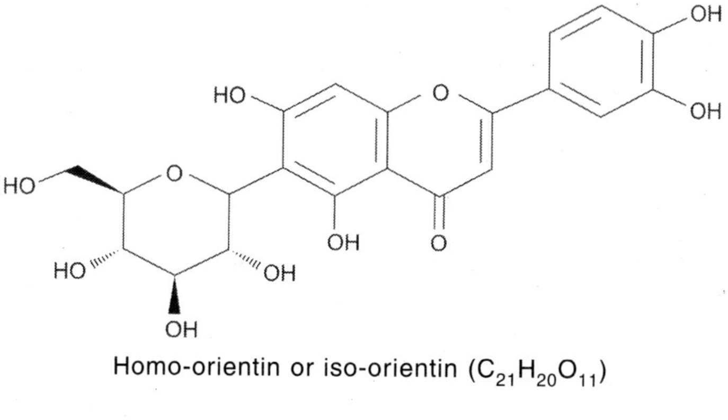

Homo-orientin or iso-orientin ($C_{21}H_{20}O_{11}$)

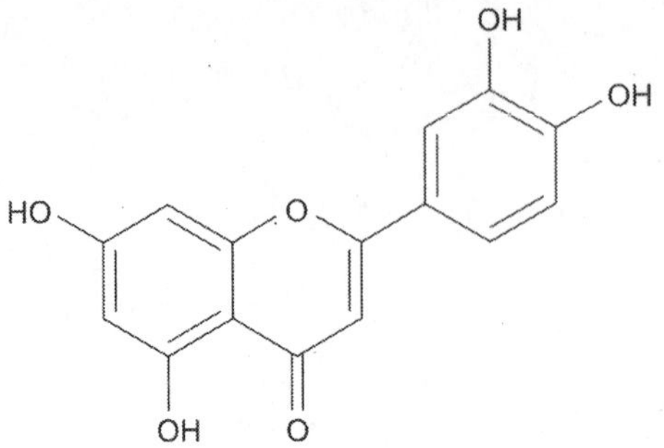

Luteolin ($C_{15}H_{10}O_6$)

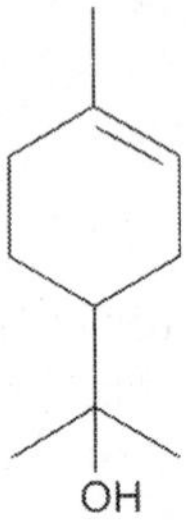

Terpineol ($C_{10}H_{18}O$)

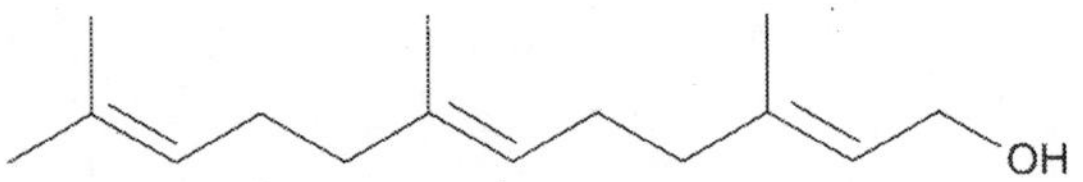

Farnesol ($C_{15}H_{26}O$)

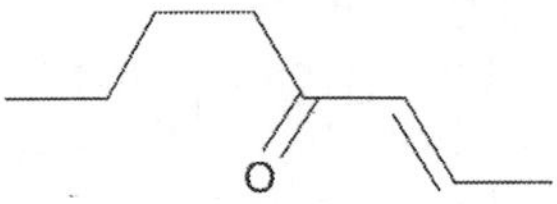

Methylheptenone ($C_8H_{14}O$)

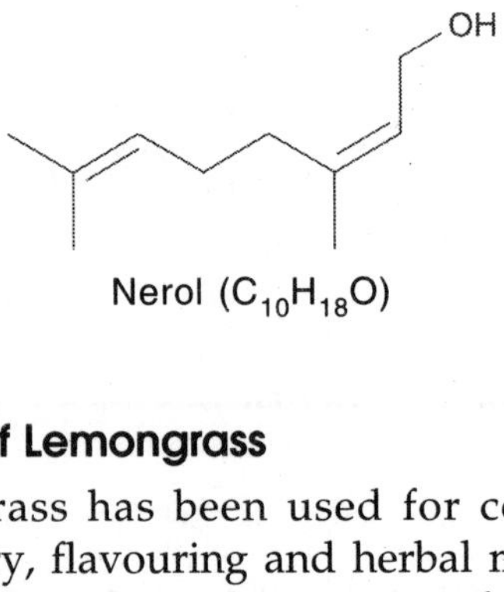

Nerol ($C_{10}H_{18}O$)

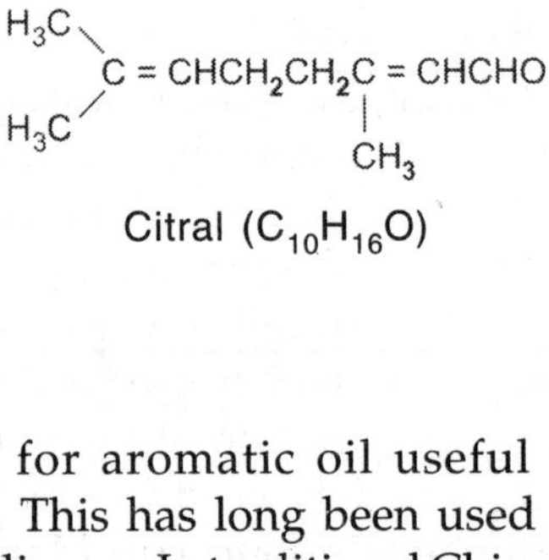

$$H_3C - C = CHCH_2CH_2C = CHCHO$$
$$CH_3$$

Citral ($C_{10}H_{16}O$)

History of Lemongrass

Lemongrass has been used for centuries for aromatic oil useful in perfumery, flavouring and herbal medicine. This has long been used in traditional Indian medicine to treat fever and disease. In traditional Chinese medicine, it is used to treat rheumatism, headache, stomach ache, cold, abdominal pain and rheumatic pain. It is used to lower high blood pressure and as an anti-inflammatory in Cuban medicine. It is used as a sedative (tea called '*abafado*'), for treating the gastrointestinal problems and for fever in Brazilian medicine. In South American folk medicine, an infusion prepared by pouring boiling water on fresh or dried leaves is widely used as an antispasmodic, antiemetic, analgesic and to treat the nervous and gastrointestinal disorders as well as fever.

Medicinal Uses

The oil is a stimulant, diaphoretic, antispasmodic and carminative. The infusion of the leaf is an excellent stomachic in children. Along with ginger, suar and cinnamon, it is given in fevers as a diaphoretic, and with black pepper, it is useful in irregular menstruation and congestive and neuralgic dysmenorrhoea and dropsy due to chronic malaria. It also acts as a tonic to the mucous membrane of the intestine and thus used in vomiting and diarrhoea. The infusion of the leaves mixed with pudina, black pepper, dried ginger and suage candy is useful in relieving colic, flatulence, fevers and catarrh. Lemon grass oil is analgesic, antimicrobial, antiseptic, astringent, bactericidal, carminative, deodorant, insecticidal, sedative and a nervine tonic. The volatile oil is useful in spasmodic affections of the bowels, gastric irritability and cholera. The oil mixed with an equal quantity of coconut oil is a good liniment for lumbago, chronic rheumatism, neuralgia, sprains, etc. It is also used against ringworm. The oil has antifungal properties. The modern research indicates that the grass induces programmed cell death in cells of cancer due to citral. It is used in low dilution in massages and as a mild depressant. It helps in the detoxification of the organs like pancreas, kidney, bladder and liver, helps cutting down the cholesterol, uric acid and toxins, helps in the stimulation of digestion, circulation, and helps in the treatment of gastroenteritis, indigestion and minimising the acne and pimples on the face. Lemongrass is to be avoided in individuals with known allergy because its oil may cause skin reactions.

Culinary Uses

In kitchen, the grass is widely used in the preparation of beverages, soups, teas, and other dishes. It mixes well with coconut milk, chicken, seafood, pickles, etc. The popular recipes of Thailand and Sri Lanka are represented by *Taro*, roast *Kabocha* soup, Thai coconut soup, Mussels broth, Jasmine tea soufflé, Cornmeal crusted skate, on-the-half-shell and Skewered shrimp. The grass is widely used in Asian cuisine either fresh or dried and powdered in the preparation of tea, soup or curries in addition to fish and seafood. This is widely used in savoury dishes and meat, seafood and vegetable curries in Indonesian, Malaysian, Sri Lankan, Vietnamese and Indian cooking. The stem is used in the preparation of tea and in pickles.

Other Uses

Large quantities of lemon-grass oil are used for the extraction of citral from which α-ionine is prepared for the synthesis of vitamin A. The oil has other uses such as a bactericide and an insect repellent against fleas, lice, ticks and mosquitoes. The oil is used as a pesticide and a preservative on the ancient palm-leaf scripts which maintains the natural fluidity of the leaf and keeps the manuscripts dry as such the text is not lost or decayed due to its hydrophobic nature. It is widely used in the production of perfumes, soaps, deodorants, skin care products, fragrances, candles and for aroma therapy. The oil is used in the form of a spray to prevent dogs from excessive barking. This is one of the most important essential oils because citral is the starting material for the production of many of the man-made aromatics at present. As the oils add shine and lustre to dull hair, the oil is used in hair care formulations.

CARAWAY

Synonyms

Carum, Caraway seed, Fructus Carvi, Wild cumin, Meridian fennel, Meadow cumin, Persian cumin (English), Kummel (German), Cumin des pres, Carvi, Lus dearg (French), Karo, Karvi (Greek), Careum, Carvum (Latin), Tmin (Russian), Alcaravia (Portuguese), Karavi (Sanskrit), Karaway, Karawiya (Arabic), Ziya (Burmese), Geluzi (Chinese), Shia jeera, Vilayati jira (Hindi), Shah Jeeru (Gujarati), Sajiragam, Sajirakam (Malayalam), Vamu (Telugu).

Biological Source

Caraway consists of the dried, ripe fruits of *Carum carvi* L. (Family: Apiaceae). The name *Carum* is derived from the Latin, *cuminum* and the Greek, *karon* adapted into Latin as *carum*, meaning *caraway*. The Sanskrit

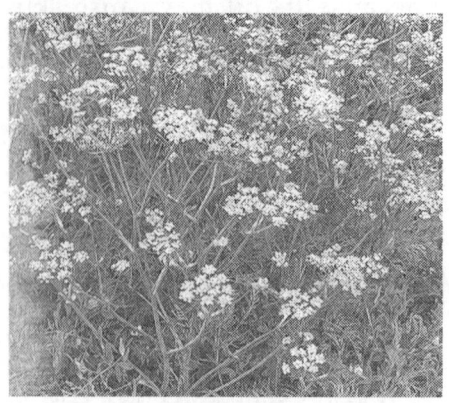
Carum carvi

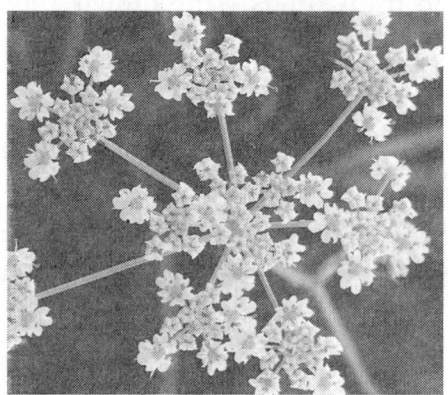
Inflorescence

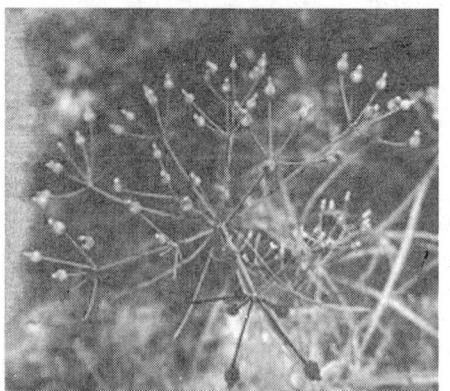
Young inflorescence

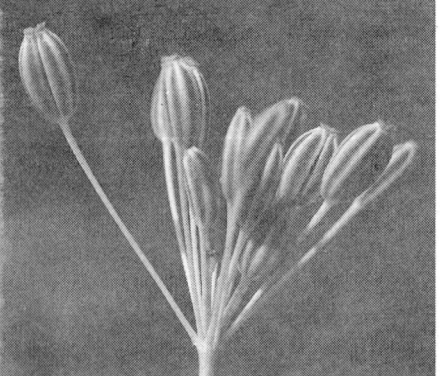
Young fruits

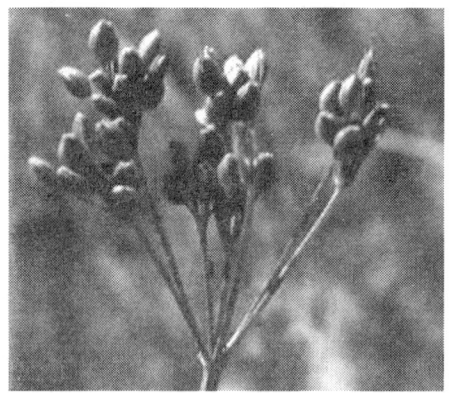

Ripe fruits

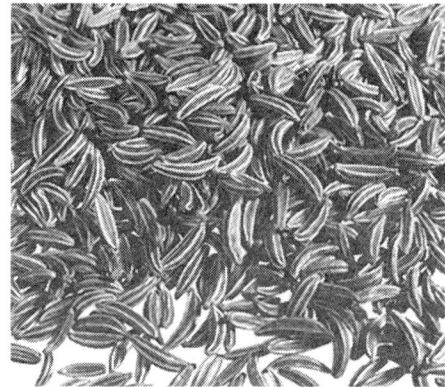

Dry fruits

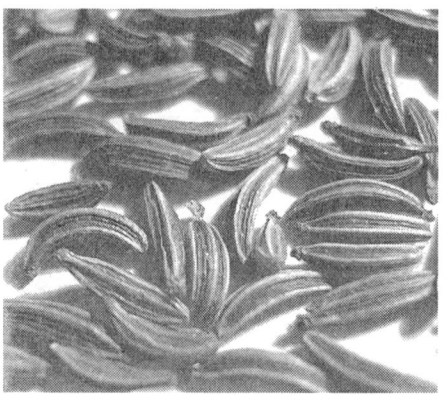

Fruits-closeup

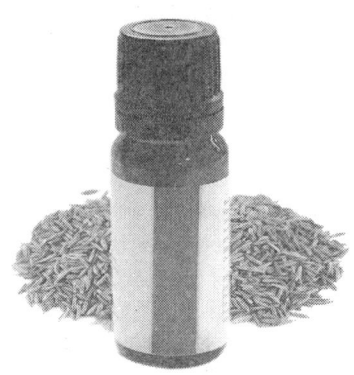

Caraway oil

word, *karavi* may sometimes be translated as *caraway*. The term, *caraway* in English dates back to at least 1440 and is believed to be of Arabic origin, *al-karawya* from the Latin, *carum*.

Geographical Source

The habitat of the plant is Asia and Europe. The plant is native to Western Asia, Europe and Northern Africa but is naturalised in USA and Canada. It is indigenous to Europe, Siberia, Turkey, Persia, India and Northern Africa. The plant seems to occur wild and has long been cultivated in Central and Northern Europe like The Netherlands, Finland, Denmark, Germany, Holland, Russia, Finland, Poland, Morocco, Spain, Norway, Hungary and England and to a lesser extent in the northern parts of USA. The plant is grown on a commercial scale in Germany, Austria, France and parts of Spain.

Collection and Preparation

The plants are mowed when the oldest fruits are ripe. After threshing and mechanical cleaning, the fruits are re-dried in the field until they have lost most of their moisture to 10–12% moisture. The fruits are thrashed, dried, cleaned, packed and stored in bags. The drug should be stored in containers which are tightly closed in dry, cool and dark place in order to retain the aroma as long as possible. The shade dried seed contains more oil content than the sun dried seed. The fresh seed should be taken to an oil extraction unit for recovery of the essential oil content. The oil is extracted by steam distillation from the dried ripe seeds.

Characters

Macroscopic Characters

The biennial plant appears like a carrot plant and possesses finely divided feathery leaves on the stem 50–60 cm high. The peduncle is 40–60 cm in length with white to pink flowers in umbels. The drug consists of mericarps separated from the pedicels. The mericarps are slightly curved and shaped like a crescent, brown, glabrous, 3–7 mm long, 1.5–2 mm broad, tapered at both ends, crowned with a stylopod. The fruit has the typical structure with six vittae and five primary ribs in each mericarp. There is a small schizogenous secretory canal in each rib just above the vascular bundle. The large endosperm is oily with a small embryo in its upper end. The odour and taste of the crushed fruits is agreeable and aromatic with a pungent anise-like flavour due to its oils, carvone and limonene. The oil has a sweet, spicy herbal odour and a slight peppery smell. It is soluble in alcohol and insoluble in water. It has a specific gravity of 0.90–0.91, a refractive index of 1.4790–1.4952, a boiling point of 193–231°C and a flash point of 134°F. It has a shelf-life of 24 months or more and is stored in cool dry place in tightly sealed containers protected from heat and light. It is very toxic to aquatic organisms.

Microscopic Characters

The outer epidermis of the pericarp is glabrous and has striated cuticle. The cells are tangentially elongated with thick outer walls. The mesocarp consists of more or less collapsed parenchyma and lacks the reticulated cells. The elliptical brown vittae lined by small epithelial secretory cells bear the oil. The inner endocarp consists of a single layer of elongated cells, arranged more or less parallel to one another. There is a layer of collapsed brown cells called the spermoderm. The endosperm consists of moderately thick-walled parenchyma containing the droplets of fixed oil and aleurone grains with rosette aggregates of calcium oxalate.

Chemical Constituents

Caraway yields 3–7% of volatile oil by distillation of the home-grown fruits, preferably from Dutch, Norwegian and Russian varieties. The principal constituents of the oil are carvol (oxygenated oil), carvone, a hydrocarbon (50–85%) and limonene (20–30%). They also contain carveol, dihydro-carveol, alpha and beta-pinene, furfurol, sabinene and perillyl alcohol in addition to proteins (20%) and fixed oil in the endosperm and yield about 6% of ash.

Perillyl alcohol ($C_{10}H_{16}O$)

Sabinene ($C_{10}H_{16}$)

Furfurol ($C_5H_4O_2$)

Beta-Pinene ($C_{10}H_{16}$)

Alpha-Pinene ($C_{10}H_{16}$)

Dihydrocarveol ($C_{10}H_{18}O$)

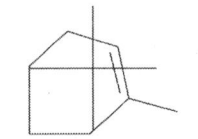

Carveol ($C_{10}H_{16}O$)

Carvone ($C_{10}H_{14}O$)

History of Caraway

The use of caraway dates back to the Stone Age. The archaeologists discovered the seeds among the refuse areas of prehistoric communities in Southern Europe and this indicates that the plant was a part of the daily life of early man. The roots of caraway have been thought to have formed the 'Chara' of Julius Caesar, consumed by the soldiers of Valerius when mixed with milk and made into bread. It was well known in classic days and it is believed that the use of caraway originated with the ancient Arabs who called it as 'Karawaya'. Pliny believed that the name Carvi was derived from Caria, in Asia Minor where the plant was found originally. It was thought that Dioscorides (40–90), the ancient Greek Physician and a pharmacologist and a botanist, during the time of Nero, advised pale-faced girls to take the oil of caraway. Caraway was very popular in the Middle Ages and in Shakespeare's time. During Elizabethan times, it was used as a condiment, and is also mentioned in Henry IV, Part II of Shakespeare. In Germany, the peasants use this to flavour their cheese, cabbage, soups and bread while in Norway and Sweden, caraway bread is largely eaten. The Russians and the Germans prepare 'Kummel', a liquor and cordial. In the olden days, it was used as a gift of retention in case of theft, formed an ingredient of love potions as a useful aid to prevent fickleness and was also fed to chicken and pigeons to prevent them from wandering off. Earlier, the fruit and the oil are stimulant and carminative, used for dyspepsia and symptoms that followed hysteria. In German folklore, it was learnt that the parents placed caraway seeds in a dish underneath their children's beds to be protected from witches.

Medicinal Uses

The tea from the seeds is a remedy for colic, loss of appetite, disorders of the digestive system and to expel the worms. The volatile oil obtained from the fruits is a stimulant, condiment and carminative. Caraway is an antiseptic, antispasmodic, antihistaminic, astringent, cardiac, disinfectant, diuretic, carminative, digestive, emmenagogue, galactogogue, expectorant, stomachic, antiparasitic and vermifuge. It has been used to stimulate the production of milk in nursing mothers, to relieve period pains in women and to treat colic in infants. The oil is used to calm the nerves and soothe mental fatigue. It is used in colic, flatulence and gastric spasm. It helps to clear bronchitis, bronchial asthma and cough as well as sore throat and laryngitis. It is an effective tissue regenerator, reduces boils, cleans infected wounds, relieves itching skin and clears acne and scalp problems.

Culinary Uses

The fruits are used as a spice in rye bread. It is also used in liquors and curries with particular reference to the European cuisine. It is also used to flavour cheese. The oil is used to flavour soaps, lotions and perfumes. The root is cooked as a vegetable. The exhausted seed is used as a cattle feed.

Adulteration

The drug is adulterated with ergotized caraway, Mogador Caraway from Morocco and Cumin, the fruit of Cuminum cyminum (indigenous to North-west Africa).

CUMIN

Synonyms

Cumin fruit, Fructus Cumini, Green cumin, White cumin, Cummin, Cumin seed (English), Al-kamuwn (Arabic), Anisacre or Cumin officinale (French), Venedischer kummel or Mutterkummel or Kreuzkummel (German), Kyminon (Greek), Latin (Cuminum), Cumino bianco (Italian), Umazeri (Japanese), Kimyon (Turkish), Kominho (Portuguese), Duru (Sinhalese), Djinten (Dutch), Ziran (Chinese), Kemun (Ethiopian), Kamoun (Arabic), Jeeraka, Jirana, Hrasvanga, Kunchika, Sugandhan, Udgaarshodan, Ajmoda, Ajaji, Jita (Sanskrit), Safed Jeera or Jeera (Hindi and Bengali), Jeera or Jira (Nepalese, Punjabi and Assamese), Zeera (Persian), Ziya (Burmese), Safed Jiru or Jiru (Gujarati), Jeelakarra or Jilakara (Telugu), Jeeragam or Jeerakam or Nallajirakam (Malayalam), Jeeragam or Seeragam (Tamil), Jeerige or Jirige (Kannada), Jeera (Konkani and Maharashtrian), Zira (Urdu).

Biological Source

Cumin consists of the dried ripe fruits and seeds of *Cuminum cyminum* L. (= *Cuminum odorum* Sahib. *C. officinale*: Family: Apiaceae). The English word, *cumin* is derived from the French word, *cumin*, borrowed from the

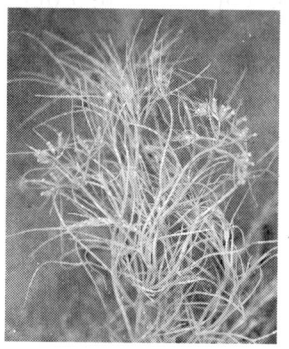

Cuminum cyminum

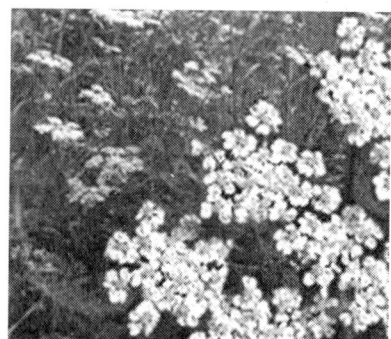

Inflorescence

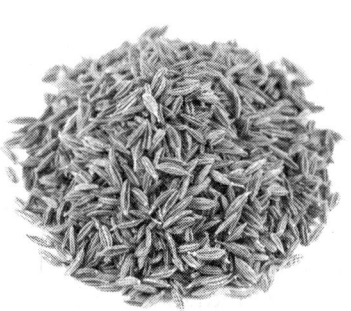

Cumin fruits

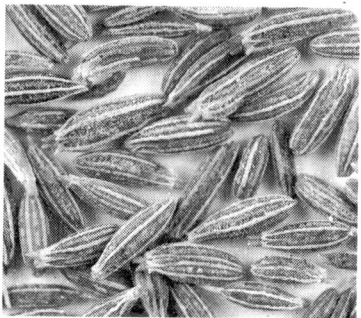

Closeup

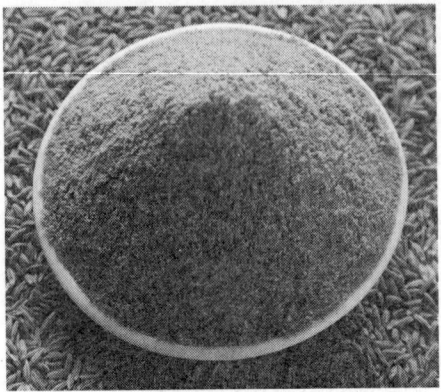

Powder

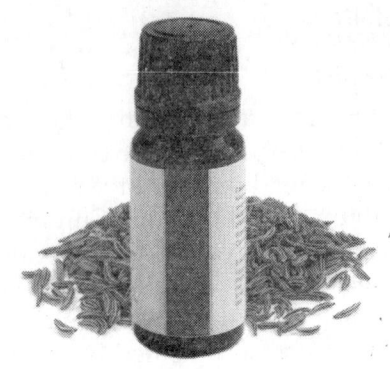

Cumin oil

Arabic, *kammun* via the Spanish word, *comino* in the 15th century. Some suggest that the word is derived from Latin, *cuminum*, and Greek term is borrowed from the Arabic.

Geographical Source

Cumin is indigenous to Egypt and a native to Syria and extends from the East Mediterranean to East India. It is widely cultivated in North Africa, Mediterranean, Middle East, Central Asia, and Indian Subcontinent, particularly in Iran, Turkey, Morocco, Egypt, Syria, Mexico and Chile. Spain and Egypt are the major cumin oil producers. The main producers of cumin are China and India, which produce 70% of the world supply and consume 90% of that. Mexico is another major producer.

Collection and Preparation

The fruits are harvested by hand and the seeds are harvested about 4 months after planting when the plant begins to wither and the seeds change from dark green to a brown yellow colour. The seed is small and boat-shaped with nine ridges along the length. The seeds are harvested by removing the whole plant from the ground. The plants are dried in the sun or in the partial sun. The seeds are beaten out by threshing the dried plants with sticks. These are further dried to 10% moisture content by placing them on mats or trays in the sun or by using a drier if it is too humid. The dried seeds are winnowed to remove the dirt, dust, leaves and twigs. The seeds are available as whole seeds and ground powder. The seeds are packed in polythene bags of different sizes according to the demand. The bags are sealed to prevent the entry of the moisture. The labels should be applied. The dried seeds must be stored in moisture proof containers away from direct sunlight. The oil is extracted by steam distillation from the dried ripe seeds.

Characters

Macroscopic Characters

The plant is a herbaceous annual which grows to a height of 30–50 cm. The leaves are 5–10 cm long, pinnate or bipinnate. The flowers are small, white or pink in umbels. Cumin fruits are 4–6 mm long and about 2 mm thick. The fruits are elongated and tapering at both ends. The cremocarp separates into mericarps. Each mericarp has four dorsal vittae and two commissural ones, brown coloured and aromatic. The odour is characteristic and aromatic while the taste is spicy and unpleasant.

Microscopic Characters

Under the microscope, mericarp shows an oily endosperm along with six vittae, four on the dorsal surface and two ventral. It also shows the large pluriserial hairs.

Chemical Constituents

Cumin yields 2.5–4% of volatile oil, 10% fixed oil, resin, mucilage, gum, malate and proteins. Pinene and the volatile oil contain 25–35% of aldehyde (cuminic or cuminaldehyde about 56%), cymene, cymol and α-terpinol. The volatile oil is colourless to pale yellow with a strong, warm, aromatic odour.

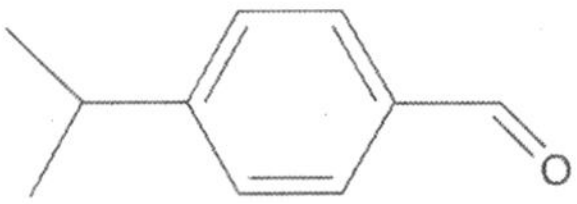

Cuminaldehyde $(C_{10}H_{12}O)$

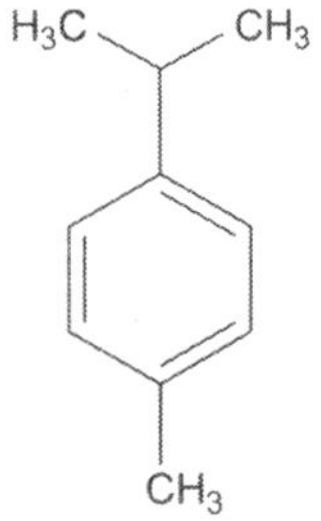

Cymol $(C_{10}H_{14})$

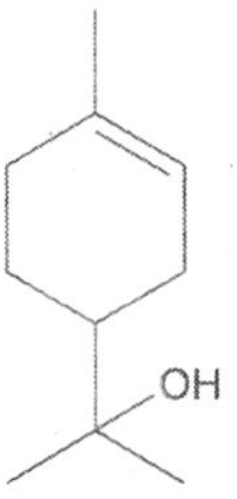

Alpha-terpinol $(C_{10}H_{18}O)$

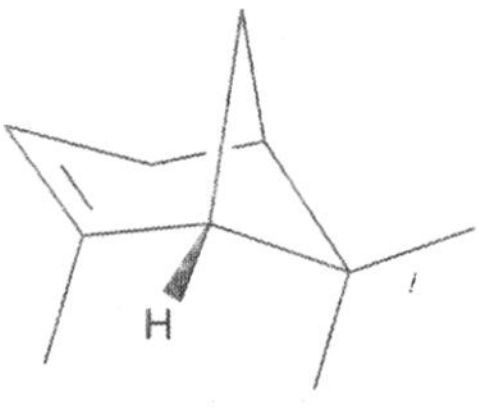

Pinene $(C_{10}H_{16})$

History of Cumin

Cumin has been in use since ancient times and the seeds which were excavated from Tell ed-Der, Syria date back to 2nd millennium BC, and have also been reported from ancient Egyptian archaeological sites. A mention of cumin appears in the Bible, in both the Old Testament (Isaiah 28:27) and the New Testament (Matthew 23:23), mainly used for its digestive properties. It was also known to be a favourite in ancient Greece and Rome and the Greeks kept cumin at their dining tables and this practice continues in Morocco even today. Egyptians used it as a cure against headaches. It was introduced to America by Spanish and Portuguese colonists. According to folklore during the Middle Ages, it was used to keep the chicken and lovers from wandering off, and the feudal lords used it as money where the serfs were paid with cumin for their services and the Pharisees used it to pay their taxes.

Medicinal Uses

Cumin seeds are used as stimulant, carminative, astringent, stomachic and used in chronic diarrhoea, hoarseness of voice and dyspepsia. The seeds are antioxidant, antiseptic, antispasmodic, antitoxic, aphrodisiac, bactericidal, depurative, diuretic, larvicidal, and nervine tonic. The seeds have a cooling effect and are used in the prescriptions for gonorrhoea. They are applied as a poultice to relieve pain and irritation of intestinal worms. The powder of the seeds mixed with honey, salt and clarified butter is applied to scorpion sting. The seeds with lime juice are used to alleviate nausea in pregnant women. The seeds are internally taken by the mother immediately after childbirth to increase the secretion of milk. The tea of dry cumin seeds is used to distinguish the false labour due to gas from real labour in pregnant women in South Asian countries. The teas are also used in Sri Lanka to soothe acute problems of the stomach. The seeds kindle appetite, digest the food, reduce flatulence or heaviness of the stomach, purify blood, reduce inflammation of the uterus, increase production of milk in lactating mothers, and reduce itching of the skin. The oil is warming oil which helps to relieve muscular pains and osteoarthritis. It also acts as a tonic and has beneficial effect on headaches, migraine and nervous exhaustion.

Culinary Uses

Cumin is the second most popular spice next to black pepper. The seeds are used as a spice in Indian, Pakistani, North African, Middle Eastern, Sri Lankan, Cuban, Western Chinese and North Mexican cuisine. It can be used either ground or as whole seeds and traditionally added to curries, chutneys, masalas, pickles, meat, etc.

DILL

Synonyms

Dill fruits, Fructus anethi, Anethum, European Dill, The Dill (English) Misariya and Satapushpa (Sanskrit), Anethum or Anetum (Latin), Persil des marais or Fenouli batard (French), Endro or Aneto (Portuguese), Garter dill (German), Ukrop (Russian), Aneto puzzolente (Italian), Eneldo (Spanish), Sova or Sowa (Hindi and Punjabi), Soyi (Dukkhanese), Shepu (Maharashtrian), Soi biol (Kashiri), Sof (Nepali), Sulpha or Dill (Bengali), Suva-nu-bi (Gujarati), Shatapushpamu or Vakataraha (Telugu), Shatakuppi-virai or Shatakuppi-sompa or Sataguppi or Guppai (Tamil), Sabbasigi soppu or Sabbasige bija (Kannada), Chatukuppa (Malayalam), Enduru or Shatapushpa or Sadakupa (Ceylonese), Sain (Burmese), Adaspudas (Malaysian), Samin (Burmese), Shiluo (Chinese), Dille or Stinkende vinke (Dutch), Anitho or Anitos or Athenon (Greek).

Biological Source

Dill consists of the dried, ripe fruits of *Anethum graveolens* (=*Peucedanum graveolens* (L.) C. B. Clarke., *Anethum sowa*): Family: Apiaceae), the sole species of the genus *Anethum*. The word, *dill* comes from the Old English, *dile*, thought to have originated from a Old Norse of Anglo-Saxon word, *dylle* or *dilla* which means 'to lull' or 'to soothe', as the plant possesses the property of relieving the gas and thus, the stomach pain in babies. In slang, *dill* implies a 'limited mental capacity'. The name of the genus *Anethum* is derived from Greek, *aneson* or *aneton* and the name of the species *graveolens* (Latin: *gravis*=heavy and *olens*=smelling) means strong smelling.

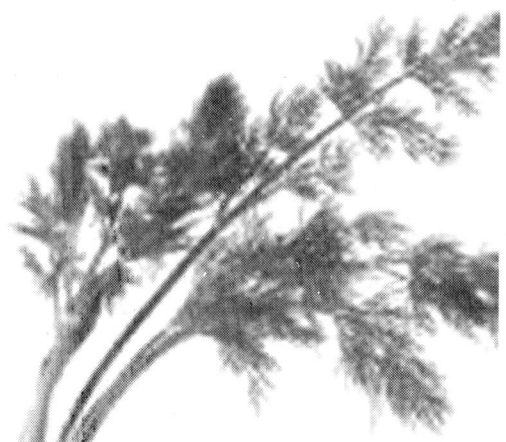

Anethum graveolens

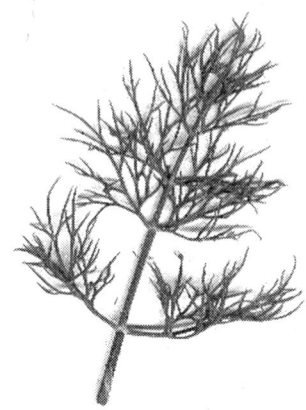

Closeup of a branch

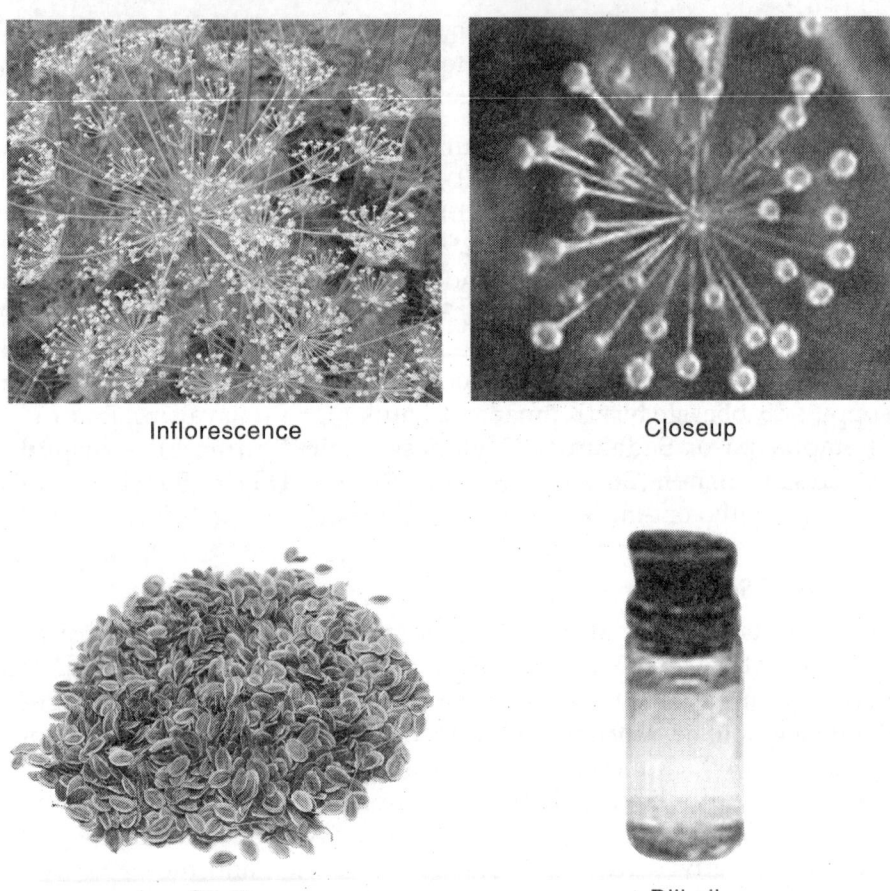

Inflorescence	Closeup

Seeds	Dill oil

Geographical Source

The plant is a native of South-Western Asia and is now naturalised in many parts of Central and Eastern Europe, Northern USA and Egypt. It is cultivated in Indian gardens for culinary use and also in U.K., Germany and Romania. It is mostly imported from Egypt, Eastern Europe and Mediterranean countries.

Collection and Preparation

For cultivation, the plant requires warm to hot summer and prefers rich and well-drained soil. The seeds remain viable for 3–10 years and the plants should not be grown near fennel as they can hybridise easily. The seed heads are allowed to develop and dry completely before harvest. Dill is best harvested in the early morning. The seed is harvested in hot weather when they begin to turn brown, 2–3 weeks after the flowers have been formed, by cutting their flower heads when the seed begins to ripen. The seed can be easily collected by hand. The seeds are placed upside in a bag in a warm dry place for one week to favour easy separation from the stems and finally stored in air tight containers.

Characters

Macroscopic Characters

The plant is intermediate between anise and caraway. The plant grows to 40–60 cm in height, the stem is slender and the leaves are alternate, finely divided and 10–20 cm long. The flowers are white to yellow and are produced in small umbels. The drug usually consists of separate, broadly oval mericarps, about 4–5 mm long, 2–3 mm broad and 1 mm thick. The fruits are slightly curved, compressed dorsally, the two central ridges being prolonged into membranous wings, while the dorsal ones are inconspicuous. The fruits have an aromatic odour and taste similar to those of caraway. All parts of the plant are strongly aromatic. The seed is very pungent and tastes bitter.

Microscopic Characters

Each mericarp has four vittae on the dorsal surface and two on the commissural. The outer epidermis has a striated cuticle, and the mesocarp contains lignified, reticulate parenchyma. The endosperm is much flattened.

Chemical Constituents

The dried ripe fruits yield volatile oil and a fixed oil. Leaves yield about 0.35% of essential oil while the fruits yield 2–4% of oil. The volatile oil of the fruit contains anethene, carvol (43–63%), limonene (40%) and a hydrocarbon. It also contains traces of dihydrocarvone, D-limonene, phellandrene, carveol and terpenenes. The leaf contains carvone (30–40%), limonene (30–40%), phellandrene (10–20%) and other monoterpenes in addition to dill ether. Volatile oil of dill is a colourless liquid. Indian species (*Anethum sowa*) contains phenylpropanoid dill apiole.

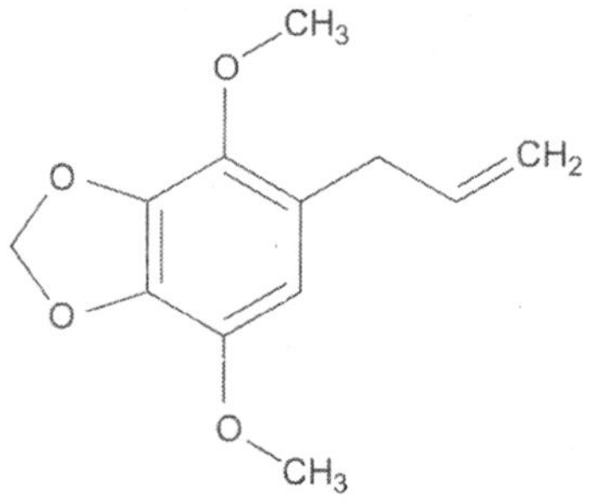

Apiole ($C_{12}H_{14}O_4$)

History of Dill

Dill has its origin in Eastern Europe and the wild type is widespread in the Mediterranean basin and in West Asia. The earliest archaeological evidence for Dill cultivation comes from late Neolithic lake shore sediments in Switzerland, and traces have also been found in Roman ruins in Great Britain. Several twigs of dill were found in the tomb of Amenhotep II. The earliest record of the plant as a medicinal herb was found in Egypt 5000 years ago and the plant was referred to and used as a 'soothing medicine' by the Egyptian doctors. Before the beginning of the Egyptian empire, dill was used as a digestive and an antiseptic. The Bible also states that the Pharisees were in the habit of paying the tithes in the form of dill and that Jesus rebuked them for tithing. The presence of dill was an indication of prosperity to the Greeks. The ancient Greeks and Romans used it as a medicinal herb and the soldiers often used the burnt dill seeds and placed them on their wounds to promote healing. The Roman gladiators were fed with meals covered with dill as it was hoped that it would grant them valour and courage. It is learnt that dill was used to relieve hiccups at the banquets by Charlemagne (8th century) and it was used as a love potion and was also believed to keep the witches away in the Middle Ages. Because of its strong smell, it was believed that dill provided protection from witchcraft and the charms were made and hung around the houses or worn on the clothing. It was often added to love potions and aphrodisiacs and the plant was believed to show its effect on the marriages and brought out happiness and good fortune. The brides in Germany and Belgium attach dill to their wedding gowns or carry it in their bouquets to be blessed. The use of dill dates back to more than 2000 years and the seeds are a household remedy for many digestive problems. It is a favourite of Russians in kitchen. As far back as the 17th century, dill seeds were used for pickling.

Medicinal Uses

Dill is used as a stimulant, carminative, stomachic, diuretic, resolvent, antispasmodic, anthelmintic, anodyne, anti-inflammatory, cardiotonic, febrifuge, antispasmodic, antidysenteric, emmenagogue and a galactogogue. It is useful in colic, dyspepsia, intestinal worms, insomnia, hiccoughs, cough, asthma, bronchitis, fever, ulcers, skin diseases, haemorrhoids and cardiac debility. It also stimulates lactation. The volatile oil is also used in flatulence, hiccup, colic and abdominal pain in infants and children along with distilled water. It is also given as a drink to women after confinement. Dill mixed with fried methi seeds in butter and the oil checks diarrhoea. The seeds boiled in water and mixed with the roots can be applied externally in rheumatism and swellings of the joints. The leaves upon moistening with the oil and warmed and applied to boils and abscesses hasten suppuration. The oil of dill is used in the preparation of dill water, gripe water mixtures and also as flavouring agent. The oil is believed to lower the glucose levels by normalising the levels of insulin and supporting the pancreatic function. It helps in bronchial catarrh, liver deficiency and vomiting. The oil is anticoagulant and helps in the risks due to coronary thrombosis and also acts against parasites causing diarrhoea.

Culinary and Other Uses

The plant is acrid, aromatic, bitter, digestive and a stimulant. The aromatic leaves are used to flavour foods, soups, pickles, etc. Traditionally, the seeds are used as a spice as they are known to soothe the stomach following a meal. In Lao cuisine, it is used in steamed fish and coconut based curries containing the fish or prawn. It is also an essential component of Vietnamese dishes like *chaca* and *canh ca thi la*. It is used with rice in the preparation of *shevid polo* in Iran. Dill is indispensable in Russian and Scandinavian cuisine. It is used to flavour potato salads, egg salads, vinegars, sauces and other vegetables. The sprouted seed is used in bread, soup and salad dressing. The oil is used as a flavouring agent in food industry. The seed infusion is a potent remedy for gripe in babies and flatulence in young children. The oil is known to relieve intestinal spasm and colic. It is a good cough, cold and flu remedy, it is also used to relieve the period pains, to increase the flow of milk in nursing mothers and to prevent the colic in the babies. In France, Germany and England, dill is a common feature in many dishes.

In the gardens, dill is the main larval food for many species of butterflies. The flower heads which are dried remain attractive in floral arrangement. The oil is used as a perfume in soaps. It is known to increase the effectiveness of insecticides when added to them.

CLOVE

Synonyms

Flores caryophylli, Caryophyllus, Cloves (English), Clou de girofle or Clous aromatiques (French), Gewurznelke or Gewurznelkev or Nagelein (German), Craveiro-da-India (Portuguese), Chiodo di garofano (Italian), Gvozdika (Russian), Kariofilla or Garyfallo (Greek), Kruidnagel (Dutch), Karabu nati (Sinhalese), Cariofilum (Latin), Karanaphul or Kabsh qaranful (Arabic), Mekjaka (Persian), Lay-hnyin (Burmese), Ding Xiang or Ting hsiang (Chinese), Lavanga or Shrisanjnan (Sanskrit), Laving (Gujarati), Lavang (Marathi), Loung (Urdu), Lavanga (Kannada), Laung (Hindi and Punjabi), Rong (Kashmiri), Karambu or Graambu (Tamil), Lavangalu or Lavangam (Telugu), Labango or Lang (Bengali), Grampu or Karampoo or Karayampu (Malayalam).

Biological Source

Cloves are the dried flower buds of *Syzygium aromaticum* (L.) Merr. et Perry (= *Eugenia caryophyllata* Thunb., *Caryophyllus aromaticus* L., *Eugenia aromatica* (L.) Kuntze. *Jambosa caryophyllus* (Spreng.) Nied. *Myrtus caryophyllus* Spreng: Family: Myrtaceae). The English name, *cloves* is derived from Latin word, *clavus* meaning 'nail' and French word, *clou* meaning the 'nail' as the buds

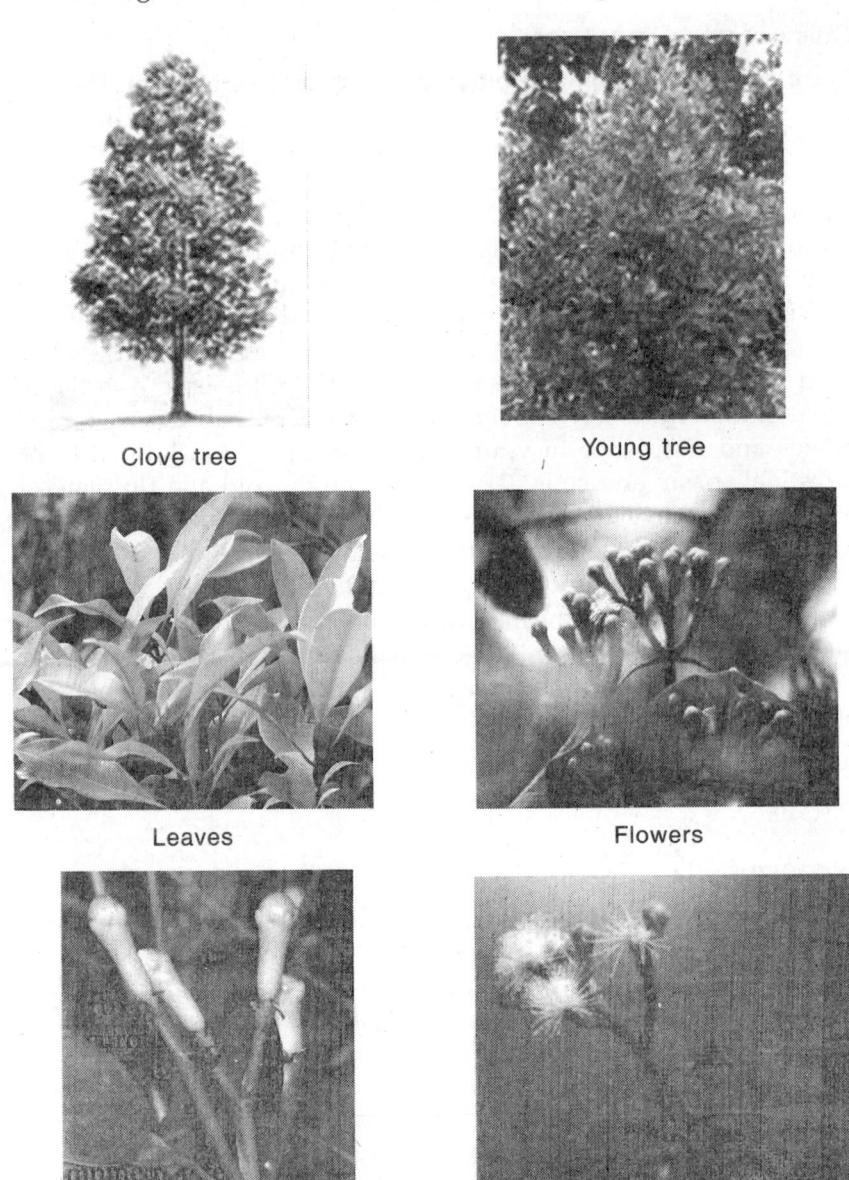

Clove tree

Young tree

Leaves

Flowers

Young buds

Mature flower

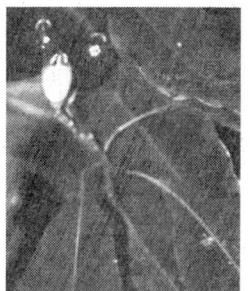
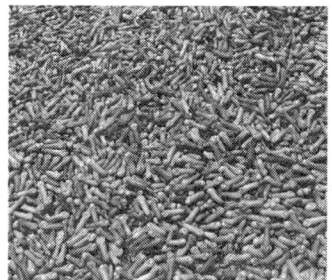
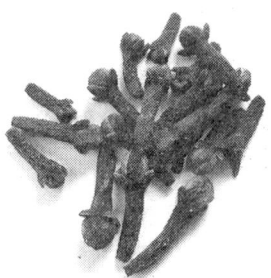

Ripe fruit   Fresh cloves

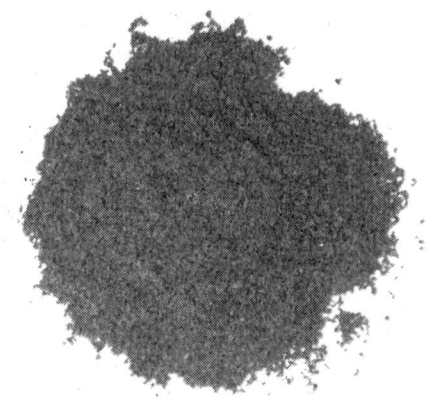
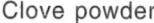
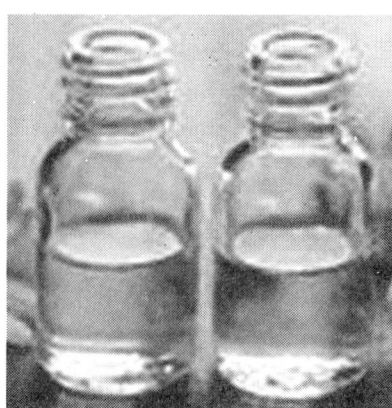

Clove powder   Clove oil

resemble small irregular nails in their shape. The generic name of the binomial *Syzygium* is derived from Greek words, *syn* meaning 'together' or 'with' and *zygon* meaning 'join', which refers to the petals merged into a cap-like structure.

Geographical Source

The plant is a native of Molucca Islands (Spice Islands or Clove islands) and the tree is endemic in the North Moluccas (Indonesia). The island of Pemba and Zanzibar are the leading producers of cloves in the world today. The Sultanate of Zanzibar and Pemba contains two clove buds on its flag. It is exotic and is primarily cultivated in Malaysia, India, Indonesia, Zanzibar, Pakistan, Java, Pemba, Madagascar, Sri Lanka, Brazil, Haiti, Kenya, Mauritius, Mexico, Seychelles, Tanzania and Carribbean Islands. It is used as a spice in cuisines all over the world. Cloves are cultivated in Seychelles, Mauritius to a lesser extent and grown in Tamil Nadu, Coorg and Kerala. The finest cloves (large, plump and reddish-brown) come from Penang, Malaysia.

Collection and Preparation

Clove grows well in rich, loamy soil of humid tropics. The unopened flower buds are of a pale colour at first, later they become green and finally into a bright red and are harvested when they begin to turn pink. At this time, they are less than 1.5–2 cm long and consist of a long calyx ending in four spreading sepals, four unopened petals and form a small ball in the centre. The opened flowers are not valued as a spice. Harvesting should be done using step ladders or hand-picked without damaging the branches, as it adversely affects the succeeding growth. It is a common practice among the growers not to leave the trees to bear fruits (mother clove), as it has an adverse effect on subsequent growth. The harvested flower buds are separated from the cluster by hand and spread in the drying yard for drying in the sun. Sometimes, they are artificially dried and garbled. The correct stage of drying is when the stem of the bud becomes dark brown and the rest of the bud lighter brown. Well-dried cloves are only one-third the weight of the original and about 11,000–15,000 dried cloves weigh one kilogram. The berry when it is nearly ripe is collected and sold as 'Mother of Cloves'. The clove oil is extracted by steam distillation.

Characters

Macroscopic Characters

The dried flower buds are about 10–17.5 mm length with a crown and a stalk. The crown or the head has four projecting teeth of calyx and a membranous corolla, which enclose the inflexed stamens. The stalk is the hypanthium. The cloves are purplish-crimson (fresh) or dark brown, reddish-brown or brownish-black in colour. They are strongly aromatic in odour, intensively fragrant and fiery burning taste.

Microscopic Characters

The powder contains part of hypanthium, sepals, petals and stamens. The epidermis is cutinized with anomocytic stomata. Masses of small, biconvex, triangular, smooth walled, immature pollen can be seen. The parenchymatous columellar cells contain the large oil reservoirs and crystals of calcium oxalate in clusters. The middle wall layers of the anther are fibrous and lignified which appear like beads in the surface view. Bits of aerenchyma are present outside the central columella. Cloves are heavier than water.

Chemical Constituents

The dried flower buds consist of 14–21% of a heavy volatile oil, 6% of camphor resin, in addition to small amounts of tannin (10–13%), woody fibres, gum, etc. The volatile oil (*Oleum caryophylli*) consists of 50–85% of eugenol (85–92% a potent antiseptic and anaesthetic), 3% of acetyl eugenol and such sesquiterpenes as β-caryophyllene, eugenin, vanillin, crategolic acid, gallotannic acid, kaempferol, rhamnetin, eugenitin, oleanilic acid, stigmasterol, campestrol, furfural, methyl-amyl-ketone, capsaicin, etc. The caryophyllin occurs as silky stellate needles. The volatile oil is colourless to pale yellow with a medium to watery viscosity and becomes visible when clove is pressed strongly between the thumb and finger.

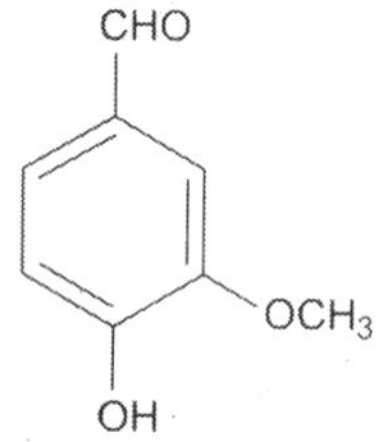

Vanillin $(C_8H_8O_3)$

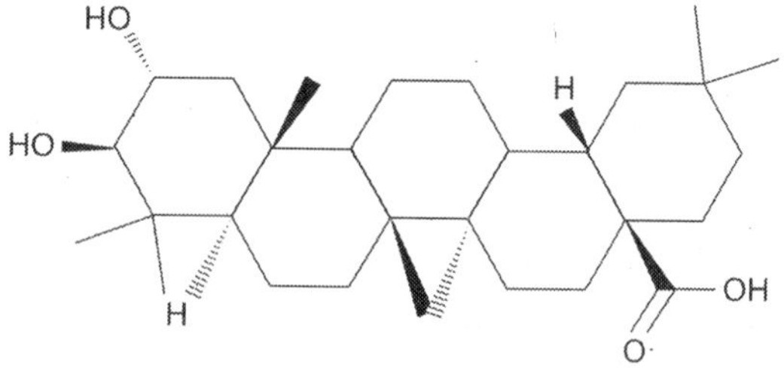

Crategolic acid or Maslinic acid $(C_{30}H_{48}O_4)$

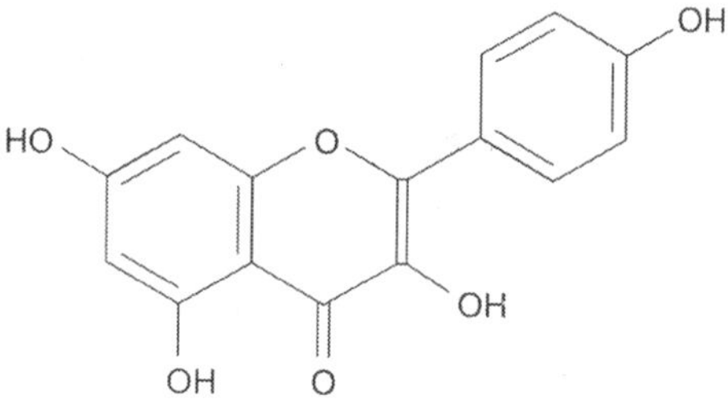

Kaempferol $(C_{15}H_{10}O_6)$

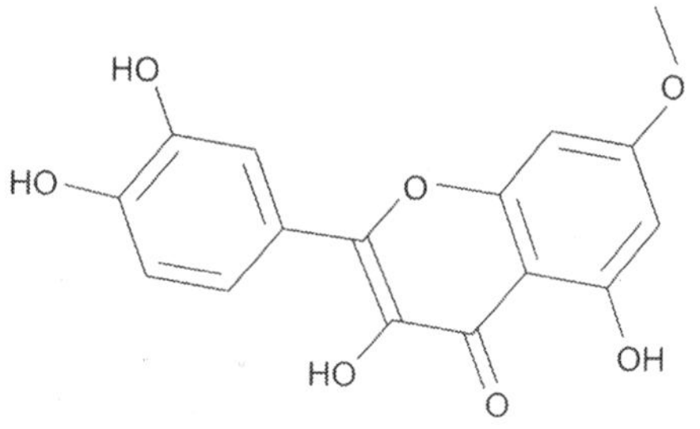

Rhamnetin $(C_{16}H_{12}O_7)$

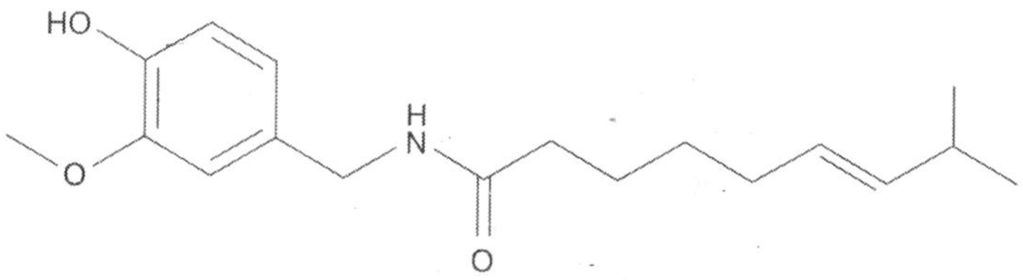

Capsaicin $(C_{18}H_{27}NO_3)$

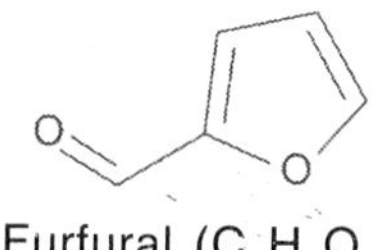

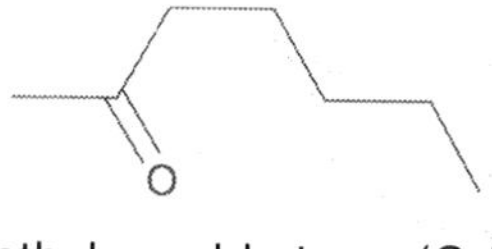

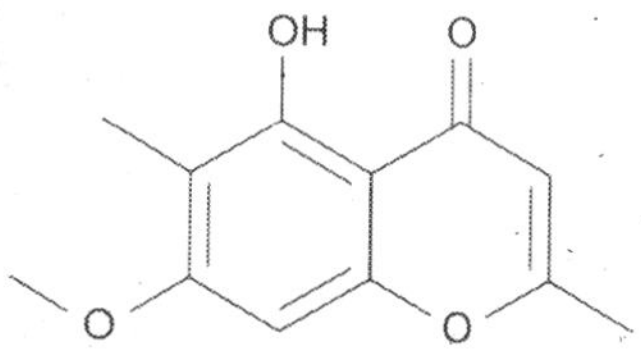

Furfural $(C_5H_4O_2)$ Methyl-amyl-ketone $(C_7H_{14}O)$ Eugenitin $(C_{12}H_{12}O_4)$

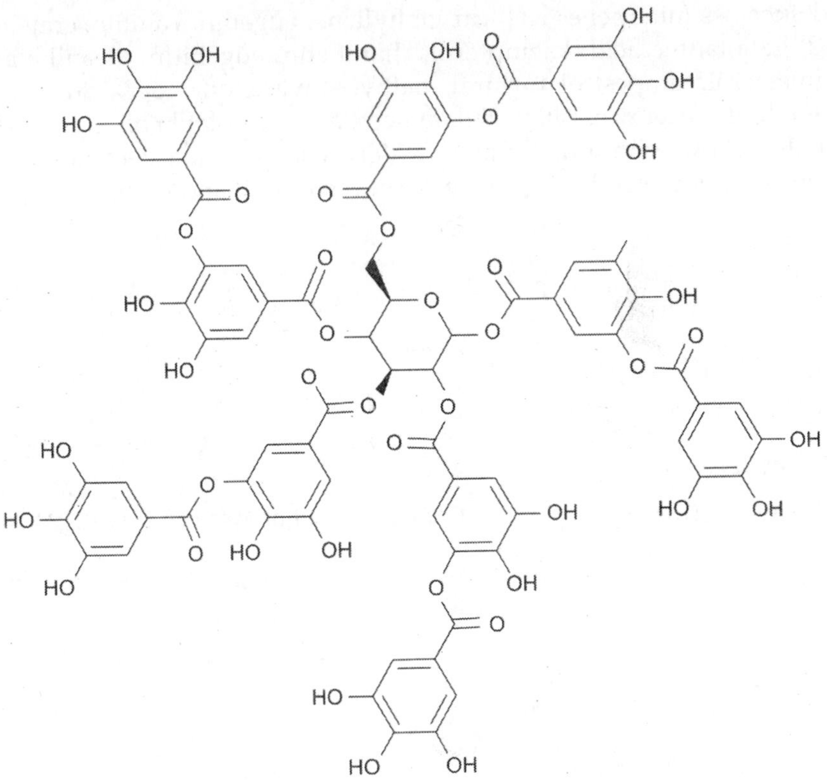

Gallo-tannic acid ($C_{76}H_{52}O_{46}$)

History of Cloves

Historically cloves were cultivated in the Spice (Molucca or Malaku) islands and the islands of Ternate, Tidore, Bacan and the west coast of Halmahera. They found their way to the Middle East and Europe before the 1st century AD. Cloves appear to have been cultivated in China as early as 266 BC. Archaeologists could unearth a ceramic vessel in Syria containing cloves dating back to 1721 BC. Cloves were highly prized during Roman times according to Pliny, the Elder. In the Middle Ages, Arabs traded the cloves in the Indian Ocean trade until late 15th century to be taken over by the Portuguese who brought large quantities to Europe from Molucca islands being the one of the most valuable spices. This trade later in the 17th century became dominated by the Dutch. In 1770, clove tree was introduced into Mauritius and this followed their cultivation in Guiana, Brazil, West Indies and Zanzibar. All ancient Sanskrit scriptures of India contained the description of cloves. It has been used as a masticatory after meals in all the rituals and had a wide popularity as a condiment as well as a therapeutic agent since the days of Ramayana. Charaka has mentioned it as *agnimandya nasaka* as it alleviates anorexia. Charaka also cited it as one of the ingredients of *tambula*. It is widely used as an adjunct in the preparation of many confections in Ayurveda. Susruta in his *Susruta Samhita*, Sutra, A-16, has mentioned its use after food to alleviate kapha and thirst. The courtiers of Han dynasty (207 BC–220 AD) in China used cloves to sweeten their breath before talking to their emperor. The Chinese physicians used it traditionally to treat indigestion, diarrhoea, hernia, ringworm, athlete's foot and other fungal infections. Traditional Ayurvedic physicians used it to treat respiratory and digestive disorders. It reached Europe around 4th century AD and the medieval herbalists used it as an antigout mixture. It was also used to treat infertility, warts, worms, wounds and toothache in Europe. The Eclectic physicians of Early America used it to treat digestive disorders and they were the first to extract clove oil from the buds and used it to relieve toothache.

Medicinal Uses

Cloves are used in Ayurvedic medicine, Chinese medicine, and Western herbalism and dentistry in which the essential oil is used as an anodyne in dental emergencies. Cloves are carminative and increase hydrochloric acid in the stomach and improve peristalsis. Cloves are anthelmintic. In toothache, the use of cloves decreases the pain and infection in the teeth and cavities in decayed teeth, as it is antiseptic. In Chinese medicine, cloves are acrid, warm and aromatic, used for hiccoughs and for fortifying the kidney. It is also used in the formulations for impotency and to clear the vaginal discharge, for morning sickness, for vomiting and diarrhoea due to coldness (hypochlorhydria) of spleen and stomach. The oil is used in skin afflictions like acne, pimples, severe burns, irritation of skin, etc. In Tibetan medicine, the oil is used topically for hypotonic muscles and for multiple sclerosis. The cloves are aromatic, stimulant, stomachic, antiseptic, antispasmodic, rubifacient, carminative and local anaesthetic. They are used in toothaches, dyspepsia and gastric irregularity and also to increase the flow of saliva. When taken internally, they increase circulation, promote the digestion of fatty food, promote nutrition and relieve the gastric and intestinal pains and spasms. They are used to correct gripping by purgatives, relieve flatulence and increase the flow of saliva. They also stimulate the skin, salivary glands, kidneys, liver and bronchial mucous membranes. The excess oil is excreted in breath, sweat, bile, milk and urine. The clove oil is externally applied in rheumatic pains, sciatica, lumbago, headaches, toothaches, etc. The juice relieves the sore throat and strengthens the gums. Popularly, the paste is applied to the forehead and to the nose bridge to relieve headache and coryza. The oil can be used for acne, bruises, burns and cuts and it is effective against vomiting, diarrhoea, flatulence and spasms. The oil relieves many respiratory problems like bronchitis, asthma and tuberculosis. Since ages, it is used as a masticatory to remove bad breath and as a freshener of mouth and throat. The application of cloves as a paste on the forehead relieves headaches, chewing removes the toothaches, and the oil as a massage alleviates pain in rheumatic joints, backache and sciatica. Cloves ameliorate hyperacidity, excessive thirst, flatulence and have a mild anticolic and antidiarrhoeal activity. It acts as a blood purifier and a stimulant to heart and also works as lactodepurant and galactogogue. It is a constituent of aphrodisiac preparations to curb the premature ejaculation. As an ophthalmic topical preparation (*anjana* or *kátuka*) it is beneficial in epilepsy and hysteria to regain consciousness. It helps relieve nausea, control vomiting and prevent intestinal worms and parasites. The powder is nontoxic to healthy, nonpregnant, non-nursing adults. Contraindications have not yet been identified. The pregnant and lactating mothers should avoid the use of cloves.

Culinary Uses

Cloves have been historically used in both North Indian and South Indian cuisine, as an ingredient of *garam masala* and *biryani*. In Gujarat, the dried cloves are used in the preparation of Indian *masala chai*. These are called *clavos de olor* in Mexican cuisine and used along with cinnamon and cumin. Cloves are often used to season *pho* broth in Vietnam. In the Netherlands, cloves are used in cheeses and are components of speculaas and stews like *hachee* of the Dutch. Cloves are employed in Chinese cuisine, Sri Lankan cuisine and Moghul cuisine as well as those of Middle East, Arab countries, Northern Africa and the greater part of Asia for meat dishes. The cloves are also used as condiment in food. Cloves are also used in baked apples, apple pie, desserts and cakes.

Other Uses

Cloves are very rarely used in Moluccas cuisine though Indonesians use up nearly 50% of the world's production. They use cloves for smoking and flavoured cigarettes called *kretek* are popular and every male enjoys them. They are also used in the production of many perfumes. In some European countries, these are used to make pomanders to hang around the house during Christmas time. The oil is insect repellant. The oil of clove is rich in phenols (80–90%) and sesquiterpenes and small amounts of ketones and alcohol and as such the strong oils are used in the manufacture of vanillin, while mild ones are used in pharmacy. Clove is an important incense in Chinese and Japanese culture. The essential oil is used in aroma therapy.

Adulterants

The cloves are adulterated with over ripe fruits of clove (Mother of Clove), fully opened flowers of cloves and exhausted cloves which are inferior in quality. The powdered cloves are adulterated with stalks of the cloves, coconut shells, olive pits and cereal flours.

FENNEL

Synonyms

Foeniculum, Fennel fruit, Fennel seed, Fructus foeniculum, Sweet cumin, Biscuit root, Indian Sweet Fennel (English), Fenchelsamen or Fenchel (German), Fenouli (French), Finocchio selvaggio (Italian), Funcho (Portuguese), Hinojo (Spanish), Finokio or Maratho (Greek), Finiculum or Foeniculum (Latin), Fennikel (Danish), Xiao hui xiang (Chinese), Maduru or Mahaduru (Sinhalese), Fenneru (Japanese), Madhurika or Mathica (Sanskrit), Badi saunp (Maharashtrian), Shoap (Marathi), Mouri or Mauri (Bengali), Sopu or Sompu or Pedda jilakarra (Telugu), Shombu or Sombu or Perunjiragam or Peruncheeragam (Tamil), Perujirakam or Perumjeerakam (Malayalam), Variyali (Gujarati), Badesopu or Dodde jirige (Kannada), Badi Saunf or Moti saunf or Bari saunf (Hindi), Mauti saunf (Urdu), Samong-saba (Burmese), Saunph (Punjabi).

Biological Source

Fennel consists of the dried ripe fruits of cultivated varieties of *Foeniculum vulgare* (Gaert.) Mill. (=*Anethum foeniculum*: Family: Apiaceae), treated as the sole species in the genus. The word, *fennel* developed from Middle

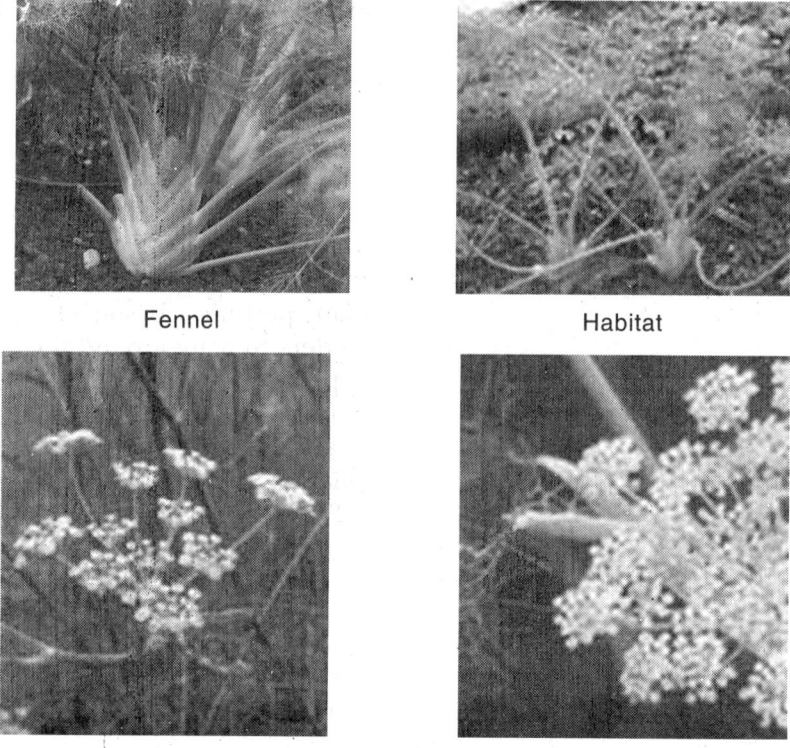

Fennel   Habitat

Flowers in umbels   Closeup

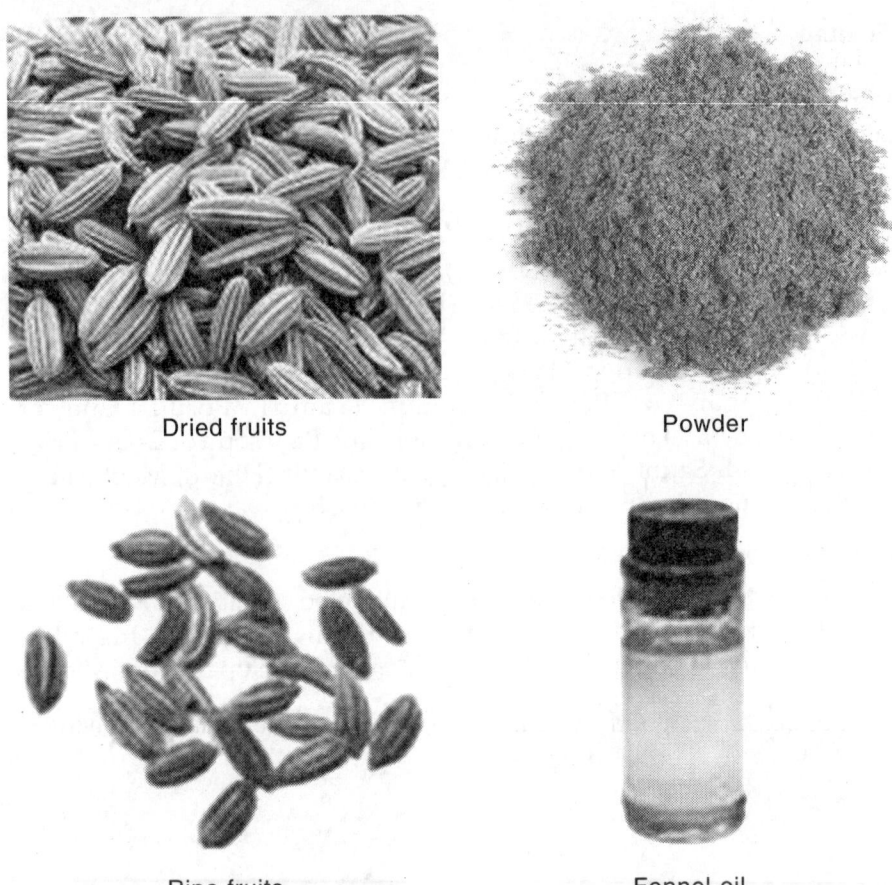

Dried fruits

Powder

Ripe fruits

Fennel oil

English word, *fenel* or *fenyl* which was derived from Old English, *fenol* or *finol*, in turn from the Latin, *feniculum* or *foeniculum*, the diminutive of *fenum* or *foenum*, meaning 'small hay' and *vulgare* means 'common'.

Geographical Source

The plant is indigenous to Mediterranean and the habitat of the plant is Southern Europe and Asia Minor. It is widely naturalised in Northern Europe, USA, Southern Canada and Australia, and cultivated on a large scale in many parts of Europe, India, China, Germany, Persia, Spain, Italy, Russia, France, Romania, Japan and Egypt.

Collection and Preparation

Fennel requires cool and dry climate for its cultivation. The crop matures in 170–180 days. All the umbels do not mature at the same time, so plucking of umbels is done when seeds are fully developed but still green. Harvesting is completed by plucking twice or thrice at 10 day intervals. After ripening, the umbels are dried in sun for 1–2 days and then in shade for 8–10 days and the fruits are separated by thrashing. The German large varitey which is green is preferred most. Indian, French and Italian fennels are yellow in colour.

Characters

Macroscopic Characters

Fennel is a biennial herb that grows to a height of 2.5 m with hollow stems. The leaves are up to 40 cm long, finely dissected with final thread like segments. The yellow flowers are produced in compound umbels. The drug consists of partly of whole cremocarps and partly of separated mericarps. Some of the cremocarps have pedicel attached to them. The fruits are glabrous at the top of which is a stylopod. The mericarps are 5–10 cm long and 2–4 mm broad. They are yellowish-green to grayish-brown, straight, elliptic or slightly curved with 5 ridges. The drug has an aromatic odour and strongly aromatic taste.

Microscopic Characters

The epicarp consists of outer epidermis, the cells of which are tabular and tangentially elongated. The mesocarp contains five bicollateral vascular bundles below each of the primary ridge. Lignified reticulate parenchyma is present above and below the vascular bundles. Four vittae are present on the dorsal surface and two vittae on the commissural (ventral surface). Endosperm consists of wide polyhedral thick-walled cells which contain fixed oil and aleurone grains with globoid and minute microcrystals of calcium oxalate.

Chemical Constituents

The flavour comes from anethole and the taste and aroma is similar to anise but not as strong. The fruits contain 3–6% volatile oil (*Oleum foeniculi*). The principal constituents of the oil are anethole (phenolic ether trans-anethol or anise camphor of about 50–80%) and the ketone fenchone (12–22%) in addition to limonene (5%), estragole (methyl chavicol), safrole, alpha-pinene (0.5%), camphene, beta-pinene, germacrene-D, beta-myrcene and *p*-cymene as well as anisaldehyde and calcium oxalate.

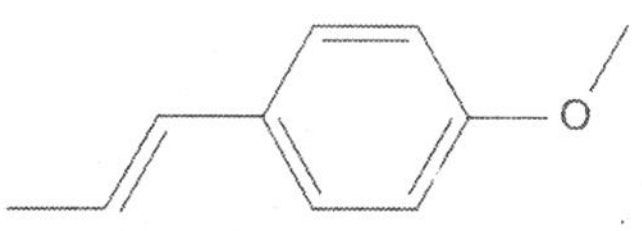

Anethole ($C_{10}H_{12}O$) 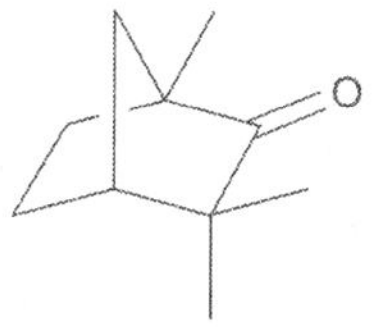   Fenchone ($C_{10}H_{16}O$)

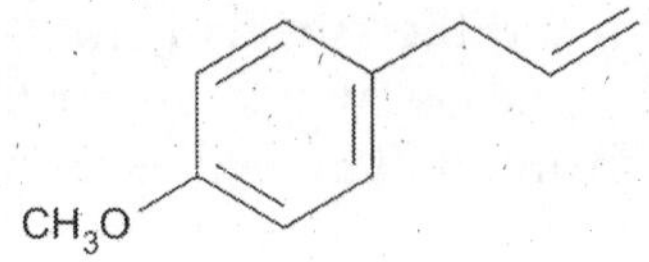

Estragole (Methyl chavicol $C_{10}H_{12}O$)

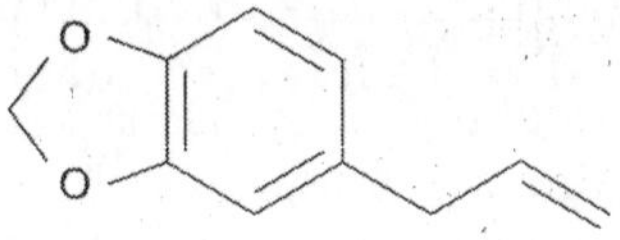

Safrole ($C_{10}H_{10}O_2$)

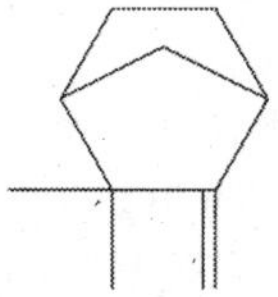

Camphene ($C_{10}H_{16}$)

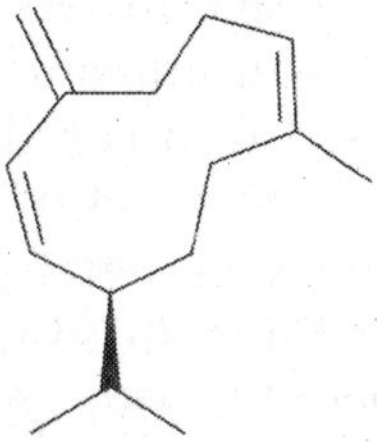

Germacrene-D

History of Fennel

In Greek mythology, Prometheus used the stalk of a fennel plant to steal fire from the gods. One report says that fennel has bestowed immortality in the Greek legend of Prometheus. Hippocrates (3rd century BC) mentioned it as a diuretic and emmenagogue and prescribed fennel for the treatment of colic in infants and also to sharpen the eyesight. Dioscorides (7th century) recommended it to nursing mothers to boost milk production and also referred to it as a suppressant of appetite. Pliny, Roman naturalist, described that fennel can be used for about 22 remedies including problems of the eye, blindness and jaundice and also observed that snakes eat it when they cast their old skins and also sharpen their eyesight with the juice by rubbing against the plant. The effect on improving the eyesight has been also upheld by many older herbalists. Ancient Romans cultivated fennel for its aromatic fruits and edible, succulent stems. Ancient Romans regarded the plant as the herb which can improve the sight and the extract of the roots was often used to clear the cloudy eyes. The anecdotes in history indicate that fennel is a galactogogue which improves the supply of milk in a breastfeeding mother. During the middle ages, it was grown in monasteries. During the middle ages, the plant was hung over the doors to ward off the evil spirits. Fennel has also been mentioned in Anglo-Saxon cookery and medical recipes prior to the Norman conquest and also in Arabic and Persian materia medica. Fennel water and the seed are mentioned in ancient record of Spanish agriculture dating back to 961 AD. Fennel has been mentioned in Eber's papyrus (1600 BC) and has been grown for 1000s of years in China (490 BC) as a culinary herb.

Medicinal Uses

Fennel and its volatile oil are used as an aromatic, stimulant, diuretic, emmenagogue, stomachic, pectoral, diaphoretic and carminative. It is also an expectorant and a galactogogue. It is a proven remedy for respiratory congestion and a common addition to baby formulations to aid in digestion. Fennel is also useful in irritable bowel syndrome. Volatile oil has a potent hepatoprotective action against carbontetrachloride induced hepatic damage in rats (Ozbek *et al.,* 2003). The root is purgative. The leaves are diuretic and increase the secretion of urine and sweat. The fruit is used as a condiment and an adjunct. The fruit juice is used to improve the eye-sight. *Aqua foeniculi* (Fennel water) is used as domestic gripe water to ease flatulence in infants and to treat babies with colic and painful teething. In adults, tea made of fennel seeds relaxes the intestines and reduces bloating. A hot fruit infusion is good for amenorrhoea and in cases of suppressed lacteal secretion. The oil is useful in flatulence and griping of purgatives. The seed or the fruit in the form of a paste is used as a cooling drink in fever and scalding of urine. Fennel is an effective diuretic and is a potent drug of hypertension. Recent studies indicated that fennel possesses diuretic, choleretic, analgesic, antipyretic and antimicrobial properties. Traditionally, it is a proven eyewash, remedy for gas, acidity, gout, cramps, spasms, etc. The ground seeds made into tea are good for snake bite, insect bites and food poisoning. It has been proven to be useful for obesity, promote the flow of urine, promote menstruation, facilitate birth, increase libido, relieve the pains of menopause in older women and estrogenic. The oil used as topical application over painful joints reduces the pain and also used as a gargle for hoarseness and sore throat. Adverse effects have not been reported. The seeds possess laxative, aphrodisiac, anthelmintic, alexiteric properties and are used in eye diseases, fever, thirst, wounds, dysentery, leprosy, etc. The fruit is used for venereal diseases and for the regulation of the periods. Leaves are diuretic and roots are purgative.

Culinary Uses

Fennel is used as a flavouring agent in pork, fish, sauces, salads, stuffings, butters and dressings. The seed is used as spice, in breads. It is also used as a flavouring agent and a condiment. The fruits are used for flavouring soups, meat dishes, sauces, confectioneries and pickles.

Other Uses

It is a food plant to the larvae of many Lepidopteran insects like Mouse Moth and Anise Swallowtail. Fennel is also used for cattle and the powder drives away fleas from kennels and stables. Fennel can also be used as a decorative border in the gardens.

Adulteration

Fennel is often adulterated with the fruits of other Apiaceae like *F. piperitum* (Italy), fruits of grasses, cereals, weed seeds, undeveloped and exhausted fruits of fennel, moldy fruits and dirt.

BLACK PEPPER

Synonyms

Fructus piperis nigri, Pepper, Peppercorn (English), Schwarzer Pfeffer or Gruner Pfeffer (German), Poivre noir or Poivre vert (French), Pepe (Italian), Pimienta (Spanish), Kosho or Peppa (Japanese), Fulful or Filfil (Arabic), Perets (Russian), Pimenta-do-reino or Pimenta (Portuguese), Piper (Latin), Peper (Dutch), Koino piperi or Piperi (Greek), Ngayok-kaung or Nga-youk-kuan (Burmese), Hu-chiao or Hei hu jiao (Chinese), Miris (Sinhala), Marica or Vella or Krishnan or Krishnadi (Sanskrit), Kali-mirch, Golmarich or Gulmarich or Sabuja marich (Bengali), Gol mirch or Gulki (Hindi), Kaali mirch, Habush, Vellajung (Punjabi), Martz (Kashmiri), Kala-miri (Maharashtrian), Miri (Konkani), Kalo-mirich or Lila Mari (Gujarati), Miriyalu, Miriyamu or Savyamu (Telugu), Milagu or Yavanappiriyam (Tamil), Volle-menasu or Menasu (Kannada), Kuru-mulaka or Paccha Kurumulagu or Yavanpriyam (Malayalam), Mire (Marathi), Kalu-miris (Sinhalese), Nayukon (Burmese), Ladahitam (Malaysian).

Biological Source

Black pepper consists of the dried, unripe fruits of *Piper nigrum* L. (Family: Piperaceae), usually known as peppercorns. Other closely related Asian species is *Piper caninum*. The word, *pepper* is derived from the Sanskrit word, *pippali* via the Latin, *piper* used by Romans. The English word, *pepper* is derived from Old English, *pipor*. Pepper means 'spirit' or 'energy' and this was used as far back as 1840.

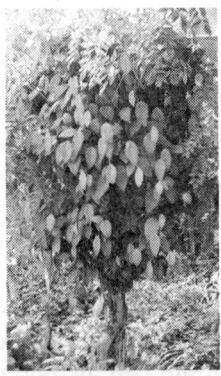

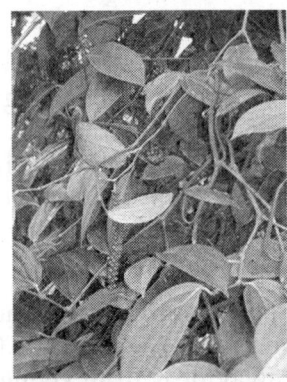

Piper nigrum on a support   Part of a shoot with leaves

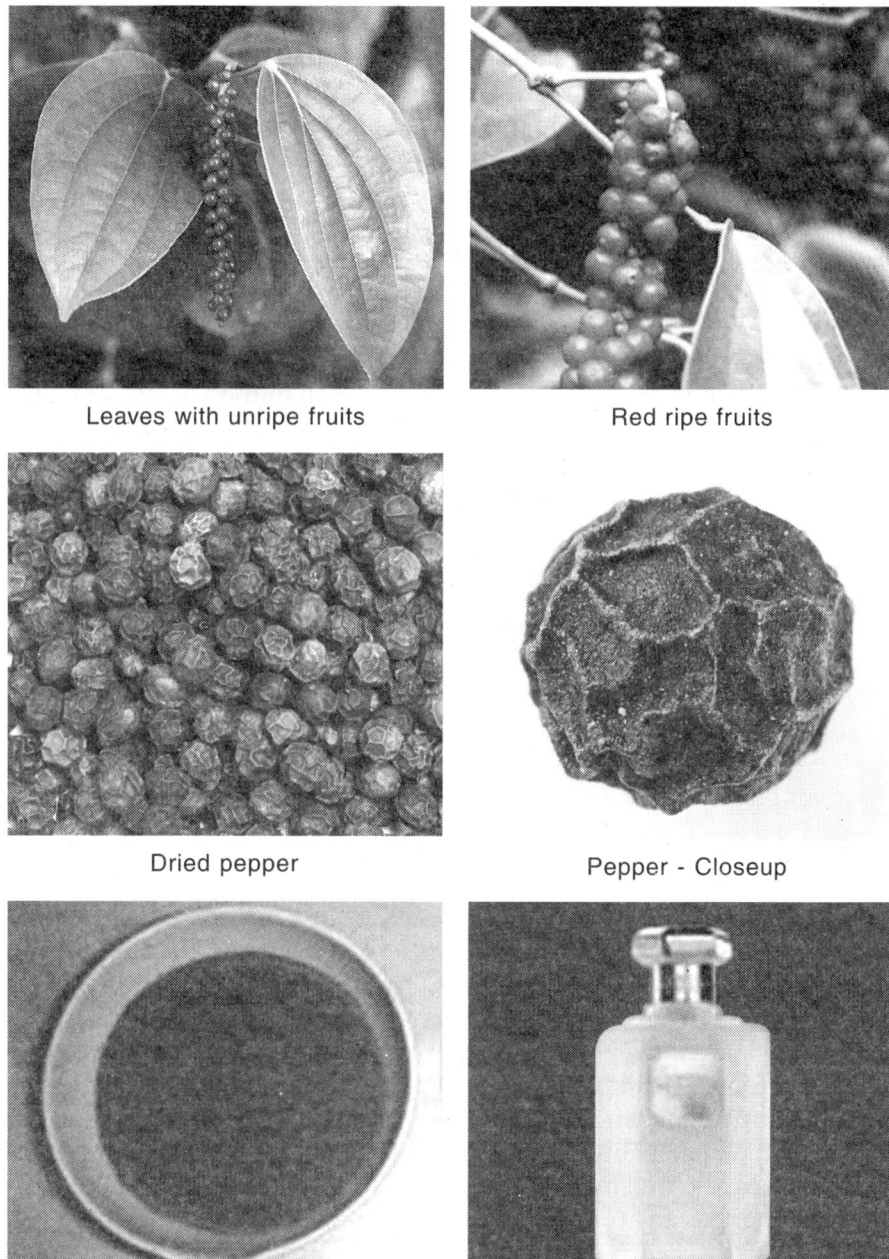

Leaves with unripe fruits

Red ripe fruits

Dried pepper

Pepper - Closeup

Pepper powder

Pepper oil

Geographical Source

Black pepper is native to Malabar in the Western Coast of Southern India and Sri Lanka and extensively cultivated there and in tropical regions. The habitat of the plant is Kerala and it is indigenous to Malabar and cultivated in South India. It is also cultivated in Sri Lanka, Indonesia, Brazil, Singapore, Penang (Malaysia), Siam, Johore, Borneo, Vietnam, Sumatra, Rioux-Lingga archipelago, South America and West Indies. Two well known types come from India's Malabar coast, Malabar pepper and Tellicherry pepper, the former is the higher grade pepper from the plants grown on Mount Tellicherry, Malabar. Vietnam is the world's largest producer (34%) and exporter of pepper as of 2008, followed by India (19%).

Collection and Preparation

Pepper is essentially a crop of wet tropics. The plant commences bearing fruit in the third year, comes into full production in the seventh or eighth year and starts declining in yield in its twenty-fifth or thirtieth year. It flowers in May-August and develops into ripe berries in another 6–8 months. The fruits that develop in the spikes are cut from the vines as soon as the lowest drupes on the axis begin to change their colour from green to red. The spikes are then dried in the sun or over fire followed by the separation of the fruits from the rachis, garbled and placed in bags. The unripe berries are cooked for sometime in hot water, to clean and prepare them for drying. The berries are dried in the sun or by machine for several days, during which time pepper around the seed shrinks and darkens into a thin wrinkled black layer. Once it is dried, the spice is called black pepper. The best grades are dried over fire and possess a smoky odour and taste and the Singapore variety seems to be the best of all.

Characters

Macroscopic Characters

Pepper plant is a perennial woody vine of 4 m height on the support and roots readily where the stem touches. The leaves are alternate, 5–10 cm long and 3–6 cm broad. The flowers are small and are produced on pendulous spikes of 4–8 cm long at the nodes. Black pepper vine is cultivated for its fruits which are almost globular and 6 mm or less in diameter, dark red when fully mature. The surface is dark brown or grayish-black and the apex shows the remains of the sessile stigmas and a basal scar. The drupes are single-seeded and the seed (peppercorn) is nearly white. Pepper has an aromatic odour and strong pungent taste. The kernel is hollow at the centre, entirely consisting of perisperm and a small endosperm and embryó.

Microscopic Characters

Transverse section of the drupe shows an epicarp of polygonal epidermal cells with a distinct cuticle followed by thin walled parenchymatous hypodermis with starch grains and chlorophyll along with scattered large secretory sacs with oil or resin contents. The inner pericarp layer, endocarp is brown and made-up of sclerenchyma. Seed coat layer is attached to endocarp and is reddish-brown. Pericarp and perisperm contain oil glands. Abundant starch grains are also present.

Chemical Constituents

The spiciness of pepper is due to a crystalline, alkaline and volatile alkaloid piperine (5–9%), a yellow balsamic volatile oil (1–2%), a colourless liquid alkaloid piperidine, a soluble pungent resin called chavicine, proteins and starch (about 30%), in addition to starch, lignin, gum, fat (1%), proteids (7%) and organic matter in the mesocarp of the fruit. Pungency and acrid taste of the fruit is due to piperine (discovered by M. Oerstadt in 1819 and accurately examined by Pelletier in 1821). The chief components of volatile oil (3%) are sabinene (15–25%), limonene (50–29%), caryophyllene (10–15%), beta-pinene (10–12%), α-pinene (8–12%), terpinene, myrcene, borneol, carvone, carvacrol, 1,8-cineol, linalool, humulene, beta-bisabalone, and acid amides. Other compounds like eugenol, myristicin and safrole are found in traces. Further, branched-chain aldehydes like 3-methylbutanal and methylpropanal are also found.

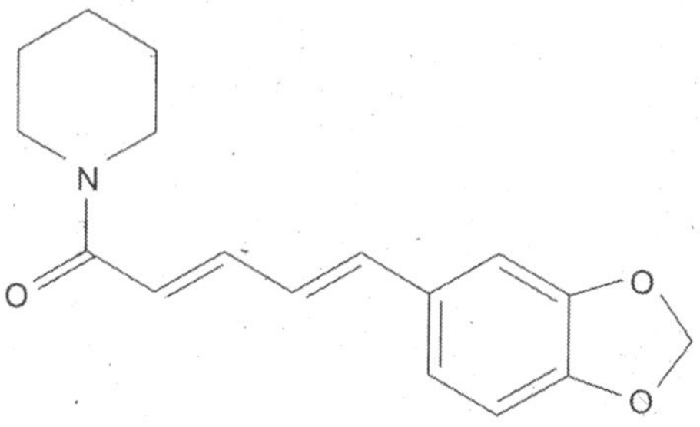

Piperine ($C_{17}H_{19}NO_3$)

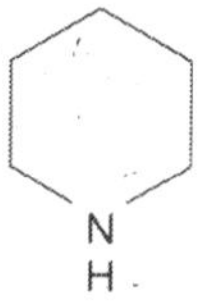

Piperidine ($C_5H_{11}N$)

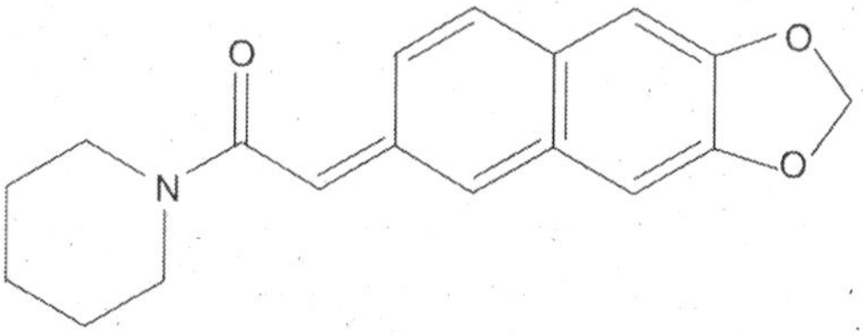

Chavicine ($C_{17}H_{19}NO_3$)

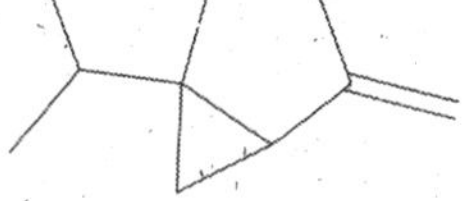

Sabinene ($C_{10}H_{16}$)

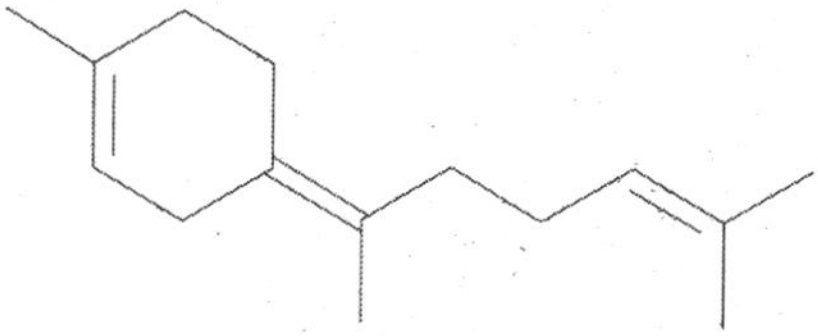

Bisabolene ($C_{15}H_{26}$)

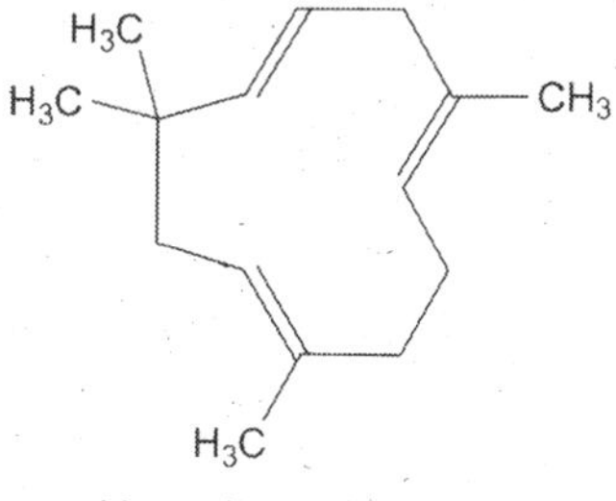

Humulene ($C_{15}H_{24}$)

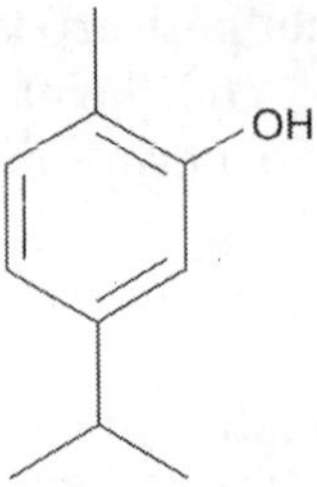

Carvacrol ($C_{10}H_{14}O$)

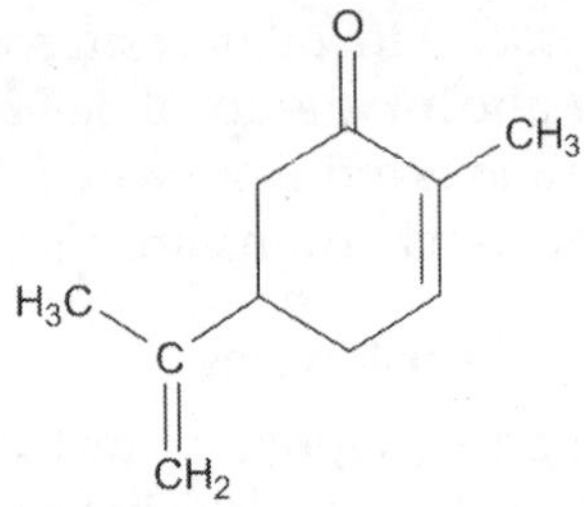

Carvone ($C_{10}H_{14}O$)

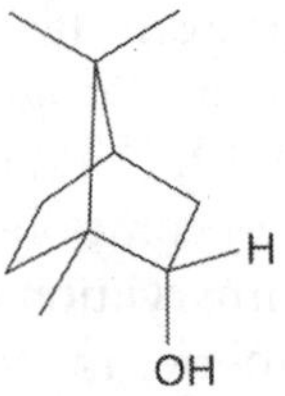

Borneol ($C_{10}H_{18}O$)

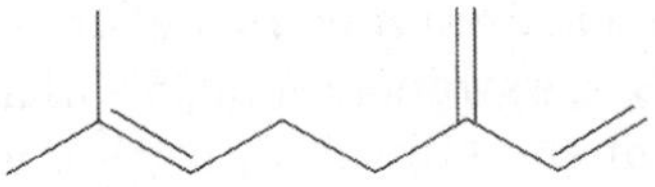

Myrcene ($C_{10}H_{16}$)

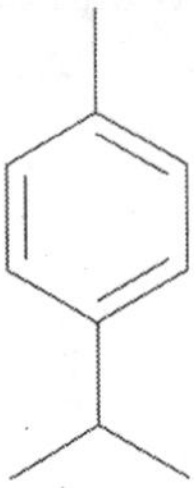

Alpha-Terpinene ($C_{10}H_{16}$)

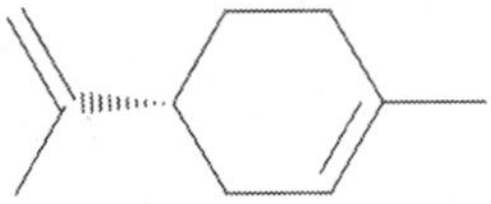

Limonene ($C_{10}H_{16}$)

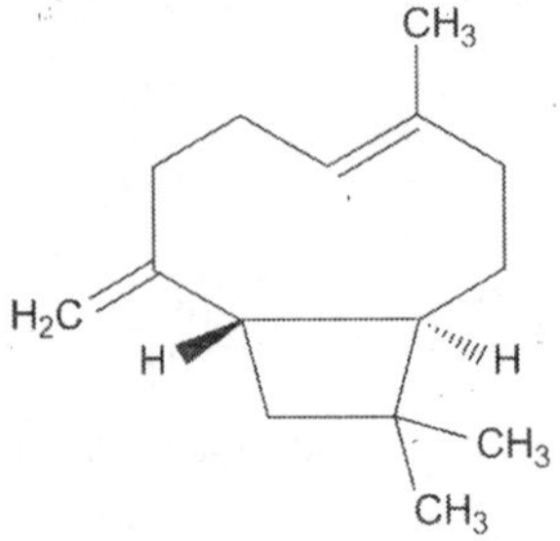

Caryophyllene ($C_{15}H_{24}$)

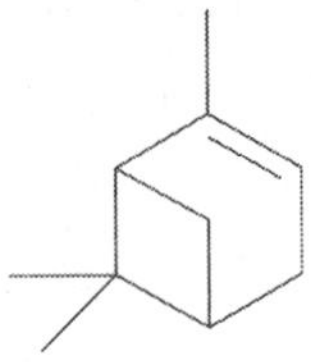

Pinene ($C_{10}H_{16}$)

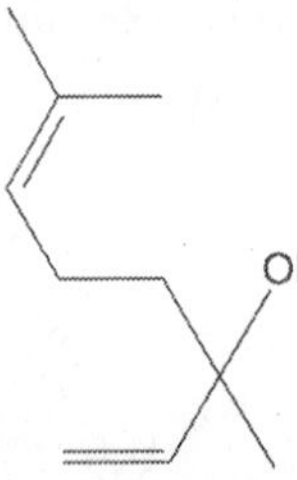

Linalool ($C_{10}H_{18}O$)

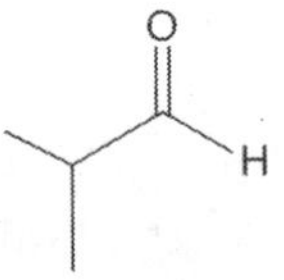

2-Methylpropanal (C_4H_8O)

History of Black Pepper

Pepper has been known from antiquity both for its flavour and use as medicine. No plant since the Apple of Eden has had a greater effect on human history than the black pepper. Pepper has been used in the Western culture for millennia with documented references dating back to 500 BC and is known as the 'King of Spices' or the 'Master Spice'. The archaeological evidence proves that humans have been using pepper and grinding peppercorns for 9000 years. The method of chewing betel nuts, betel leaves (Piperaceae) and lime powder (*tambula*) was first described by Herodotus (340 BC). This began when Alexander the Great (327 BC) invaded India and discovered the pleasure of well-seasoned food. Though pepper has been mentioned in writings that are over 3000 years old, the cultivation began in Indonesia around 100 BC. Black pepper was found stuffed in the nostrils of Ramesses II placed as a part of the mummification rituals shortly after his death in 1213 BC. Pepper was also known in Greece as early as 4th century BC. Hippocrates was known to have employed pepper in several diseases. Pliny, the Elder, in his Natural History describes the prices in Rome around 77 AD, as '*Long pepper ..... is 15 denarii per pound, while that of white pepper is 7, and of black, 4*'. This indicates that pepper was used as commodity money during the Roman time. Black pepper was well known and widespread in Roman Empire according to *Apicius' de re coquinaria*, a 3rd century cook book which includes pepper used in majority of its recipes and in '*The History of the Decline and Fall of the Roman Empire*' Edward Gibbon wrote that pepper was a favourite ingredient of the most expensive Roman cookery. It is also said that Alaric, the Visigoths (410 AD) and Attila, the Hun (408 AD), each demanded a ransom of more than 3000 pounds of pepper from Rome as a tribute when they besieged the city in 5th century, which speaks of the fact that pepper was so valuable at that time and was the collateral currency. In the Middle ages, pepper was used to conceal the taste of partially rotten meat, as the people of the time knew that eating the spoiled food would make them sick, and it is true that piperine in pepper has antimicrobial properties. Black pepper was known in China in the 2nd century BC if the reports of Tang Meng, an explorer are correct. Black pepper made its first appearance in Chinese texts as *hujiao* (foreign pepper) and by the 12th century it had become a popular ingredient in Chinese cuisine. Pepper reached South East Asia more than 2000 years ago and was grown in Malaysia and Indonesia about that time. Pepper plantations in Brazil go back to 1930. Pepper has been used in India since pre-historic times as a spice, and has been known to Indian cooking since 2000 BC. India particularly, the Malabar coast (present Kerala state) was the important source until well after the Middle ages to Europe, the Middle East, North Africa, Thailand and Malaysia. In trade, it was often referred to as 'black gold' and was used as a form of commodity money, as the

Romans knew both long pepper (*Piper longum*) and black pepper and referred them as pepper. Chapter 5 of *Samannaphala Sutta*, a Buddhist book, contains reference to pepper as one of the few medicines allowed to be always carried by a monk. By 16th century, pepper was being grown in Java, Sumatra, Madagascar and Malaysia. Thus, pepper was both a seasoning and medicinal spice historically.

Medicinal Uses

The fruits of pepper are used in indigestion, asthma, fever, cough, dysentery and haemorrhoids. It is stimulant, carminative, antiperiodic and stomachic. It is also anthelmintic, rubifacient, resolvent and antipyretic. The oil (*Oleum piperis*) is used in the treatment of pain relief, rheumastism, chills, flu, colds, exhaustion, muscular aches and fever. It is used to increase circulation, to increase the flow of saliva, to stimulate appetite, to encourage peristalsis, to tone up the muscles of the colon and as a general digestive and nerve tonic. It is used as a gargle for relaxed uvula and paralysis of the tongue. It corrects atonic dyspepsia, flatulence and nausea. It is also used in vertigo, arthritis and has been advised in diarrhoea and cholera. Externally, it is used for relaxed sore throat and skin diseases. It is also bacteriostatic and fungistatic. Pepper acts as a stimulant and accelerates the frequency of the pulse, promotes diaphoresis, excites mucous surfaces and stimulates urino-genital apparatus.

Culinary Uses

Pepper is mainly used as a culinary condiment in almost all cuisines of the world. Black pepper is popular for mild stews preferred in the cuisine of the Royal Thai Court. In Cambodia, this is a part of the table condiment called *tik marij*. Sweetmeats containing pepper were common in ancient Greece and Rome, and a few of them are still found in current European cuisine like *panforte* (Italian) and *Lebkuchen* (German). In India, pepper is used more abundantly in the preparation of *curry powder* (Anglo-Indian), *garam masala* (North Indian) and *sambar podi* (South Indian). Pepper is also popular in Arabic cuisine such as *zhoug* (Yemen), *baharat* (Coast of Gulf), *ras el hanout* (Morocco), *galat dagga* (Tunisia) and *berbere* (Ethiopia).

Other Uses

East Africans believe that the body odour after consuming substantial amounts of pepper repels mosquitoes. Gardeners use pepper spray (in warm water) against several kinds of pests like ants, potato bugs, silverfish, cockroaches and moths.

Adulteration

Pepper is adulterated with hulls (broken pieces of pericarp) of white pepper. The poorest grade is the Acheen pepper and is often mixed with pepper shells, dirt and small stones. The pepper powder is often mixed with groundnut nutshells, buckwheat hulls, cocoa shells, legume seeds, pepper stems, cereal hulls, mustard husks and seeds, juniper berries, olive pits, flax seed, ground charcoal and dust.

REVIEW QUESTIONS

1. **Essay and Short Answer Questions:**
   1. Write short notes on:
      a. Peppermint oil
      b. Uses of coriander
      c. Lemon oil
      d. Pharmaceutical uses of ginger
      e. Cardamom
      f. Tulsi
      g. Lemon grass
      h. Caraway
      i. Cumin
      j. Dill
      k. Fennel
      l. Black pepper
   2. Describe the source, collection and preparation, constituents and pharmaceutical uses of cinnamon.
   3. Describe the biological source, collection and preparation, constituents and medicinal uses of nutmeg.
   4. Describe the source, constituents and pharmaceutical uses of eucalyptus.
   5. Describe the source, collection and preparation, constituents and pharmaceutical uses of cloves.

2. **Choose the Correct Alternative:**
   1. Volatile oils are: [ ]
      a. Soluble in water   b. Insoluble in alcohol and ether
      c. Optically active   d. All the above
   2. The following is used in non-staining iodine ointment: [ ]
      a. Olive oil   b. Linseed oil
      c. Castor oil   d. Lard oil
   3. Which one of the following is a good immunomodulating agent?   [ ]
      a. Tulsi   b. Nutmeg
      c. Mentha   d. Cumin

4. The synonym of eucalyptus oil is: [ ]
   a. American worm seed oil   b. Chenoposan
   c. Indian melissa oil   d. Dinkum oil

5. Eucalyptus oil is used as: [ ]
   a. Counter-irritant   b. Antiseptic
   c. Both a and b   d. None

6. The following is used as a dental analgesic and in the preparation of cigarettes: [ ]
   a. Tulsi   b. Cloves
   c. Cardamom   d. Fennel

7. The number of vittae present in the fruit of coriander: [ ]
   a. 12   b. 8
   c. 6   d. 4

3. Fill in the Blanks:

1. .... method is used for the extraction of volatile oils from the crude drugs.

2. Lemon grass is an example for...volatile oils.

3. .... oil is a strong bactericidal agent.

4. The cathartic property of castor oil is due to irritant action of ....

5. The chief constituent of caraway volatile oil is ....

6. .... is used for citral content and for the synthesis of vitamin A.

7. Olive oil is extracted by .... method.

8. .... oil has blood cholesterol reducing property.

9. The crude eucalyptus oil produced is rectified again after treatment with ....

10. The fat of nutmeg is also known as ....

11. Cinnamon bark contains a sweet substance known as ....

12. *Mentha piperita* is a hybrid of a cross between .... and ....

13. The nutlets of *Mentha* have an aromatic odour and taste followed by a cooling sensation on drawing in breath due to ....

14. The glandular hairs on the mid rib and the veins in *Mentha* contain the ....

4. True or False Statements:

1. Coriander is cultivated only as a kharif crop. [True/False]
2. Dill volatile oil is used in the gastric disturbances of infants and children. [True/False]
3. Linseed oil is obtained from *Garcinia indica*. [True/False]
4. Castor oil is used as an emollient. [True/False]
5. Freshly harvested volatile oil containing plants should be dried in sunlight [True/False]
6. Volatile oils have a low refractive index and optically inactive. [True/False]
7. Cloves is an example for oxide volatile oils. [True/False]
8. Linseed oil is used in medicines. [True/False]
9. The synonym of lemongrass oil is Indian Melissa oil. [True/False]
10. Beta-ionine which is the starting material for vitamin A synthesis is obtained from citral. [True/False]
11. The synonym of olive oil is lanolin. [True/False]
12. Cinnamon is the first spice to be mentioned in the old testament. [True/False]

5. A. Match the following:

1. Carminative	[ ]	a. Mentha oil
2. Aromatic	[ ]	b. Caraway
3. Gripe water	[ ]	c. Cinnamon
4. Toothpaste	[ ]	d. Coriander
5. Spice	[ ]	e. Dill

B. Match the following:

1. Queen of spices	[ ]	a. Black pepper
2. Mace	[ ]	b. Stylopod
3. King of spices	[ ]	c. Lysigenous cavities
4. Cremocarp	[ ]	d. Aril
5. Lemon oil	[ ]	e. Cardamom

C. Match the following:

1. Ocimum	[ ]	a. Antiparasitic and vermifuge
2. Caraway	[ ]	b. Mother of cloves
3. Aqua foeniculi	[ ]	c. COX-2 inhibitor
4. Dill fruits	[ ]	d. Domestic gripe water
5. Ripe berry of clove	[ ]	e. Emmenagogue and galactogogue

General Tests for Detection of Drug Components

GENERAL TESTS FOR THE IDENTIFICATION OF CARBOHYDRATES IN DRUGS

Introduction

Carbohydrates (saccharides some of them have sweet taste and hence are called sugars) are the most abundant organic compounds found in the living organisms which are composed of carbon, hydrogen and oxygen. These act as primary source to provide the energy for the functioning of the living organisms. These substances hydrolyze to yield polyhydroxy aldehydes and ketones. Carbohydrates (hydrates of carbon) derive their name from their basic empirical formula $(CH_2O)_n$. They occur as trioses $(CH_2O)_3$, tetroses $(CH_2O)_4$, pentoses $(CH_2O)_5$ and hexoses $(CH_2O)_6$, etc. Their chemical properties are built-up the distinguishing features of carbohydrates such as: the number of alcoholic groups, both primary $(-CH_2OH)$ and secondary $(=CHOH)$ make the molecule highly water-soluble. These groups can interact between themselves and form a glycoside linkage $(-HC-O-CH-)$, which gives rise to the possibility of forming a disaccharide, trisaccharide, polysaccharide, etc. The $-OH$ groups can also react with $-NH_2$ groups to give rise to amino derivatives found in biological systems. The aldehyde group at one end of the molecule is highly reactive and a powerful reducing agent which gets itself oxidised to a carboxyl group. This reducing power is very useful in the estimation of sugars. The carbohydrates with aldehyde groups are called aldoses. There is also a possibility for the formation of numerous isomers. The presence of the asymmetric carbon atoms (the 4 valencies of the carbon getting linked to four different groups) makes the carbohydrates optically active (when a beam of plane polarised light passes through a solution containing an optically active substance, the plane gets rotated). Normally, in the biological material, the d-series of carbohydrates occur.

Carbohydrates are one of the most important components in drugs. They may be present as isolated molecules or may be physically associated with or chemically bound to other molecules of the drug. The individual molecules can be classified as *monosaccharides, oligosaccharides or polysaccharides* according to the number of monomers that they contain. The molecules in which the carbohydrates are covalently attached to the proteins are known as the *glycoproteins,* while those in which they are covalently attached to the lipids are called the *glycolipids.*

Monosaccharides are water-soluble, crystalline compounds which are aliphatic aldehydes or ketones containing one carbonyl group and one or more hydroxyl groups. Natural monosaccharides are either pentoses or hexoses. Common hexoses are glucose, fructose and galactose while common pentoses are arabinose and xylose. The reactive centres are the carbonyl and hydroxyl groups.

Oligosaccharides are low molecular weight polymers of monosaccharides (with less than 20 carbons) that are covalently bonded through glycosidic linkages. Disaccharides consist of two monomers while the trisaccharides consist of three monomers. Most common oligosaccharides contain glucose, fructose and galactose monomers.

Polysaccharides are high molecular weight polymers of monosaccharides (with more than 20 carbons). If the monosaccharides are same, these are called *homopolysaccharides,* and those which contain a mixture of more than one type of monomer are called *heteropolysaccharides.* The former are represented by starch, cellulose and glycogen while the latter are represented by pectin, hemicellulose and gums. Most polysaccharides contain 100 to several 1000 monosaccharides. Some exist as linear chains while others as branched chains. Some are digested by humans like starch, while others are indigestible like cellulose, hemicellulose and pectin. The former are useful as an important source of energy while the latter form *dietary fibre* like lignin. The consumption of different types of dietary fibres has beneficial physiologically functional properties for humans, such as prevention of cancer, heart disease and diabetes. The consumption of dietary fibre helps to protect against colon cancer, cardiovascular disease and constipation. The major components of the dietary fibre are cellulose, hemicellulose, pectin, hydrocolloids and lignin. Major components of the dietary fibre are cell wall polysaccharides of plants (cellulose, hemicellulose and pectin) and non-cell wall polysaccharides (hydrocolloids like guar gum, gum arabic, tragacanth gum and agar) commonly used as gelling agents, stabilisers and thickeners.

QUALITATIVE TESTS FOR STARCHES (CARBOHYDRATES)

1. **Iodine test:** This is a general test for the presence of carbohydrates. The iodine test is used to test for the presence of starch. 2–3 drops of Lugol's iodine (Lugol's solution—first made in 1829, named after a

French Physician, J. G. A. Lugol: also called iodine-potassium iodide, markodine, strong solution, aqueous iodine solution) is added to 5 ml of the solution to be tested in a test tube. Lugol's iodine reagent is elemental iodine (5 g) dissolved in an aqueous (85 ml of distilled water) solution of potassium iodide (10 g) with a total iodine content of 150 mg/ml. A positive test for starch is blue-black colour. A positive test for glycogen is a brown-blue colour. A negative test is the brown-yellow colour of the regent. The reagent reacts with starch producing a blue black colour which is more intense. The amylose produces a dark blue/black colour while the amylopectin results in an orange colour/yellow hue. When starch is broken down into smaller units, blue-black colour is not produced. Glycogen produces brown-blue colour which is less intense. Other polysaccharides and mono-saccharides yield no colour change and the test solution remains brown-yellow (the colour of the regent). It is thought that iodine ions (I_3^- and I_5^-) fit inside the coils of amylose and the charge transfers between the iodine and the starch, and the energy level spacings in the resulting complex correspond to the absorption spectrum in the visible light region. The strength of the resulting blue colour depends on the amount of amylose present (iodine forms coloured complexes with polysaccharides).

2. **Molisch's test:** This is a general test (common) for the presence of carbohydrates larger than tetroses. This test is based on the dehydration of carbohydrate (pentose and hexose) by the acid. Molisch reagent is a solution of alpha-naphthol in 95% ethanol. This test helps in detecting glycoproteins and as such a negative result indicates the absence of carbohydrates. 2 drops of Molisch reagent (5% solution of alpha-naphthol in alcohol) is added to 2 ml of the sugar solution in a test tube and mixed thoroughly. The tube is inclined and 5 ml of concentrated sulphuric acid is gently added down the walls of the test tube. A purple (reddish-violet) coloured ring at the interface of the sugar and the acid (junction of the two liquids) indicates a positive test. If it appears green, the solution is discarded. The qualitative test is performed on 0.2 M solutions of starch, sucrose, glucose, lactose, galactose, ribose and ribulose. The compounds are dehydrated to furfural or hydroxy-methyl-furfural in the presence of sulphuric acid. Furfural is derived from the dehydration of pentoses and pentosan, while hydroxy-methyl-furfural is produced from hexoses and hexosans. Oligosaccharides and polysaccharides are hydrolyzed to yield their repeating monomers by the sulphuric acid. The alpha-naphthol reacts with the cyclic aldehydes to form the purple coloured condensation product. If the test is positive, a carbohydrate is present in the protein molecule.

3. **Benedict's test (for reducing sugars—monosaccharides):** This is a test for the presence of the reducing sugars in alkaline solution. The reagent is prepared by dissolving 17.3 g of sodium citrate and 10 g of sodium carbonate in about 75 ml of water and filtered if necessary. In a separate container, in about 20 ml water, 1.73 g of copper sulphate ($CuSO_4.7H_2O$) is dissolved and slowly added with stirring to a solution of alkaline citrate. The volume is made-up to 100 ml. Benedict's solution (the reagent is more stable) is an alkaline solution containing cupric ions which oxidise the aldehyde to a carboxylic acid and in turn the cupric ions are reduced to cuprous oxide which forms a red precipitate. The reagent is composed of copper sulphate, sodium carbonate and sodium citrate with a pH of 10.5. The citrate will form soluble complex ions with Cu^{++} preventing the precipitation of copper carbonate in alkaline solutions. 15 drops of the 1% solution to be tested (glucose, fructose, sucrose, lactose and maltose) is taken into separate, labelled test tubes (12 × 75 mm) and to each of the tubes is added 1 ml of Benedict's solution and the tubes shaken. The tubes are kept in a boiling water bath (40–50 degrees Celsius) and heated for 5 minutes, and later allowed to cool. The formation of green, red or yellow precipitate is a positive test for the reducing sugars. The alkaline conditions in which the test is carried cause isomeric transformation of the ketoses to aldoses (all monosaccharides and most of the disaccharides) which reduces the blue Cu^{2+} ion to cuprous oxide, a brick red-orange precipitate. This is normally used in the clinical laboratories for testing urine.

4. **Barfoed's test (for reducing monosaccharides):** This is a test for the presence of the reducing sugars in an acidic solution. This determines whether the carbohydrate is a monosaccharide or a disaccharide. This is a slight modification over Benedict's test and Fehling's test, as the reduction of copper is carried out in mild acidic conditions which make it somewhat specific for monosaccharides. The reagent is prepared by dissolving 13.3 g copper acetate in 200 ml of water and adding 1.8 ml of glacial acetic acid to it. The reagent reacts at a faster rate with monosaccharides to produce cuprous oxide than disaccharides do. Barfoed's reagent is copper acetate in dilute acetic acid with a pH of 4.6. The colour changes are same as in the Benedict's test. 15 drops of the 1% carbohydrate solutions to be tested (glucose, fructose, sucrose, lactose and maltose) is taken into separate, labelled test tubes (12 × 75 mm) and to each of the tubes is added 1 ml of Barfoed's reagent. The tubes are kept in a boiling water bath and heated for 10 minutes, and later allowed to cool. The formation of a green, red, or a yellow precipitate is a positive test for the reducing monosaccharides. If the tubes are heated longer than 3 minutes, a positive test can be obtained for disaccharides. The acidic condition

allows the oxidation of the monosaccharides but does not oxidise the disaccharides. If the time of heating is carefully controlled, the disaccharides do not react while the reducing monosaccharides give the positive result (red cuprous oxide precipitate). Ketoses fail to isomerise with this reagent.

In addition to Benedict's test and Barfoed's test, the other tests for the detection of the reducing monosaccharides in the sample, are:

a. *Picric acid test (for reducing monosaccharides):* 3 ml of the sample solution is taken in a test tube and to it is added 1 ml of saturated picric acid solution and 1 ml of 1% or 4% sodium hydroxide solution, and the tube is warmed. The test is positive if red colour appears due to the formation of picrylic acid which indicates the presence of a reducing monosaccharide in the sample.

b. *Tommer's test (for reducing monosaccharides):* 2 ml of 0.5% copper sulphate solution is taken in a test tube and to it is added 2 ml of the sample solution and mixed. To this mixture is added 2 ml of 40% sodium hydroxide solution, and is boiled and cooled. A red or a yellow precipitate of cuprous oxide indicates that the test is positive. This is an indication that the sample contains reducing monosaccharide.

c. *Nylander's test (for reducing monosaccharides):* 5 ml of the sample solution is taken in a test tube, and to it is added 0–5 ml of Nylander's reagent, and boiled for 3 minutes and cooled. The development of a black precipitate (bismuth nitrate reduced to black bismuth) indicates that the test is positive, and that the sample contains reducing monosaccharide.

d. *Methylene blue test (for reducing monosaccharides):* 3 ml of distilled water and 0.5 ml of 40% sodium hydroxide solution are taken in a test tube, and to it is added a drop of methylene blue, and boiled and cooled. The solution remains blue in its colour and to it is added 1 ml of the sample solution, and boiled and cooled. The disappearance of the blue colour (methylene blue reduced to leuco-methylene blue which is colourless) indicates that the test is positive and an indication that the sample contains reducing monosaccharide.

e. *Potassium ferricyanide test (for reducing monosaccharides):* 3 ml of 1% potassium ferricyanide solution is taken in a test tube and to it is added 1 ml of 40% sodium hydroxide solution. The mixture is boiled and to it is added 10 drops of the sample solution (drop by drop) and the boiling is continued. The yellow colour of ferricyanide decolourises which is an indication that the test is positive and that the sample contains reducing monosaccharide.

5. **Lasker and Enkelwitz test (for ketoses):** This is a test for the presence of the ketoses. The test utilises Benedict's solution but the reaction is carried out at a much lower temperature. The colour changes are the same as with the Benedict's test. Dilute sugar solutions of 0.02 M concentration are to be used. 1 ml of the solution to be tested is added to 5 ml of Benedict's solution in a test tube and mixed well. The tube is heated in a 55°C water bath for 10–20 minutes. Ketopentoses give a positive reaction within 10 minutes, while ketohexoses give a positive reaction in 20 minutes. The aldoses do not give a positive reaction. The reagent uses copper ions to detect the reducing sugars in an acidic solution.

6. **Bial's test (for pentoses):** This is a test for the presence of pentoses. The reagent is prepared by dissolving 150 mg of orcinol in 50 ml of concentrated hydrochloric acid. Bial's reagent uses orcinol (5-methyl-resorcinol), hydrochloric acid and a small amount of ferric chloride catalyst. The dilute sugar solutions of 0.02 M concentration are to be used with this test. 2 ml of the solution to be tested is added to 5 ml of Bial's reagent in a test tube. The tube is gently heated to boiling and later allowed to cool. The formation of a green coloured solution or precipitate denotes a positive reaction (before 10 minutes). During the reaction, the pentoses are converted to furfural by the reagent and form a blue-green colour with orcinol. This test is generally used to distinguish the pentoses from hexoses. Furfural generated by the dehydration of pentose and pentosans forms the coloured condensation products with orcinol.

7. **Mucic acid test (for galactose):** This is a test for the presence of galactose. 1 ml of concentrated nitric acid is added to 5 ml of the solution to be tested in a test tube, and mixed well. It is heated on a boiling water bath until the volume of the solution is reduced to about 1 ml. The mixture is removed from the water bath and cooled at room temperature overnight. The presence of insoluble crystals in the bottom of the tube indicates a positive reaction that is the presence of mucic acid. This is due to the oxidation of galactose by nitric acid. Oxidation of most monosaccharides by nitric acid yields soluble dicarboxylic acids. But, the oxidation of galactose yields an insoluble mucic acid. Lactose will also yield a mucic acid due to hydrolysis of the glycosidic linkages between its glucose and galactose subunits.

8. **Seliwanoff's test (for fructose):** This is a test for ketoses or ketohexoses. Seliwanoff's reagent contains resorcinol in 6M hydrochloric acid. The reagent is prepared by dissolving 50 mg of resorcinol in 100 ml of dilute hydrochloric acid (either 3N or 1 : 2 dilutions). 1 drop of the respective sugar solution and 1 drop of water blank is added to about 3 ml of Seliwanoff's reagent in a clean test tube

and mixed well. The test tube is placed in the boiling water bath with sufficient water and heated for 3 minutes after the water begins to boil. The ketohexoses like fructose and disaccharides with a ketohexose like sucrose form a cherry-red precipitate as a product of condensation. This is a positive test. Sugars other than ketohexoses produce a product of yellow to light pink colour. The positive reaction is due to the condensation of hydroxy-methyl-furfural (formed due to dehydration of the hexose on heating) with resorcinol to give a red product. The reagent is caustic and if gets in contact with the skin or clothing, it is to be thoroughly rinsed. After the test, the solution is to be discarded in the sink and rinsed in plenty of water.

9. **Fehling's test (for carbohydrates):** This is the reduction test of carbohydrates. Fehling's solution is prepared by dissolving 7 gm of copper sulphate ($CuSO_4.7H_2O$ – Fehling's solution A) in water and making up to 100 ml. 24 gm of potassium hydroxide (KOH) and 34.6 gm of sodium potassium tartrate (Fehling's solution B) are dissolved in a separate container and made-up to 100 ml in water. The two solutions are mixed prior to use. The solution contains cupric ions in the form of a stable complex along with tartrate. To 2 ml of this solution, a few drops of the test solution is added and boiled. If the carbohydrate possesses a reducing group, the cupric ion will be reduced to cuprous ion or even copper and shows up as a rusty brown colour or a red (yellow or brownish-red) precipitate.

10. **Anthrone test (for carbohydrates):** This is a general test for all carbohydrates (like glucose, sucrose and starch). In this test, carbohydrate gets dehydrated when it reacts with conc. sulphuric acid to form furfural, which reacts with anthrone (0.2% anthrone in conc. sulphuric acid) to give a bluish-green coloured complex. 200 mg of anthrone reagent is dissolved in 100 ml of concentrated sulphuric acid. To 2 ml of this solution in a test tube, 2 drops of the test solution is added and mixed well. If there is no immediate colour change, it is boiled in a water bath for 10 minutes and observed. The colour changes to bluish-green indicating that the test is positive.

11. **Osazone test (for ketoses and aldoses):** This test is used for the identification of sugars, and it involves the reaction of monosaccharide with phenylhydrazine. All the reducing sugars form osazones with excess of phenylhydrazine when kept at boiling temperature. Each sugar has a characteristic crystal form of osazones. Sucrose is a non-reducing sugar and it does not form osazone crystals, and upon hydrolysis, the products, glucose and fructose form needle-shaped crystals. Both the ketoses and aldoses react with phenylhydrazine to produce a phenylhydrazone which further reacts with two other molecules of phenylhydrazine to yield osazone. The

yellow needle-shaped crystals of osazone are produced by glucose, fructose, and mannose; rhombic plate-shaped crystals are formed by galactose; powder puff-shaped crystals are formed by lactose; and mushroom-shaped crystals are formed by lactosazone. The crystals of different shapes will be shown by different osazones.

12. **Tollen's test (silver-mirror test for aldehydes):** This is a qualitative laboratory test which is used to distinguish between an aldehyde and a ketone. This is due to the fact that the aldehydes are readily oxidised while the ketones are not. Tollen's reagent is a colourless, basic, aqueous solution of silver ions coordinated to ammonia (ammoniacal silver nitrate solution). The reagent is prepared by a 2-step process: Aqueous silver nitrate is mixed with aqueous sodium hydroxide, and aqueous ammonia is added drop-by-drop until the precipitated silver oxide completely dissolves. The reagent oxidises an aldehyde into the corresponding carboxylic acid. The reaction is accompanied by the reduction of the silver ions in the reagent into metallic silver, if the test is carried out in a clean glass test tube which forms a mirror on the inner walls of the test tube. On reacting with carbohydrate, elemental silver is precipitated out of the solution, occasionally onto the inner surface of the reaction tube or vessel, which produces a silver mirror on the inner wall of the tube. The treatment with a ketone does not result in a silver mirror.

13. **Foulger's test (for fructose):** 0.5 ml of the sample (fructose) solution is taken in a test tube and to it is added 3 ml of Foulger's reagent. The mixture (0.5 ml of the sample + urea + sulphuric acid + stannous chloride) is boiled and the tube is shaken gently. If the test is positive (in the presence of fructose), blue colour appears.

14. **Moore's test (for glucose):** This test is based on the liberation of aldehydes which subsequently polymerise to form the resinous substance, 'caramel'. 4 ml of the sample solution is taken in a test tube and to it is added an equal volume of 2% sodium hydroxide solution and boiled. If the test is positive, the solution turns yellow in the beginning and reddish brown later due to the formation of caramel, a condensed product of glucose. This indicates that the sample contains glucose. The test is positive to glucose, galactose, maltose, fructose and lactose; and is negative to sucrose, glycogen and starch.

15. **Colour tests for disaccharides and polysaccharides:**
    a. *Iodine test (colour test for glycogen):* 2 ml of the sample solution is put in a test tube, boiled and cooled at room temperature. To it is added 1 or 2 drops of Iodine solution. The appearance of red or wine red colour is an indication that the sample contains glycogen and the test is positive.

b. *Iodine test (colour test for starch):* A 2% potassium iodide solution in alcohol is prepared in a test tube. To this, a sufficient amount of iodine crystals are added to colour it deep yellow. A small amount of starch is placed in the depression of a porcelain test plate, and to it is added 1 to 3 drops of dilute iodine solution. The test solution turns blue indicating the formation of the iodine complexes which is a positive test for starch.

GENERAL TESTS FOR THE IDENTIFICATION OF PROTEINS AND AMINO ACIDS IN DRUGS

Introduction

Proteins are important macronutrients that are essential for the survival of organisms. They are the constituents of all the cells in the living bodies. 10–35% of calories should come from the proteins, and these are found in meat, poultry, fish, meat substitutes, cheese and milk, etc.

Proteins are the most complex and functionally diverse molecules of the living organisms. The enzymes, blood cells, muscle tissue, etc. are composed of proteins. The base elements of proteins are carbon, hydrogen, oxygen and nitrogen. The monomers of the proteins are 20 different amino acids (alpha-amino acids—the amino group is attached to the alpha-carbon which exist as zwitter ions and are crystalline in nature) and these are bonded together in unique combinations to create a polypeptide chain, the protein polymer. The chain is then folded into a unique functional protein. The backbone of a protein is made of –CO–NH– linkage called the peptide linkage which is common to all proteins. The properties of the proteins are governed by the different R (residual) groups of the amino acids. The interaction between the various R groups help in giving a 3-dimensional structure or conformation to the protein as a whole. The –CO–NH– groups are capable of forming weak hydrogen bonds within the chain as such the a-helical structure of proteins is stabilised. The bonds which help in the formation of 3-dimensional structure are weak and can be easily disturbed by the changes in pH, temperature, surface tension, etc. as such the structure is lost and the protein gets denatured. Hence, the proteins should always be kept in a buffered solution and at a low temperature (0–4°C). The response of the extra ionisable groups in glutamic acid and lysine to pH changes confers the electrical changes to proteins.

Amino acids are the basic building units of proteins. There are 20 amino acids (both essential and nonessential) which occur commonly in biological systems. They are: Glycine (*Gly* – nonessential – C_2H_3NO), alanine (*Ala* – nonessential – C_3H_5NO), valine (*Val* – essential – C_5H_9NO), leucine (*Leu* – essential – $C_6H_{11}NO$), isoleucine (*Ile* – essential and ambiguous

– $C_6H_{11}NO$), serine (*Ser* – nonessential – $C_3H_5NO_2$), threonine (*Thr* – essential – $C_4H_7NO_2$), tyrosine (*Tyr* – essential – $C_9H_9NO_2$), phenylalanin (*Phe* – essential – C_9H_9NO), tryptophan (*Trp* – essential – $C_{11}H_{10}N_2O$), asparagine (*Asp* – nonessential and ambiguous – $C_4H_6N_2O_2$), glutamine (*Glu* – nonessential and ambiguous – $C_5H_8N_2O_2$), lysine (*Lys* – essential – $C_6H_{12}N_2O$), arginine (*Arg* – nonessential – $C_6H_{12}N_4O$), histidine (*His* – essential – $C_6H_7N_3O$), cysteine (*Cys* – nonessential – C_3H_5NOS), methionine (*Met* – essential – C_5H_9NOS), aspartic acid (*Asp* – nonessential – $C_4H_5NO_3$), glutamic acid (*Glu* – nonessential – $C_5H_7NO_3$) and proline (*Pro* – nonessential – C_5H_7NO). The basic chemical structure of an amino acid is $R—CH—NH_2—COOH$. The R- in the formula represents a residual group (different chemical groups in each amino acid) which determines the individuality of the amino acids. The most common feature is that they possess a minimum of two ionisable groups, the acidic carboxyl group ($–COOH = COO^- + H^+$) and the basic amino group ($–NH_2 + H^+ = –NH_3$) on the same carbon atom, called the α-carbon atom and because of this, the amino acids undergo the reactions. H^+ takes part in these ionisation reactions and the processes are pH dependent. At low pH value, ionisation of $–COOH$ will be pushed backwards and that of $–NH_3$ forward. As pH increases, the carboxyl group will start ionising. At a particular pH called pK_1, the two species will be of equal concentrations. Any further increase in pH will result in a steady decrease of the former which eventually disappears at the point pI or the *isoionic point*.

Depending on the number of amino acids involved in the condensation reaction, the proteins are classified as: Dipeptides, tripeptides, and polypeptides. Dipeptides are the products formed by the condensation of two alpha-amino acids; tripeptides are formed by the condensation of three alpha-amino acids; and polypeptides are the products of condensation of a large number of amino acids. A polypeptide having a molecular mass greater than 10,000 is called a protein. The proteins may be primary, secondary, tertiary or quaternary.

QUALITATIVE TESTS FOR AMINO ACIDS/PROTEINS

1. **Millon's test:** This is a test for any compound containing a phenolic hydroxy group. Millon's reagent is a mixture of mercuric and mercurous nitrates and nitrites, which on heating with compounds containing the phenolic groups (such as tyrosine), produce a red colour. The reaction involves mercuration and nitration or nitrosation. Tyrosine gives this test in its free state as well as in combined state.

   15% solution of mercuric sulphate in 15% sulphuric acid is prepared. 1 ml of the test solution in a test tube is added to a few drops of this reagent and heated for 10 minutes at 100°C, in a boiling water bath for about 5 minutes. Later, the tubes are cooled and observed for the colour change. Pink to dark red colour is a positive test for tyrosine and this is probably due to a mercury salt of nitrated tyrosine. A white coloured precipitate is formed first which then changes to brick red on boiling. Millon's reagent is highly toxic and highly corrosive. Hence, gloves are used and the test is carried out in fume hoods. The colour produced in Millon's test is due to the derivatives of benzene in which a hydrogen ring has been replaced by a hydroxyl group, and this reaction serves as a test for the presence of tyrosine. Gelatin does not give a positive result.

2. **Ninhydrin test:** The compounds that contain the free amino groups (such as amino acids, peptides or proteins) give this test. When such compounds are treated with ninhydrin (triketohydrindene hydrate) and heated, they produce deep blue to violet pink or even red colour. Ninhydrin undergoes an oxidation-reduction reaction with the free amino groups, by oxidatively deaminating them to carbonyl groups and ammonia. The reduced form of ninhydrin then couples with ammonia, and the residual ninhydin (oxidised) to give rise to a blue-violet or even red dye. Due to the lack of alpha-amino group, the proline and hydroxyproline give yellow colour with ninhydrin.

   This test is used to detect the presence of amino acids and proteins containing free amino groups. When heated with ninhydrin, these give characteristic deep blue coloured or occasionally pale yellow coloured complexes. 1 ml of casein, 2% egg albumin and 0.1 M glycine are placed into separate, labelled test tubes (12 × 75 mm). 4 drops of 0.1% of ninhydrin solution is added to each of the tubes. A boiling chip is added to each of the test tubes and the tubes are heated in a hot water bath for about 5 minutes. Later, the tubes are cooled and observed for the colours. A deep blue or pale yellow colour is a positive test for glycine and other two go negative. Ninhydrin is a carcinogen and direct contact with it should be avoided.

3. **Sulphur (lead sulphide) test:** The presence of sulphur-containing amino acids such as cysteine can be determined by converting sulphur to an inorganic sulphide through cleavage by a base. The resulting solution is combined with lead acetate, a black precipitate of lead sulphide results. The positive test is due to the presence of either disulphide (–S–S–) or –SH group. To 2 ml of test solution, 2 ml of 40% aqueous sodium hydroxide is added. The reagent, sodium plumbate is prepared by mixing 5 ml of 0.1 N sodium hydroxide with 2 ml of 0.1 M lead acetate and heated till the white precipitate disappears. 0.5 ml of this reagent is added to the test solution. The tubes are stoppered and shaken before heating in a boiling water bath for 5 minutes. Later, they are cooled and colours are noted. A black precipitate or brown

colouration is a positive test for cysteine, and no colour is negative which indicates the absence of sulphur. If the result is in doubt, the solution should be filtered and the filter paper is examined. The precipitate, which is lead sulphide, is formed as a result of the decomposition of the cystine by the alkali.

4. **Biuret test:** The substances that contain 2 or more peptide linkages produce a blue-violet colour with dilute copper sulphate solution in a strong alkali. This is called biuret reaction, after the compound called biuret which gives the positive test. The colour is developed due to the formation of a complex between the cupric ion and two adjacent peptide chains.

   This test is used to detect the presence of the peptide bond. When treated with copper sulphate solution in the presence of an alkali (NaOH or KOH), the protein reacts with copper (II) ions to form a violet-coloured complex called biuret. The biuret reagent is a blue coloured solution and contains copper ions and these reflect off closely clustered amide groups of protein casting a pink-purple (violet) colour to a solution containing proteins. The violet colour is a positive reaction in a biuret test. 40 drops of liquid to be tested is taken into a test tube and 3 drops of biuret reagent is added to it and gently shaken to mix. The proteins if present will turn the solution pink or purple. Excess of the addition of copper sulphate must be avoided in making the reagent, since the colour of the salt prevents the recognition of the colour produced in the reaction. The presence of ammonium salts interferes with the test. In applying the reaction to the solutions containing these salts, a large excess of sodium hydroxide must be present. The compounds which give the biuret test must contain at least 2–CO–NH– groups. The colour formed in the reaction varies in shade with the complexity of the molecules.

5. **Xanthoproteic test:** This is an identification test of the protein and it gives a positive result with those proteins with amino acid carrying an aromatic group. When the protein is treated with hot conc. nitric acid, a yellow coloured substance is formed, and the colour is due to xanthoproteic acid which is formed by the nitration of certain amino acids present in the protein (tyrosine and/or tryptophan).

   To the material to be tested, either a solid (1 or 2 gm) or an aqueous solution (2 cc), 5 drops of concentrated nitric acid is added and heated to boiling. The change in the colour is observed. The solution is cooled and made alkaline with dilute ammonia or sodium hydroxide. If yellow colour appears first, it will turn to orange colour. The colour is produced as a result of the formation of the nitro-derivatives of the compounds which contain a benzene ring, e.g. tyrosine.

6. **Hopkins Cole test (Adamkiewicz test):** To the material to be tested, either a solid (1 or 2 gm) or an aqueous solution (2 cc), 5 drops of a solution of glyoxylic acid (obtained by exposing glacial acetic acid to sunlight for a few minutes) is added. 2 ml of concentrated sulphuric acid is added with caution pouring it down the sides of the test tube until two layers are formed. If no colour is generated, it is put aside for a few minutes and examined. A violet ring at the junction of the two layers is a positive test for tryptophan. The colour produced is due to the formation of a compound from the glyoxylic acid in the reagent and the tryptophan in the protein. A similar colour is produced when sulphuric acid is added to a protein solution in the presence of a trace of formaldehyde. The reaction is used as a test for formaldehyde in milk.

7. **Pauly's test:** When diazotised sulphanilic acid is added to the alkaline solution of histidine and tyrosine, a red product is obtained. This is due to the coupling of histidine and tyrosine with diazotised sulphanilic acid to form the azo dyes.

   1 ml of sulphanilic acid (1% solution in 10% hydrochloric acid) and 2 ml of the test solution are mixed in a test tube and cooled in ice. To this, is added 1 ml of 5% sodium nitrite solution. After 5 minutes, 2 ml of 1% sodium carbonate solution is added and the colour change if any is observed. The test is positive for tyrosine, histidine and tryptophan.

8. **Ehrlich's test:** This test is specific for indoles. This is a biochemical test performed on the species of bacteria to detect the ability of the organism to degrade the amino acid tryptophan to produce indole. The reagent consists of 10% p-dimethyl-amino-benzaldehyde in 10% hydrochloric acid. 1 ml of test solution is added to 1 ml of the reagent in a test tube. The red or pink coloured ring is a positive test for tryptophan as it contains an indole nucleus. No colour change after the addition of the reagent is taken as negative. Along with the differentiation of enteric bacteria (like *E. coli*), this test can also be used for the differentiation of the species such as *Proteus*, *Klebsiella* and *Citrobacter*.

9. **Sakaguchi reaction:** When arginine is treated with alpha-naphthol and sodium hypochloride or hypobromide, it develops a red colour. This test is specific for the guanidine group of arginine and also non-amino acids like creatine. 3 ml of the test solution is added to 1 ml of 40% sodium hydroxide solution and 2 drops of a-naphthol (1% alcoholic solution) is added to it. A few drops of bromine water (a few drops of bromine to 100 ml of water added with caution) are also added, and the colour change if any is observed. The red colour is a positive test for arginine.

10. **Nitroprusside test:** This test is specific for the amino acid, cysteine, the only amino acid containing a sulphydryl (-SH) group. This group reacts with nitropruisside in alkaline solution to yield a red complex. To 2 ml of the protein solution to be tested, 1 ml of 2% sodium nitroprusside ($Na_2Fe (CN)_5NO$) solution and then 2–3 drops of 40% ammonium hydroxide solution are added. A deep purple-violet or red colour is produced. Free sulphydryl groups as in cysteine, some proteins and glutathions (in its reduced form) give this test. The disulphide groups (as in cysteine) give a positive reaction only after reduction to sulphydryl groups.

11. **Folin's phenol test:** When the proteins containing tyrosine or tryptophan with alkaline solution are added to Folin's phenol reagent (a phospho-molybdo-tungstic acid), a blue colour is obtained due to the reduction of Folin's reagent.

12. **Bromine water reaction:** This is carried out only when tryptophan is found in its free form rather than in a combined form. In a weakly acidic solution, free tryptophan produces a pink colour with bromine water due to halogenations of tryptophan.

13. **Coagulation test:** The proteins are first acidified with acetic acid and then heated for a short time. Coagulation occurs which confirms the presence of simple proteins (such as albumins).

GENERAL TESTS FOR THE IDENTIFICATION OF LIPIDS IN DRUGS

Introduction

Lipids form a heterogeneous group of compounds which possess the common property of not dissolving in water but dissolve in organic solvents like alcohol, acetone, chloroform, benzene, ether and hexane. This property of specific solubility is made use of in the extraction of lipids from the tissues, free from any water-soluble matter but further analytical methods are largely individualistic. For the general extraction of almost all lipids from the biological samples, either a mixture of ethanol or ethyl ether or a mixture of chloroform and methanol is used. The lipids are generally bound to the proteins in biological systems and such lipoproteins cannot be efficiently extracted by nonpolar organic solvents alone. The methanol or ethanol helps in breaking the bonds between the lipids and the proteins.

Lipids are hydrophobic (nonpolar), soluble in organic solvents and are much harder to breakdown for energy. Lipids contain more energy per unit weight. Lipids are fat molecules. The basic elements of a fat are carbon, hydrogen and oxygen. Their varied biological functions include energy source, energy storage, cell membrane structural components, hormones, vitamins, vitamin adsorption, protection and insulation. There are four main groups of lipids namely: Fatty acids—saturated and unsaturated, glycerides, nonglyceride lipids and complex lipids like lipoproteins and glycolipids. These can also be broadly divided into saponifiable lipids (triglycerides, glycolipids, sphingolipids, some types of waxes and phospholipids) and nonsaponifiable lipids (steroids, prostaglandins, leukotrienes and terpenes).

QUALITATIVE TESTS FOR THE IDENTIFICATION OF LIPIDS

The fats and oils are concentrated source of the energy, and certain percentage of the body weight of human being is fat and about 20–35% of calories should come from the fat. The fats in diet are essential for good health and are needed for body growth and also the processing of the vitamins required. The fats make-up part of all the cells in the body and these help to maintain the body temperature. They also form the fatty tissue around the delicate organs of the body to protect them from injury.

Chemically, the fats and oils are the trimesters of glycerol and higher fatty acids, and these are of either animal or plant origin (e.g. *Desi ghee* is the animal source while vanaspati is the plant source). The fats are solids while the oils are liquids at ordinary temperature. Both the fats and the oils may be either saturated or unsaturated.

The saturated fats contain only single bonds within the carbon chain, while the unsaturated fats contain the double bonds within the carbon chain. The former are of animal origin and are usually present in a solid form, and these increase the level of the blood cholesterol (e.g. meat fat, butter, etc). The unsaturated fat is found in fishes like salmon and tuna, nuts and seeds, etc. Coconut oil and palm oil also contain the saturated fat.

The three main tests for the identification of lipids are: the general tests for lipids, the solubility test for lipids and the emulsification test for lipids.

1. **Sudan III test:** Sudan III stain is a red, fat-soluble dye that is used in the identification of the presence of the lipids, triglycerides and lipoproteins in liquids as it stains the fat cells red. Equal parts of the test liquid (0.5 ml of ether or chloroform) and water about half-full is taken in a test tube and to it is added 0.5 ml of the sample drop by drop till the sample (oil) is fully dissolved. To it is added, 1 to 3 drops of Sudan III reagent and gently shaken to mix. Since, the oil is less dense than water and insoluble in water, the oil will form a red layer or globules above the water in the test tube. A red stained oily layer will separate out and float on the surface of water if fat is present (positive test).

2. **Test with ruthenium red:** This is a red staining dye. It is a poly-cationic cell biology reagent that tightly binds to tubulin dimers and a

potent inhibitor of intracellular Ca^{2+} get released from ryanodine-sensitive intracellular stores at nanomolar concentrations through membrane channels. The inorganic dye, ammoniated ruthenium oxychloride (chemical name—sometimes also called ruthenium red) is used in histology to stain aldehyde-fixed mucopolysaccharides and stains the sugar portions of the glycoprotein molecules. In microscopy, it is used for differential staining and also as a diagnostic reagent. In research work, this is used to study the changes in cytoplasmic concentrations of calcium. It is also known to block the Ca^{2+} uptake and release from mitochondria. It also blocks the cell membrane, locates capsaicin-activated cation channels and voltage-sensitive Ca^{2+} channels to inhibit the neurotransmitter release. Its molecular formula is $H_{42}Cl_6N_{14}O_2Ru_3$ or $[(NH_3)_5RuORu(NH_3)_4ORu(NH_3)_5]^{6+}6Cl^-]$. Its molecular weight is 786.35 and is soluble to 50 mM in water.

When the stain solution is added to the test solution, a colour change is observed and this is a positive test for many compounds. Isabgol powder becomes pink indicating the presence of mucilage. Similarly, when a solution of ruthenium red is added to powdered agar, the particles become red or pink indicating the presence of mucilage. Gum acacia and guar gum fail to show a red colour.

3. **Solubility test for lipids:** This test is based on the property of solubility of lipids in organic solvents and insolubility in water. The oils and fats are soluble in chloroform, alcohol, ether, benzene, etc.

   Five test tubes marked as A, B, C, D and E are taken, and 5 ml of water, absolute alcohol, ether, chloroform and benzene are put one in each of the test tubes. 3 to 4 drops of sample is added in each test tube and the test tubes are shaken thoroughly and are allowed to stand for some time. Upon observation, drops of oils are seen floating on the surface of water in the test tube A (which contains water); the drops of oil are observed to settle at the bottom of the alcohol in test tube B; and the same is seen to get mixed up in the tubes C, D and E which contain ether, chloroform and benzene respectively. In test tube A, the sample contains fat (positive test) as it is not soluble in water; while in test tubes B, C, D and E as the sample is soluble only in organic solvents; and it sinks to the bottom in test tube B which contains the absolute alcohol.

4. **Translucent spot (grease-spot) test:** The fats and oils have higher boiling points at room temperature, and as such they cannot absorb enough heat to evaporate. When the fat or oil is placed on a sheet of paper, it diffracts light, and this light can pass from one side of the paper to another side to produce a translucent spot.

A filter paper is taken and four areas were labelled on it as—castor oil, lecithin, water and dichloroethane. Later, a drop of each sample was placed in the corresponding areas of the filter paper by a pipette. Then, the filter paper is subjected to heat by placing it on a hot-plate adjusted to its lowest setting. The translucence of the lipid samples were observed (positive test).

5. **Acrolein test:** This test is used to detect the presence of glycerol or fat. Pure glycerol (sample) or a small solid lipid is taken in a dry test tube, and a few crystals of potassium hydrogen sulphate (dehydrating agent) are added to it and heated over a Bunsen burner for a few minutes by holding it with a test tube holder. It was allowed to cool for observation. When fat is treated strongly in the presence of a dehydrating agent (like potassium bisulphate) the glycerol portion of the molecule gets dehydrated (removal of water) to form an unsaturated aldehyde, acrolein that has a very pungent irritating odour (burnt cooking grease).

About 0.5 gm of powdered sodium bisulphate ($NaHSO_4$) or potassium bisulphate ($KHSO_4$) is taken in a clean dry test tube, and to it is added 3 to 4 drops of the sample. This is mixed thoroughly and heated. An irritating smell of acrolein is felt if fat is present. This is a positive test.

6. **Baudoin test (sesame oil):** This is normally used to detect the presence of sesame oil. This oil gives a characteristic rose red colour with conc. hydrochloric acid and furfural solution. *Vanaspati ghee* contains about 5% sesame oil while the *pure desi ghee* does not contain the same. Hence, this test can be applied to find out whether the given sample of *desi ghee* contains *vanaspati ghee* or not.

7. **Huble's test (unsaturation):** This test is used to detect the degree of unsaturation in oil or fat. This reagent reacts with the alcoholic solution of iodine which contains some mercuric chloride. The violet colour of iodine fades away during the reaction if the oil or fat is unsaturated. If the oil or the fat is saturated, the violet colour of iodine does not fade away.

8. **Emulsification test:** The oil or the liquid fat becomes finely divided and gets dispersed in water when it is shaken with water to get emulsified. Emulsification is permanent and complete in the presence of an emulsifying agent. The important emulsifying agents are the bile salts, proteins, soaps, monoglycerides and diglycerides. The emulsifying agents lower the surface tension of the liquid. Thus, they are important in the processes of fat digestion in the intestine.

Two clean and dry test tubes are taken and 2 ml of water is added in one test tube and 2 ml of dilute bile salt solution in the other. 2 drops of mustard oil is added to each tube and the tubes are shaken vigorously for 1 minute. The tubes are allowed to stand for 2 minutes to note that in one tube with water, oil is broken in small pieces to float on the surface of water, while in the second tube with bile salt solution, the oil can be seen in minute droplets which remain suspended in the liquid (after permanent emulsification). An emulsion is formed (as the acid neutralises the alkali forming the soap). The test sample contains fat and this is a positive test.

9. **Saponification test:** Saponification is a process which involves the conversion of fat (or oil) into soap and alcohol by the action of heat in the presence of an aqueous alkali (e.g. sodium hydroxide). Soaps are the salts of fatty acids while the fatty acids are saturated monocarboxylic acids that have long carbon chains (e.g. $CH_3 (CH_2)_{14} COOH$).

The vegetable oils and animal fats are the traditional materials that are saponified. These materials are called the triglycerides, and are the mixtures derived from diverse fatty acids. The triglycerides can be converted into soap either in a one-step or two-step process. In the former method, the triglyceride is treated with a strong base (e.g. lye) which cleaves the ester bond to release the fatty acid salts (soaps) and glycerol. This is the main industrial method to produce the glycerol.

The saponification value is the amount of base required to saponify a fat sample. The soap makers formulate their recipes with a small deficit of lye to account for the unknown deviation of saponification value between their oil batch and the lab averages.

The reaction of fatty acids with base is the other main method of saponification. The reaction involves the neutralisation of the carboxylic acid. This method is used to produce the soaps industrially (those derived from magnesium, the transition metals and aluminium). This method is ideal for the production of the soaps derived from a single fatty acid, which leads to soaps with predictable physical properties (by engineering applications).

The esters can be hydrolyzed by the alkali to yield a parent alcohol and the salt. When the fatty acid possesses a long chain, the salt formed is a soap (which we commonly use). This is called saponification. Both the oils and fats usually contain long chain fatty acids and as such they are the starting materials for the preparation of the soap.

One ml of the oil is taken in a test tube and to it is added an equal amount of alcoholic potassium hydroxide solution. Both are thoroughly mixed and the mixture is warmed by shaking it up gently with a little distilled water. The appearance of some oil drops indicates the incomplete saponification. The oil drops disappear after complete saponification.

Glossary of Medical Terms Used

Spermicidal	–	A substance which kills the sperm.
Abortifacient	–	An agent that induces the expulsion of the foetus (abortion).
Abscess	–	A painful swollen area where pus is formed, often accompanied by high temperature.
Acne	–	Blackheads appear on the skin, usually on the face, neck and shoulders, due to the inflammation of the sebaceous glands which later become infected (**Acne vulgaris**).
Acrid	–	An agent that produces the irritation on the tongue.
Adhesive	–	A binder used in wet granulation process or an agent that binds.
Adjunct or Adjuvant	–	An agent that helps in the administration of another substance.
Alexipharmic	–	A medicine that neutralises the poison.
Alexiteric	–	A condition where the patient cannot understand printed words
Alleviate	–	To relieve (a pain).
Alterative	–	A medicine that restores the normal function of an organ or a system without any impression on any of the body organs.
Ameliorate	–	To make get better or improve.
Amenorrhoea	–	The absence of one or more menstrual periods, normal during pregnancy and after the menopause, but otherwise abnormal in adult women.
Anaesthetic	–	The substance that produces loss of sensation and consciousness from its effects on the brain and spinal centres.

Analgesic	–	A medicine that relieves pain by depressant action on the nerve centres or by impairing the conductivity of nerve fibres.
Anodyne	–	An agent that gives relief from pain.
Anorexia	–	A condition where a person refuses to eat because of the fear of becoming fat (in girls).
Anthelmintic	–	An agent that kills or expels the intestinal parasites or worms.
Anthrax	–	A disease of cattle and sheep caused by *Bacillus anthracis* which can be transmitted.
Anti-allergenic	–	An agent which will not aggravate allergy (cosmetics).
Antibacterial	–	An agent which destroys bacteria.
Antibiotic	–	An agent which stops the spread of bacteria, developed from living organisms.
Antidiarrhoeal	–	An agent which stops diarrhoea.
Antidote	–	A substance that counteracts the action of a poison.
Antiemetic	–	A substance that relieves nausea thus preventing emesis.
Antifungal	–	A substance which kills or controls fungi.
Antihistaminic	–	A drug used to control the effects of allergy.
Anti-inflammatory	–	Drug which reduces inflammation.
Antimalarial	–	A drug which is used to treat malaria.
Antimicrobial	–	An agent which destroys microorganisms.
Antioxidant	–	An agent that reduces oxidation (biological).
Antiperiodic	–	An agent which acts against the poison, in the periodic disorders like ague, neuralgia, etc.
Antipruritic	–	A substance that relieves the sensation of itching.
Antipyretic	–	An agent that reduces the temperature due to fever.
Antiseptic	–	An agent that prevents putrefaction/sepsis (formation of pus) or the bacteria responsible for it.
Antispasmodic	–	A substance that relieves convulsions or spasmodic pains.
Antistress	–	An agent that relieves stress.
Antitoxic	–	A substance that relieves the toxicity (immunising agent) in the body.
Antitubercular	–	A medicine that is used against tuberculosis.

Antitussive	–	A drug used to reduce coughing.
Anxiolytic	–	A medicine that relieves the anxiety (the state of being worried and afraid).
Aphrodisiac	–	A substance that arouses/stimulates the sexual desire.
Aphthae/Aphthous ulcers	–	Ulcers that develop in the mouth.
Aromatherapy	–	A treatment to relieve tension in which fragrant oils containing plant extracts are massaged into the skin.
Aromatic	–	An agent characterised by fragrant, spicy odour and taste and stimulates gastrointestinal mucous membrane.
Arteriosclerosis	–	A condition where the walls of the arteries become thick and rigid due to the deposits of fats and minerals, making the blood difficult to pass and thus cause high blood pressure, stroke and coronary thrombosis.
Arthritis	–	A painful inflammation of a joint.
Asthma	–	Narrowing of bronchial tubes wherein muscles go into spasm and the patient has difficulty in breathing.
Astringent	–	An agent that stops bleeding thereby making the skin tissues contract and harden.
Atherosclerosis	–	A condition where fats and minerals get deposited on the walls of an artery, thus preventing the blood to flow easily.
Atonic dyspepsia	–	A condition where the patient feels pains or discomfort in the stomach due to lack of tone or tension in the muscles.
Atrophy	–	The wasting of a body part or organ.
Bactericide	–	An agent that destroys bacteria.
Bacteriostatic	–	Agent that stops bacteria from multiplication but does not kill them.
Binder	–	A substance that makes materials more firm (production of tablets).
Blennorrhoea	–	The discharge of watery mucus as in gonorrhoea.
Borborygmus	–	A rumbling noise in the abdomen due to gas in the intestine.
Bronchitis	–	An inflammation of the mucous membrane of the bronchi.

Bronchopneumonia – An infectious inflammation of the bronchioles which may lead to the general infection of the lungs.

Bruise – A dark painful area on the skin with blood under the skin

Bubo – A swelling of a lymph node in the armpit or groin.

Cachexia – An ill health with wasting and general weakness.

Cardiac – Related to the heart.

Carminative – An agent that soothes by relieving the pain from flatulence, which relieves colic or indigestion.

Catarrh – An inflammation of the mucous membranes in the nose and throat creating an excessive amount of mucous.

Cephalagia – A pain in the head.

Chapping – Cracking of the skin due to cold.

Chemotherapy – The use of chemical drugs (antibiotics, painkillers, etc.) to fight a disease especially in cancer.

Cholagogue – Agent which promotes the secretion/excretion of bile.

Cholera – A serious bacterial disease spreading through food or water which has been infected by *Vibrio cholerae*.

Choleretic – An agent that increases the production of bile.

Chorea – A sudden severe twitching of the face and shoulders, a disease of the nervous system.

Chronic fatigue syndrome – See postviral syndrome or myalgic encephalo-myelitis or postviral fatigue syndrome.

Chronic hydro-cephalus – A diseased condition of excessive quantity of cerebrospinal fluid in the brain lasting for a longer time.

Coagulation – Action of clotting of the blood.

Colitis – An inflammation of the colon.

Colostomy – A surgical operation to make an opening between the colon and the abdominal wall to allow faeces to be passed out without going through the rectum.

Conjunctiva – A membrane covering the front of the eyeball and inside of the eyelids.

Constipation – Difficulty in passing enough faeces often.

Coronary heart disease – A disease affecting the coronary arteries leading to strain of the heart or a heart attack (CHD).

Coryza	– Common cold or nasal catarrh—an inflammation of the nasal passage where the patient sneezes and coughs with a blocked and running nose.
Cramps	– Painful involuntary spasms in the muscles where the muscles may stay contracted for sometime.
Cystitis	– An inflammation of the urinary bladder where a patient passes water very often accompanied by burning sensation.
Debilitated	– Patient made weak by a disease.
Decongestant	– Agent which reduces congestion and swelling (used to unblock the nasal passages).
Delirium tremens	– State of mental disturbance which includes hallucinations, trembling and excitement (usually in chronic alcoholics).
Demulcent	– A substance that soothes or protects the mucous membranes.
Denture	– A set of false teeth fixed to a plate fitting into the mouth.
Deodorant	– An agent which prevents unpleasant smell.
Depressant	– An agent that reduces the activity of a part of the body (tranquiliser).
Dermatitis	– An inflammation of the skin due to disease.
Detergent	– A cleaning substance which removes bacteria and grease.
Detoxification detoxication	– The removal of toxic substance from the body to make a poison harmless.
Diaphoresis	– An excessive perspiration.
Diaphoretic/ Sudorific	– A substance that increases perspiration/sweating.
Diarrhoea	– A condition where a patient frequently passes liquid faeces.
Digestive	– An agent that promotes digestion.
Digestive atony	– A condition where the patient feels discomfort in the digestive system due to lack of tone or tension in the muscles.
Diphtheria	– An infectious disease of children by *Corynebacterium diphtheriae* marked by fever and the formation of a fibrous growth in the throat restricting breathing and swallowing.
Disintegrant/ Disintegrator	– Any substance which favours disintegration (to become pieces).

Diuretic	–	A substance that increases the secretion and flow of urine.
Dysentery	–	An infection and inflammation of the colon causing bleeding and diarrhoea.
Dysmenorrhoea	–	Experiencing pain during menstruation.
Dysuria	–	Difficulty in passing urine.
Eczema	–	An inflammation of the skin with itchy rash and blisters which is noncontagious.
Ejaculation	–	A process during which semen is sent out of the penis.
Emetic	–	A substance that induces vomiting.
Emmenagogue	–	An agent that stimulates the menstrual flow.
Emollient	–	An agent that softens the skin on external application or soothes the irritated or inflamed surface by internal usage.
Emulsifier	–	A substance which favours the formation of an emulsion (mixture of liquids which do not mix—such as oil and water).
Enema	–	A liquid put into the rectum for the introduction of a drug into the body or to wash the colon before an operation.
Enteralgia (colic)	–	Pain in any part of the intestinal tract.
Enteritis	–	An inflammation of the mucous membrane of the intestine.
Eosinophilia	–	A condition of having an excess of eosinophils in the blood.
Epilepsy	–	Nervous system disorder with convulsions and loss of consciousness due to the discharge of cerebral neurones.
Eructation (belching)	–	A process during which the air in the stomach is allowed to come up through the mouth.
Erysipelas	–	A contagious skin disease caused by *Streptococcus pyrogenes* where the skin on the face becomes hot, red and painful.
Estrogenic (oestrogenic)	–	An agent used to treat the conditions which develop during menopause.
Excipient	–	A substance added to a drug so that it can be made into a pill or a tablet.
Exhaustion	–	An extreme tiredness or fatigue or physical exertion.

Expectorant	–	An agent that promotes expectoration (cough).
Febrifuge	–	An agent that reduces the fever.
Fibromyalgia	–	A condition where the patient experiences pain in the fibrous muscles.
Flatulence	–	A condition in which gas or air collects in the stomach or intestine causing discomfort.
Fungistatic	–	Any agent which stops multiplication of fungi.
Galactagogue	–	Any agent that increases the secretion of milk in the breasts.
Gangrene	–	A condition of the patient where the tissues die and decay associated with the loss of blood supply to the arteries as a result of bacterial action, through an injury or a disease.
Gargle	–	A mild antiseptic solution used to clean the mouth (mouthwash).
Gastritis	–	An inflammation of the stomach.
Gastroenteritis	–	An inflammation of the membrane that lines the intestine and stomach accompanied by diarrhoea and vomiting due to viral infection.
Germicide	–	An agent that destroys the germs, microbes, worms.
Gingivitis	–	An inflammation of the gums due to bacterial infection.
Glossitis	–	An inflammation of the surface of the tongue.
Goitre	–	An excessive enlargement of the thyroid gland caused by lack of iodine, as a swelling round the neck.
Gonorrhoea	–	A sexually transmitted disease (STD) caused by *Neisseria gonorrhoeae*, that produces painful irritation of the mucous membrane and a watery discharge from the vagina or the penis.
Gout/Podagra	–	A diseased condition in which abnormal quantities of uric acid is produced and precipitated as crystals in the cartilage around joints.
Griping	–	Experiencing pain in the abdomen.
Grippe	–	Influenza
Haematuria	–	The presence of blood in the urine due to injury or a disease of the kidney or the bladder.
Haemorrhage	–	The loss of blood in a large quantity due to bursting of a blood vessel.

Haemorrhoids/Piles – A condition where the veins get swollen in the anorectal passage.

Haemostatic – An agent that arrests/stops bleeding.

Halitosis – A condition where a person's breath smells unpleasant.

Hallucinogenic – An agent which produces hallucinations.

Hiccup (hiccough or singultus) – A sudden inhalation of breath followed by the closure of the glottis which makes a characteristic sound due to a spasm in the diaphragm.

Hyperacidity – An increase of acid in the stomach.

Hypertension – A condition where the pressure of the blood in the arteries is too high (high BP).

Hypnotic – An agent that induces sleep.

Hypoglycaemic – Suffering from hypoglycaemia (lack of sugar).

Hysteria – A state where the patient is unstable, and may scream or wave the arms and slow to react to the outside stimuli.

Impotency – An inability to have an erection or ejaculation and have sexual intercourse in a male.

Influenza – An infectious disease of the upper respiratory tract transmitted by a virus with fever and muscular aches.

Insecticide – A substance that destroys insects.

Insomnia – Sleeplessness or inability to sleep.

Irritable bowel colon/Spastic colon – An inflammation of the mucous membrane in the intestine, where the patient suffers pain caused by spasms in the muscles of the walls of the colon.

Irritant – A substance that induces irritation or inflammation.

Jaundice (icterus) – A diseased condition with an excess of bile pigment in the blood where it is deposited in the skin and the white of eye to give yellow colour.

Larvicidal – An agent which kills the larvae.

Laryngitis – An inflammation of the larynx.

Laxative – An agent which causes the bowel movement or substance that loosens the motion (as in constipation).

Leprosy/Hansen's – An infectious bacterial disease of the skin and peripheral nerve tracts caused by *Mycobacterium leprae* which destroys the tissues and cripples the patient if no treatment is given.

Leucorrhoea/Whites – A condition where there is an excessive discharge of white mucus from the vagina.

Libido – Sexual urge.

Liniment – An oily liquid used for rubbing on the skin to ease the stiffness of a sprain or pain.

Lipogenesis – Production of fat deposits.

Lipolytic – An ability of a substance to break lipids.

Lithotomy – Removal of a stone from the bladder by surgery.

Lumbago – Pain in the lower back due to rheumatism or strain.

Marasmus – A wasting disease which affects small children who have difficulty in absorbing the nutrients (suffering from malnutrition).

Masticatory – A substance when chewed increases the secretion of saliva.

Menopause – Period usually between 45 and 55 years of age when a woman stops menstruating and can no longer bear children.

Menstruation – Bleeding from the uterus in a woman each month when the lining of the womb is shed because of the absence of the fertilised egg.

Migraine – Severe recurrent headache accompanied by vomiting and visual disturbance.

Multiple sclerosis – A disease of the central nervous system which gets progressively worse in which the patches of nerve fibres lose their myelin resulting in numbness in the limbs, weakness and paralysis.

Narcotic poison – An agent which makes a patient sleep or become unconscious to help in pain relief.

Nausea – Feeling sick or want to vomit.

Nervine – An agent that calms the nervous excitement and acts on nervous diseases.

Neuralgia – Pain running along a nerve in spasms.

Oligomenorrhoea – A condition of a patient with infrequent menstruation.

Ophthalmia – An inflammation of the eye due to the disease.

Ophthalmopathy – Suffering of the eye due to disease.

Osteoarthritis (osteoarthrosis) – A degenerative disease where the joints are inflamed to become stiff and painful in the middle aged and elderly people.

Paralysis	–	A condition where muscles of the body (of a part) become weak and cannot be moved due to damaged motor nerves.
Pastille	–	A sweet jelly containing medication in it, which can be sucked into relieve a sore throat.
Pectoral	–	A substance that is useful in diseases of the respiratory tract.
Pelvic cellulitis	–	Bacterial inflammation of the connective tissue or subcutaneous tissue of the pelvis (internal space inside the pelvic girdle).
Pericarditis	–	Inflammation of the pericardium, membrane which surrounds and supports the heart.
Peristalsis	–	Movement like waves produced by alternate contraction and relaxation of muscles along an organ (intestine or oesophagus) which pushes the contents along it automatically.
Peritonitis	–	Inflammation of the peritoneum (membrane covering the organs) due to bacterial infection.
Phthisis	–	Old term referring to tuberculosis.
Pleuritis	–	Inflammation of the pleura, membranes covering the lung, usually in pneumonia.
Pneumonia	–	Inflammation of the lung, wherein the alveoli of the lung become filled with fluid.
Postpartum	–	After the delivery or birth of a child.
Postviral syndrome	–	Condition affecting the nervous system where the patient feels tired and depressed experiencing pain and weakness in the muscles (myalgic encephalomyelitis or postviral fatigue syndrome).
Poultice	–	Pressing of the infected part with hot water to draw out pus, to relieve pain and favour circulation (fomentation).
Protective	–	Agent which protects against a disease.
Psoriasis	–	Inflammatory skin disease in which red patches are covered with white scales.
Purgative	–	Substance that produces copious evacuation of the bowels.
Purulent	–	Producing pus (suppurating).
Refrigerant	–	Agent possessing cooling properties and that lowers the body temperature.
Resolvent	–	Agent which makes inflammation disappear.

Restorative	–	Agent that restores health and vigour.
Rheumatism	–	A general term given for pains and stiffness in the joints and muscles.
Rickets/Rachitis	–	Disease where the bones are soft and do not develop properly because of lack of vitamin D, in children.
Rubefacient	–	Agent that causes distension of the capillaries and makes the skin warm and pink or red.
Scabies	–	Irritating infection of the skin caused by a mite living under the skin.
Sciatica	–	Pain along the sciatic nerve, at the back of the thighs and the legs.
Scorbutic disease	–	Refers to scurvy, caused by lack of vitamin C or ascorbic acid.
Scrofula	–	A type of tuberculosis in the lymph nodes in the neck, now rare.
Scrophulous	–	Suffering from scrofula, a type of tuberculosis in the lymph nodes of the neck which is rare.
Scrotum	–	A bag of skin that contains the testis, epididymis and a part of the spermatic cord.
Scurvy/Scorbutus	–	A disease caused by lack of vitamin C (ascorbic acid) found in fruits and vegetables.
Sedative	–	A substance that exerts a soothing effect by lowering the functional activity.
Septicaemia	–	Condition where the bacteria and their toxins are present in the blood, multiply rapidly and destroy the tissue (blood poisoning).
Sialagogue	–	Agent that causes the flow of saliva.
Sinusitis	–	Inflammation of the mucous membrane in the maxillary sinus behind the cheek bone in the upper jaw.
Sore throat	–	A condition where the mucous membrane in the throat gets inflamed, usually because of infection.
Spasm	–	A sudden, usually painful involuntary contraction of a muscle (as in a cramp).
Spasmodic	–	An agent that produces convulsions or spasms.
Spasmodic cough	–	Cough which occurs from time to time, in spasms.
Spasmolytic	–	An agent which relieves the muscular spasms.
Spermatorrhoea	–	A condition where a large amount of semen is discharged frequently without orgasm.

Spermicidal   – A substance which kills the sperm.

Stabiliser – An agent which helps to make the condition stable.

Stimulant – A substance that excites to speed up the functions of an organ or a process in the body.

Stomachic – An agent that stimulates the activity of stomach.

Strangury – A condition where very little urine is passed caused by a disorder of the bladder or a stone in the urethra.

Styptic – An agent which stops bleeding.

Suppository – A soluble material (as glycerine jelly) containing the drug, placed in the rectum or in the vagina which gets dissolved by the body fluids (acts as a lubricant or to treat the disorders like vaginitis).

Suppuration – Formation and discharge of pus.

Syphilis – A sexually transmitted disease (STD) caused by *Treponema pallidum*, a spirochaete.

Tachycardia – A rapid beating of the heart or increase in the heart beat.

Thrombosis – Blocking of an artery or a vein by a mass of coagulated or clotted blood.

Tuberculosis (TB) – An infectious disease caused by the tuberculosis bacillus where infected lumps are formed in the tissues.

Tympanitis (Otitis) – An infection of the middle ear.

Urethritis – An inflammation of the urethra.

Uvula – A piece of soft tissue which hangs down from the back of the soft palate.

Vermifuge – A substance that expels the intestinal worms.

Vertigo – Dizziness or giddiness where the patient feels that everything is rushing round him, because of a malfunction of the sense of balance.

Virus-static – An agent which stops the multiplication of the virus.

Whitlow/Felon – An inflammation due to infection near the nail in the fleshy part of the finger.

Whooping cough/ Pertussis – An infectious disease sometimes serious, caused by *Bordetella pertussis* which affects the bronchial tubes, common in children.

Xerophthalmia – A condition where the cornea and the conjunctiva of the eye become dry, due to lack of vitamin A.

Pharmacological Terms Used for Drugs Acting on Various Body Systems

1. Drugs that act on Mouth and Salivary Glands

a. *Sialagogues/sialics:* These drugs increase the secretion of saliva, and they act either directly upon the salivary glands or their secreting nerves or they may act reflexly. These may be *directly acting sialogogues* (e.g. pilocarpine and physostigmine) or *reflexly acting sialogogues* (e.g. alcohol, acids, bitters and aromatics), or they may act through sensory nerve endings in the mouth or through the stomach (e.g. ipecacuanha and antimony).

b. *Antisialics:* These drugs diminish the secretion of saliva, by paralysing the secretory nerve endings (e.g. atropine) or acting by decreasing the irritation of the buccal mucous membrane (e.g. demulcents—these substances have the property of protecting the mucous membrane when they are irritated or inflamed (e.g. syrups, honey, mucilages and linseed tea).

2. Drugs that act on Stomach and Intestines

a. *Stomachics:* These are the drugs which increase the flow of the gastric juice. The alcohols and the bitters stimulate the gustatory nerves in the tongue and reflexly increase the gastric juice and thus increase the appetite (gentian, calamba, mustard and ginger).

b. *Gastric stimulants:* These are the drugs which produce a slight irritation of the gastric mucosa which increases the vascularity of the stomach. Most of these act as *emetics* if they are given in larger doses.

c. *Gastric sedatives:* These drugs reduce the gastric pain and control vomiting (e.g. ice and bismuth act locally while morphine acts centrally).

d. *Gastric tonics:* These drugs act by increasing the acidity of the chime, and stimulate the movement of the stomach (e.g. dilute hydrochloric acid and dilute nitric acid).

e. *Neuromuscular gastric stimulants:* These drugs increase the tone of the gastric muscles and stimulate the movement of the stomach.

f. *Carminatives:* These drugs assist in the expulsion of the gases from the stomach and the intestines (e.g. turpentine, aromatic spirit of ammonia and cardamom).

g. *Emetics:* These agents produce vomiting, and some of them act locally by irritating the sensory nerve endings while others produce emesis directly stimulating the vomiting centre (e.g. the saturated common salt can act as a local emetic while apomorphine acts centrally).

h. *Antiemetics:* These agents prevent vomiting. Some of these drugs act locally by reducing the irritation of the sensory nerve endings (e.g. *demulcents*—act centrally on the chemorecepotor trigger zone (CTZ) or on the vomiting centre (e.g. domperidone).

i. *Antacids:* These drugs correct the excessive acidity of the ingesta (e.g. alkalies like lime water).

j. *Gastric antiseptics:* These drugs are used commonly in ruminants to control the excessive fermentation in the rumen. These are also called antizymotics (e.g. oil of turpentine).

k. *Purgatives/cathartics:* These drugs cause the evacuation of the intestinal contents.

l. *Intestinal astringents:* These are the agents which limit the action of the bowel and also correct the excessive fluidity of the intestinal contents. Some of these act as *vascular astringents*—by contracting the intestinal blood vessels and lessening the amount of fluid excreted (e.g. lead salts), while the others lessen the peristaltic movement of the intestine (e.g. opium). Some of the drugs because of their antacid nature check the excessive action of the intestine by eliminating the acidity. Some others, because of the insolubility, form a coating over the intestinal mucous membrane and protect it from further irritation. Certain drugs, because of their tannic acid content coagulate the protein, which forms a protective covering over the intestinal mucosa.

m. *Intestinal antiseptics:* These agents help in diminishing the activity of the bacteria in the intestine. Sometimes, these are prescribed in diarrhoea and allied conditions which are believed to be due to the presence of the bacterial pathogens (e.g. carbolic acid and oil of turpentine, etc.)

n. *Cholagogues:* These agents help in increasing the expulsion of bile juice, and the bile juice itself acts as a direct cholagogue (e.g. ox bile). Some of the purgatives reduce the absorption of bile by increasing the intestinal action, and reflexly stimulate the contraction of the gallbladder and bile duct (these are called indirect cholagogues). These are frequently prescribed in the disorders of bile.

3. Drugs that act on Urinogenital Tract

a. *Diuretics:* These drugs increase the flow of urine. For example, potassium nitrate increases the fluidity of the blood by raising the osmotic tension of the plasma attracting water from the tissue fluid. Such increased blood volume and the excess fluid filtered by the glomeruli and reabsorption from the tubule is prevented by the presence of saline. Some volatile oils (e.g. oil of turpentine) produce diuresis by causing the dilation of the renal vessels. Some others (like digitalis) increase the blood flow through the kidneys by their action on the heart.

b. *Vesicle sedatives:* These drugs relieve the irritability of the bladder, and these are represented by alkalies like sodium bicarbonate.

c. *Lithotropic drugs:* These are the agents which prevent the deposition of the solids from the urine or promote their removal.

d. *Urinary antiseptics:* These are the agents that prevent the multiplication of the organisms in urine, mucosa of the bladder and the urinary passages (e.g. benzoic acid).

e. *Aphrodisiacs:* These drugs increase the sexual desire by increasing the general body vigour such as strychnine and yohimbine which exert their action by causing a vascular congestion of the genital organs.

f. *Anaphrodisiacs:* These drugs diminish the sexual desire (e.g. general sedatives like potassium bromide).

g. *Galactogogues:* These agents are believed to increase the secretion of milk.

h. *Antigalactogogues:* Some drugs paralyse the termination of all nerves of the secretory glands which may also produce an action on the mammary glands which may fail to produce the milk (e.g. belladonna).

4. Drugs that act on Cardiovascular System

a. *Vasoconstrictors:* These are the agents that cause constriction of the walls of the blood vessels and thus diminish their efficiency. The arterioles are specially affected by these drugs (e.g. adrenalin).

b. *Vasodilators:* These are the agents which cause dilation of the peripheral arterioles by relaxation of the unstriped muscle in them (e.g. amyl nitrate).

c. *Cardiac stimulants:* These are the agents that cause a more forcible heart beat which might be due to a direct action on the heart muscle or sometimes indirectly by raising the blood pressure (e.g. caffeine and digitalis).

d. *Cardiac depressants:* These drugs diminish the force of cardiac contraction and thus lessen the frequency of the heart beat (e.g. quinine).

    e. *Haematinics:* These are the drugs that improve the quality of the blood by increasing the number of RBCs (red blood corpuscles) as well as the amount of Hb (haemoglobin) in the blood (e.g. the iron salts).

5. **Drugs that act on Respiratory System**
   a. *Expectorants:* These drugs cause an increase of bronchial secretion and render the secretions fluidier and thus facilitate its expulsion (e.g. potassium iodide and antimony salts).
   b. *Analeptics/respiratory stimulants:* These are the agents that increase the irritation of the respiratory centre and thus increase the rate and depth of the respiration (e.g. doxapram).
   c. *Respiratory sedatives:* These drugs lessen the irritability of the respiratory centre (e.g. morphine).
   d. *Bronchial relaxants:* These are the drugs that are used to bring about the relaxation of the bronchial musculature to relieve bronchial asthma (e.g. adrenaline).

6. **Drugs that act on CNS (Central Nervous System)**
   a. *Cerebral stimulants:* These are the agents which cause an overall increase of the functional activity of the cerebrum (e.g. caffeine).
   b. *Spinal stimulants:* These are the agents which increase the reflex excitability and conductivity of the spinal cord in medicinal doses (e.g. strychnine).
   c. *Narcotics:* These are the drugs which can be used to produce deep sleep accompanied by a depression of the circulatory and respiratory mechanisms (e.g. barbiturates).
   d. *Soporifics/hypnotics:* These agents induce sleep (e.g. chloral hydrate).
   e. *Analgesics/anodynes:* These are the agents which are applied for the pain relief (e.g. morphine).
   f. *Anaesthetics:* These are the agents that are used for producing the total loss of consciousness so that the pain is no longer felt and at the same time abolishing the reflex action, especially during major surgeries.

7. **Drugs that act on the Eye(s)**
   a. *Mydriatics:* These are the drugs which cause dilatation of the pupil (e.g. atropine).
   b. *Miotics:* These are the drugs which cause the contraction of the pupil (e.g. pilocarpine).

8. **Drugs that act on the Skin**
   a. *Sudorifics/diaphoretics:* These drugs induce sweating (e.g. ammonia acetate solution).

b. *Anhydriotics/antidiaphoretics:* These agents lessen the secretion of sweat (e.g. atropine).

c. *Counter irritants:* These agents increase the irritability of the applied area and thereby increase the healing process (e.g. haematinics, vesicants, pustulants and caustics).

d. *Emollients:* These agents reduce the irritability of the applied area (e.g. vegetable oils).

9. **Alteratives:** These drugs bring about a favourable change in the process of nutrition and thus repair especially in the convalescent period (e.g. iron salts and potassium iodide).

Subject Index